Restoration of Lost Human Uses of the Environment

Other publications by the Society of Environmental Toxicology and Chemistry (SETAC):

Endocrine Disruption in Invertebrates: Endocrinology, Testing, and Assessment
deFur, Crane, Ingersoll, and Tattersfield, editors

Reproductive and Developmental Effects of Contaminants in Oviparous Vertebrates
Di Giulio and Tillitt, editors

Multiple Stressors in Ecological Risk and Impact Assessment
Foran and Ferenc, editors
1999

Linkage of Effects to Tissue Residues: Development of a Comprehensive Database for Aquatic Organisms Exposed to Inorganic and Organic Chemicals
Jarvinen and Ankley
1999

Ecotoxicology and Risk Assessment for Wetlands
Lewis, Mayer, Powell, Nelson, Klaine, Henry, Dickson, editors
1999

Uncertainty Analysis in Ecological Risk Assessment
Warren-Hicks and Moore, editors
1998

Ecotoxicological Risk Assessment of the Chlorinated Organic Chemicals
Carey, Cook, Giesy, Hodson, Muir, Owens, Solomon, editors
1998

Sustainable Environmental Management
Barnthouse, Biddinger, Cooper, Fava, Gillett, Holland, Yosie, editors
1998

Ecological Risk Assessment Decision-Support System: A Conceptual Design
Reinert, Bartell, Biddinger, editors
1998

Principles and Processes for Evaluating Endocrine Disruption in Wildlife
Kendall, Dickerson, Giesy, Suk, editors
1998

For information about any SETAC publication, including SETAC's international journal, *Environmental Toxicology and Chemistry*, contact the SETAC Office nearest you:

1010 N. 12th Avenue
Pensacola, Florida, USA 32501-3367
T 850 469 1500 F 850 469 9778
E setac@setac.org

Avenue E. Mounier 83, Box 3
1200 Brussels, Belgium
T 32 2 772 72 81 F 32 2 770 53 83
E setac@ping.be

http://www.setac.org

Restoration of Lost Human Uses of the Environment

Edited by
Grayson Cecil
Cecil Consulting, Houston, TX

From the Conference on Restoration of Lost Human Uses of the Environment
Washington, DC
7–8 May 1997

SETAC General Publications Series

SETAC Liason
Kenneth L. Dickson
University of North Texas, Denton, TX

Current Coordinationg Editor of SETAC Books
C.G. Ingersoll
U.S. Geological Survey, Columbia, MO

Publication sponsored by the Society of Environmental Toxicology and Chemistry (SETAC)

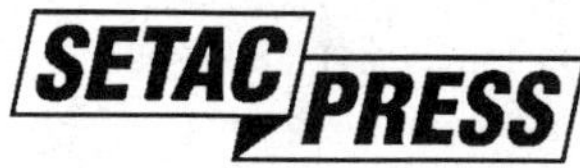

Cover by Michael Kenney Graphic Design and Advertising

Library of Congress Cataloging-in Publication Data

Conference on Restoration of Lost Human Uses of the Environment (1997: Washington, D.C.)
Restoration of lost human uses of the environment: from the Conference on Restoration of Lost Human Uses of the Environment, Washington, D.C., 7–8 May 1997 edited by Grayson Cecil.
p. cm.
Includes bibliographical references
ISBN 1-880611-21-X
1. Oil spills--Environmental aspects--Congresses. 2. Hazardous wastes--Environmental aspects--Congresses. 3. Restoration ecology--Congresses. 4. Liability for oil pollution damages--Congresses. 5. Liability for hazardous substances pollution damages--Congresses. 6. Natural resources--Valuation--Congresses. I. Cecil, Grayson, 1934– . II. Title.
TD427.P4c655 1997 98-43870
363.738'28--dc21 CIP

International Standard Book Number 1-880611-21-x
Printed in the United States of America
06 05 04 03 02 01 00 99 10 9 8 7 6 5 4 3 2 1

(∞) The paper used in this publication meets the minimum requirements of the American National Standard for Information Sciences—Permanence of Paper for Printed Library Materials, ANSI Z39.48-1984.

Reference Listing: Cecil GR. 1999. Restoration of lost human uses of the environment. From the Conference on Restoration of Lost Human Uses of the Environment; 7–8 May 1997; Washington, DC. Pensacola FL: Society of Environmental Toxicology and Chemistry (SETAC). 373 pp.

The SETAC General Publications Series

Society of Environmental Toxicology and Chemistry (SETAC) General Publications require approval by the Board of Directors to be developed. The scope of General Publications may either be narrow or broad depending on the type of publication. General Publications may or may not be developed from a SETAC-sponsored activity and may or may not need to be peer reviewed through SETAC. The conference leading to this General Publication was not sponsored by SETAC, but this publication has been externally peer reviewed through the SETAC editorial process.

The SETAC General Publications are useful to environmental scientists in research, research management, chemical manufacturing, regulation, and education, as well as to students considering careers in these areas. The series provides information for keeping abreast of recent developments in familiar subject areas and for rapid introduction to principles and approaches in new subject areas.

Contents

List of Figures

List of Tables

Conference Opening Remarks

*Grayson Cecil**

This conference was a long time in the making and is the result of many hours of planning by many people. Let me first acknowledge the enormous contribution of the sponsors of this conference. Their financial assistance was crucial to the success of the conference, but more importantly, the assistance of their representatives in the planning process was a key ingredient in any achievements we might have here in the next 2 days.

And I believe we can and will achieve much. As a general principle, I believe that cooperation in the natural resource damage assessment (NRDA) process has been accepted by all of the trustees, responsible parties, attorneys, and consultants. The alternative has been deemed by all to be unacceptable in its expense and its risks. However, having acknowledged that we all agree on cooperation, making that work in the field and on the ground is a different matter. Making cooperation work in the Superfund context is, I believe, even more difficult than in the oil spill context. To make a slight pun, oil spills are "cleaner" than toxic releases. In an oil spill, we generally know who spilled it and exactly when and where it was spilled; in addition, we are dealing with a single compound. In the Superfund context, none of these matters are that straightforward.

The group assembled here represents the leaders in the NRDA field. There are a few missing persons, but not many. The issue we have chosen to tackle is perhaps the most difficult in the NRDA regulations. For reasons too complex to mention, at least some economic models have not met with generalized acceptance. And in dealing with lost human use of the environment, we are confronting matters that may require such modeling. You will hear over the next 2 days several approaches that have the potential to achieve general acceptance. This conference is unique in that no one point of view is espoused. We have sought input from a range of disciplines and orientations and have established this conference as one to advance the state of the art and develop consensual approaches.

It is most important that a preeminent group such as that gathered here work seriously on the matters that divide us. As the Superfund and oil spill regulatory constructs move toward a single scheme, as I believe they will, we need to develop a "tool box" of assessment methods that have withstood dispassionate inquiry and have emerged as acceptable NRDA tools. If you think of the tool box analogy, it has great applications. In putting together your own tool box, you do not know what problems will be addressed, but you are selecting proven tools with wide application. You know that when the job comes along, if you have the right tools, the job will go much more smoothly. If we wait until a spill or release to undertake this assembly of tools, too many other considerations will intervene in the white hot passions of the moment

*Cecil Consulting, Houston, TX

when crucial financial and public concerns are at stake. The intellect and experience necessary to craft a solution for developing restoration programs for lost human uses of the environment are here at this moment. I invite you to consider the challenge of moving beyond what we know today to seek new solutions that are as yet undefined.

As we developed the agenda for this conference, the planning committee chose to address the restoration issue at successive levels of detail. First, we invited Dick Stewart and Marty McHugh to give an overview of the issues of lost human use. Then we selected 2 framework papers—one for selection of restoration projects and one for scaling such projects. Next, we chose 3 papers on discrete issues that arise in the compensatory restoration process, and finally, we determined to close with presentation of several diverse case studies. We hope that you will be led to consideration of the case studies at the close of the conference with new insights and new ideas for expeditious and economic restoration.

The authors and panel members will be given an opportunity to edit their remarks after the conference in order to reflect the input from the conference. We have asked a few participants to take notes on the question and answer sessions so that we might preserve the comments. We then plan to publish the proceedings with the intention that such a publication will form the tool box that we create here this week. This will present a considerable addition to the field of NRDA, and I believe each of you will feel a sense of accomplishment at being part of its creation. We can then move on to address other cogent NRDA issues in this collegial manner and ultimately create the perfect box of workable tools for both Superfund and oil spill incidents.

Remarks

Kathleen A. McGinty *

I am truly pleased to have the opportunity to address such a diverse group engaged in this focused and challenging endeavor: the restoration of our critical natural resources.

As restorationists, you have a very important and exciting charge: to come up with ways to repair, replace, and compensate for natural resources and their associated functions that have been disrupted, injured, or lost. But, before we can restore, we must fully understand what has been lost. The effort to comprehend what has been lost and to implement restoration places you on the frontier of some of the most significant technical and scientific challenges in environmental protection.

Your work in achieving natural resource restoration on the ground coincides with another process of "restoration" we have undertaken over the past 4 years: restoring the focus of our natural resource programs through reforms that advance our shared goals of stewardship while overcoming the discord, polarization, and endless court battles that have marked some of our early approaches to natural resource damages.

In this area, as in all of our natural resource programs, we have refocused our efforts so that we can more effectively meet the stewardship responsibilities imposed by statute and expected by the public. Through these efforts, our natural resource programs are once again becoming a common ground rather than another battleground. We are building an environmentalism where government acts as a partner—not just as policeman—where there is collaboration and not endless confrontation.

What have we done?

Superfund

Talk about polarization and litigation! For a long time, Superfund topped the list. At the start of the Administration, we brought all of the stakeholders in and gave them a place at the table. We produced a plan for reform that everyone—from Fortune 500 companies to local environmental justice groups—could support.

When Congress failed to enact our proposal, the U.S. Environmental Protection Agency (USEPA) undertook a series of administrative reforms that fundamentally redirected the Superfund program. With a stronger cleanup program in place, the President challenged Congress to accelerate the cleanup program, by reinstating the Superfund taxes and providing the funding needed so that two-thirds of USEPA's sites could be cleaned up in the next 4 years. The recent bipartisan budget agreement, which incorporates all the elements of the President's proposals on accelerating toxic waste cleanup, shows that he had the right idea.

We are continuing to work with the Congress on Superfund legislation that will allow us to enhance our reform effort through needed legislative change. Even today, in fact,

* Council on Environmental Quality, The White House, Washington, DC

we will provide the Congress with a clear and detailed statement of the Administration's principles for Superfund reform. This comprehensive statement provides a blueprint for Superfund reform legislation, and we are hopeful that we can move quickly toward a bipartisan bill that incorporates our approach.

In those principles and in our broader reform effort, we have recognized that there is more to addressing the legacy of toxic waste than we see in the USEPA-led cleanup program, and natural resource restoration is as important as cleanup. As we brought about real reform to the USEPA Superfund program, we also built consensus around common-sense, common-ground reforms to our natural resource restoration programs:

- We have shifted the focus of the natural resource damage programs to *restoration.* We want to abandon the approach of litigating first and planning restoration later.
- We have developed a more open process to include responsible parties and the public in damage assessment and restoration planning.
- We recognized that response or source control often has to precede restoration. So, as part of his initiative to accelerate toxic waste cleanup, President Clinton gave federal resource managers new authority to issue section 106 orders to get cleanups moving. The Council on Environmental Quality (CEQ) is now working with the agencies to finalize a memorandum of understanding (MOU) that gives everyone clear guidance about how and when this new authority will be used.
- We have worked to integrate the roles and responsibilities of federal and state response and natural resource agencies.
- Today, in response to concerns raised by some that natural resource trustees theoretically could demand a second cleanup—additional cleanup at the same facility beyond that required by USEPA or a state response agency—CEQ is initiating a second MOU among the relevant agencies to provide a more integrated and predictable approach to response and restoration.

We have also developed a legislative proposal that reflects this common-sense approach and implements our reforms. Our proposal would ensure that Superfund reform legislation strengthens our restoration programs; that significant ecological injuries are restored to baseline condition; and that restoration includes restoration of the interim losses the public has suffered until restoration is achieved.

Our proposal also would ensure that we move toward a restoration-based approach for natural resource damage and away from the litigation-first approach that has marked some of the early cases. For example, we join with our state and tribal trustees in calling for a fix to the statute of limitations. What will that do? We believe that it will reduce litigation and that at a minimum, it will move us away from premature litigation.

In our mind, this is progress on this important issue—the path to positive change. But, as the Superfund principles we release today will make clear, we will not accept just any change to this program. Specifically, we disagree with what we see as the reductionist approach to natural resource restoration. This approach would recognize only a narrow category of natural resource attributes. Under this approach, the only values that trustees could take into account when deciding the scope of restoration would be actual human uses of the natural resource that have direct market measures. The advocates of this approach would have us believe that the value of a river is measured only by the number of hikers or fishers along its bank, for example, and that significant ecosystem injury should go unrestored unless there is a demonstrable interference with human uses that, again, are measurable in market terms. But, this is a dangerous approach. If you think about it, the unstated premise of this approach is that the more pristine the natural resource, the less concerned we can be about its restoration. Now surely, that is not an approach we want to take.

It is true that human uses are important and, in fact, are often controlling factors governing our decisions about restoration. But, what are human uses? Are they only market measurements of hiking days or fishing days? What about existence values, aesthetic values, and ecosystem services that *often* have no direct market measure? Do these count? They are critically important to our health, our well being, and our overall quality of life. We now know that it may be important to restore plant and animal populations that have been injured by toxic waste even if the species is not hunted, gathered, or marketed. We now know that—even if we were to focus exclusively on human uses—we cannot capture all of the benefits to humans by focusing only on current market values. We must consider the broader values that society and science identify with preserving the integrity of our ecosystems.

Overall, what is called for is humility and caution. We have to recognize that we do not always understand the complex contributions that ecosystems make to our well being. Before we dismiss injuries as insignificant, we have to remind ourselves that the history of environmental degradation has been not merely of catastrophic events, but of incremental impacts that have had devastating and likely unforeseen cumulative effects.

We must challenge ourselves to conceive of human use with the breadth and the humility demanded by our dependence on ecosystem health. In a ground-breaking new book, *Nature's Services*, Gretchen Daily identifies the myriad of goods and services that flow from natural ecosystems as Earth's life-support systems. Think about that. Have you ever thought of yourself as a technician responsible for maintaining life's essential services? What happens when life-support systems are disrupted? The book explores from a variety of perspectives the many ways society depends on and affects natural ecosystems.

Natural resources confer countless benefits on our well-being, including

- wetlands contribute to water quality and flood control;
- healthy streams and sediments provide habitats for fisheries;
- clean waterways provide opportunities for recreation and commerce; and
- healthy forests support biodiversity and improve air quality.

Even if we look through the narrowest lens of actual human use, the case for restoration of natural resource injuries is compelling. Losses to society and the U.S. economy from the public's inability to use and enjoy natural resources are potentially enormous.

Over 76 million Americans enjoy bird watching, photography, and other nonconsumptive uses of wildlife, contributing $18 billion per year to the economy. Annually, 50 million anglers contribute nearly $70 billion to the nation's economy. Moreover, these and other Americans gain an enjoyment, serenity, and sense of community and national pride from unspoiled natural resources that transcend such economic impacts.

The natural resource damage provisions of the Comprehensive Environmental Response, Compensation, and Liability Act (CERCLA or Superfund) and the Oil Pollution Act (OPA) allow us to reclaim our environment and restore those natural resources—and their many economic and noneconomic benefits—that have been degraded or destroyed.

Under Superfund, state, tribal, and federal trustees have made significant progress toward restoring natural resources injured by hazardous substances. By working within USEPA's remedial process, trustees and responsible parties have agreed to restore habitat and injured resources at more than 25 hazardous waste sites as part of negotiated comprehensive settlements. Trustees have also obtained settlements and advanced restoration as a direct result of natural resource damage assessment activities.

In Baytown, Texas, for example, restoration is complete at the French Limited Superfund Site, where a sand pit was used to dispose of enormous quantities of sludge and contaminated sediment. Chemical residues had contaminated groundwater and subsoils near the site, injuring migratory birds, crabs, and other natural resources. Working within the USEPA cleanup process, however, federal trustees reached a settlement with the responsible parties to restore a marsh that would provide for the replacement of natural resources that had been injured, destroyed, or lost. Everyone worked cooperatively, and now, the ecosystem is springing back: animals have returned and local residents can now use the restored marshland for nature walks and fishing.

In Tacoma, Washington, efforts continue to restore and enhance habitat for fish and wildlife injured by years of pollution in Commencement Bay. Two seasons of planting have been completed at the project, converting nearly 5 acres of industrial uplands to a mix of clean, replanted upland habitat, intertidal salt marsh, and intertidal mud and sand habitats. Again, many people were brought together to this end. In October 1995, community volunteers pitched in and planted over 600 native upland trees and shrubs as part of this effort. An additional 300 trees and shrubs were planted by natural resource trustees a year later.

There are many, many other examples

What lessons do we draw from these examples? First, we see clearly that the natural resource damage provisions of our environmental laws—CERCLA, OPA, the Clean Water Act, and the National Marine Sanctuaries Act, and others—are working. The tools in current law can bring about the effective and efficient restoration of our critical natural resources. Second, we have learned that, when these tools are used properly with the federal agencies working effectively together and in partnership with the states, tribes, and local government, and responsible parties recognize their obligation to restore natural resources, restoration can be achieved through collaboration rather than litigation.

We have also learned that much remains to be done. Now is not the time to abandon our commitment to restoration in favor of the reductionist approach.

One compelling example is the Hudson River—one of the nation's most important river systems— rich with history and story and important to our environment and our economy. The *New York Times* has run a series of articles on the Hudson's recovery. Painting the progress that has been made through effective partnerships as well as through Clean Water Act enforcement, the stories also underscored that there is much yet to be done. Specifically, polychlorinated biphenyl levels are still unacceptably high and fish—while they have returned—are still too contaminated to eat.

To address these concerns, federal and state response and natural resource agencies are working in close partnership to develop both remedial and restoration plans. The Hudson thus provides a clear opportunity for us to implement an integrated approach to restoration in which the work of natural resource trustees, response agencies, responsible parties, and affected communities is fully coordinated.

The Hudson also provides a clear warning against the reductionist approach that would have us measure ecological injury only according to the actual human uses we can anticipate today. A decade ago, it might have been impossible to attribute actual human-use values to minor changes in water quality caused by wetlands loss or other natural resource injuries. Yet now we recognize that those marginal changes may very well decide whether New York municipalities will have to spend billions for additional filtration to provide communities with drinking water.

In the lower Hudson, we see another lesson. We know now, as we did not a decade ago, that the failure to address hazardous substance contamination ultimately does damage to the economy as well as to the environment. In New York Harbor, a century of irresponsible disposal has made it vastly more expensive and more difficult for port companies to safely dredge the channels and berthing areas that are vital to the region's economy.

In summary, as our understanding of the Hudson river and other ecosystems becomes more sophisticated, and unanticipated costs of natural resource injury become more plain, the case for restoration of significant injuries becomes more compelling, and the shortcomings of the reductionist approach became more apparent.

So, as you focus on the restoration of human uses, I challenge you to conceive of human "use" broadly and to understand it as one piece of a much larger picture. I also challenge you to resist the reductionist approach, by recognizing the broader array of values and services that ecosystems provide and that we are only now beginning to understand.

Finally, I challenge you to challenge us, by continuing your dialogue with us in both the legislative and administrative process of reform of our natural resource programs. We want your help as we explore new and innovative ways to enhance and improve our restoration programs, while creating incentives for private parties to step up to their stewardship obligations. Above all, we need your help in finding common ground—and move away from the battlegrounds—in our efforts to protect and restore natural resources.

Acknowledgments

The following sponsors are gratefully acknowledged for their generous financial and planning assistance for the conference.

American Bar Association–Section of Natural Resources:
Energy and Environmental Law

American Forest and Paper Association

American Petroleum Institute

National Mining Association

National Fish and Wildlife Foundation

National Park Service

Society for Ecological Restoration

United States Department of Commerce/National Oceanic and
Atmospheric Administration

United States Department of the Interior

SETAC thanks the following sponsors for their contribution to the publication:

American Petroleum Institute

National Oceanic and Atmospheric Administration

SETAC would also like to thank the external peer reviewer, Robert Gearheart with Humboldt State University, for his critique of this publication.

Abreviations

CERCLA	Comprehensive Environmental Response, Compensation, and Liability Act
CV	Contingent valuation
CVFA	Castle View Fishing Area
CWA	Clean Water Act
DFG	Department of Fish and Game
DOI	Department of the Interior
GLO	Texas General Land Office
HEA	Habitat equivalency analysis
ICRM	Interim corrective restoration measure
ITOPF	International Tanker Owners Pollution Federation
MOA	Memorandum of Agreement
MOU	Memorandum of Understanding
NEBA	Net environmental benefits assessment
NEPA	National Environmental Policy Act
NOAA	National Oceanic and Atmospheric Administration
NRD	Natural resource damage
NRDA	Natural resource damage assessment
OPA	Oil Pollution Act of 1990
PAH	Polycyclic aromatic hydrocarbon
PRP	Potentially responsible party
RI	Remedial investigation
RP	Responsible party or Revealed preference
RUM	Random utility model
SAY	Service acre year
SCM	Stated choice method
SP	Stated preference
TER	Triangle Economic Research
USR	Upper Sacramento River
WTP	Willingness to pay

Conference attendees/contributors*

Wiktor Adamowicz
Department of Rural Economy
University of Alberta
Edmonton, Alberta, Canada

Jenifer Baker
Clock Cottage, Church Street
Shrewsbury, United Kingdom

Diana Balmori
Balmori Associates, Inc
New Haven, CT

Mark Barash
Department of the Interior
Boston, MA

James Bieke
Shea & Gardner
Washington, DC

Thomas Birdsall
Putnam, Hayes & Bartlett, Inc.
Palo Alto, CA

Thomas Campbell
Campbell & Graves, LLP
Houston, TX

Robin Cantor
Law & Economics Consulting Group
Washington, DC

Steve Cary
New Mexico Office of the Natural
Resource Trustee
Santa Fe, NM

Grayson Cecil
Cecil Consulting
Houston, TX

James Connaughton
Sidley & Austin
Washington, DC

Philip Cooney
American Petroleum Institute
Washington, DC

Ralph d'Arge
University of Wyoming
Laramie, WY

Rick Dawson
National Park Service
Atlanta, GA

William Desvousges
Triangle Economic Research
Durham, NC

Kenneth Dickson
Institute of Applied Sciences
University of Texas
Denton, TX

Carol Dinkins
Vinson & Elkins
Houston, TX

John Duffy
Steptoe & Johnson
Washington, DC

Richard Dunford
Triangle Economic Research
Durham, NC

Erin Fries
Triangle Economic Research
Durham, NC

Kevin Gaynor
Vinson & Elkins
Washington, DC

Anton Giedt
NOAA
Glouscester, MA

Sara Hudson
Triangle Economic Research
Durham, NC

Michael Huguenin
Industrial Economics, Inc
Cambridge, MA

F. Reed Johnson
Triangle Economic Research
Durham, NC

Dennis King
University of Maryland
Center for Environmental Studies
Solomons, MD

Alan Maki
Exxon Corporation
Houston, TX

Kristy Mathews
Triangle Economic Research
Durham, NC

Molly McCammon
Exxon Valdez Oil Spill Trustee Council
Anchorage, AK

Kathleen McGinty
Council on Environmental Quality
The White House
Washington, DC

Martin McHugh
NOAA/HAZMAT
Chicago, IL

Gordon Robilliard
ENTRIX
Walnut Creek, CA

Robert Rowe
Hagler Bailly Consulting, Inc.
Boulder, CO

Melissa Ruby
Triangle Economic Research
Durham, NC

Leslie Sauer
Andropogon Associates, Ltd
Philadelphia, PA

Richard Stewart
New York University School of Law
New York, NY

John Wiens
Department of Biology
Colorado State University
Fort Collins, CO

Robert Unsworth
Industrial Economics, Inc
Cambridge, MA

* Affiliations were accurate at the time of the conference.

Introduction

*Craig R. O'Connor**

This volume contains papers prepared for the conference on Restoration of Lost Human Uses of the Environment, held 7–8 May 1997, in Washington, DC. The conference focused on restoration of interim losses of human uses of the environment resulting from oil spills and hazardous substance releases. The papers presented at the conference were solicited from a broad range of contributors and address the topic of restoring lost human uses of the environment in the context of natural resource damage assessments (NRDAs). Each paper was critiqued by panel members from differing disciplines, followed by an open dialogue among conference participants.

Natural resource trustees are stewards of the nation's natural resources and are mandated to manage, protect, and restore them. The natural resource damage provisions of the Clean Water Act, Comprehensive Environmental Response, Compensation, and Liability Act (CERCLA), the Oil Pollution Act (OPA), and the National Marine Sanctuaries Act, allow NOAA and other federal, state, and tribal trustees to reclaim our environment and restore those natural resources that have been degraded or destroyed. NOAA's trustee program acts on behalf of the public to restore coastal and marine resources injured by oil spills and hazardous material releases.

The papers in this collection focus on actions, and issues associated with those actions, that might be carried out to restore lost human uses of the environment following an incident covered by CERCLA or OPA. The natural resource damage provisions of both CERCLA and OPA direct natural resource trustees to recover for restoring natural resources injured by incidents and for the losses to the public and the environment of those natural resources from the time of the injury until recovery to baseline.

Harm to the public's natural resources from the improper transport and handling of oil in general and improper handling and disposal of hazardous substances at specific sites throughout the country persists to this day. Losses to society and the U.S. economy from the public's inability to use and enjoy natural resources are potentially enormous. Over 76 million Americans enjoy bird watching, photography, and other nonconsumptive uses of wildlife. Fishing contributes some $38 billion annually to the economy, hunting contributes $21 billion, and wildlife viewing contributes $27 billion. Citizens gain enjoyment, serenity, and a sense of community and national pride from unspoiled natural resources that transcend such economic impacts.

State, tribal, and federal trustees are making progress toward restoring natural resources harmed by spills of oil and releases of hazardous substances. As confirmed by the General Accounting Office (GAO) report "Status of Selected Federal Natural Resource Damage Settlements," trustees across the Nation are using funds recovered

*Craig O'Connor is Deputy General Counsel for the National Oceanic and Atmospheric Administration (NOAA). The views expressed in this article are solely those of the author, and do not necessarily represent the position of NOAA or the U.S. government.

from responsible parties for restoration. The GAO report also notes that restoration takes time and is often delayed by many factors beyond the control of the trustees. Nevertheless, the federal trustees have been working hard to effect changes that accelerate the restoration of injured resources.

Significant progress has been and is being made by state, tribal, and federal trustees toward restoring injured natural resources. By working within the U.S. Environmental Protection Agency's (USEPA) remedial process, trustees have reached agreements with responsible parties to restore habitat and injured resources as part of negotiated comprehensive government settlements. Trustees have also obtained settlements and advanced restoration as a direct result of natural resource damage assessment (NRDA) activities. To accelerate this process, natural resource trustees have adopted several changes aimed at expediting restoration. In 1994, the Department of the Interior finalized revisions to the CERCLA NRDA regulations that require trustees to focus their assessment work and base their claims on a publicly reviewed plan for restoring injured resources to their baseline condition (i.e., the condition that would have existed in the absence of the release). In January 1996, NOAA issued final NRDA regulations under the OPA that extends the restoration-based approach of the 1994 CERCLA regulations. NOAA has also proposed, in conjunction with other trustees, amendments to CERCLA's natural resource damage provisions that would, if enacted, expedite the damage assessment and restoration process.

Before trustees present a claim for an oil spill under the OPA rule, they must develop a plan not only for restoring resources to their uninjured condition, but also for restoring the services lost in the interim while the resources remain impaired. The OPA rule specifies that the trustees will no longer assess monetary damages for interim losses based on economic values for the vast majority of oil spills. Instead, the goal of the assessment is timely, cost-effective restoration of the natural resources that have been injured. Under the rule, trustees focus on developing a plan for accomplishing that restoration. Responsible parties will then have the option of either implementing the plan or funding the trustee's implementation of the plan.

This new paradigm is being used for the *North Cape* oil spill, where natural resource trustees and the responsible party continue to work cooperatively to assess the effects of the spill and to determine appropriate restoration actions for Rhode Island's coastal environment. Four teams of experts have examined impacts to salt pond communities (including fish, shellfish, and vegetation), marine communities (including lobster and surf clams), birds, and human uses (including charter boat fishing, tourism, and recreation). The restoration planning efforts of these teams are nearing completion, and a draft restoration plan is expected in 1998.

Despite these improvements, there has been controversy. For this conference on the restoration of human uses, the authors were asked to put aside the seemingly endless debates over certain issues and focus on those areas where we can work together. This approach allows us to move forward at the same time that it acknowledges that there are some issues on which we may never agree.

There have been quite a few successes in recent years on restoring injured natural resources and, through these restoration efforts, the public has been compensated for losses pending the restoration of the physical environment. There have been conferences and publications relating to restoration of the environment. What we hoped to accomplish through the conference is equal focus on what we can do to restore lost human uses of the environment. We hope this is only the beginning and wish to encourage more meetings and publications on this topic since it is an integral part in the trustees' responsibilities as managers of natural resources.

I wish to personally thank all of the speakers at this conference. Their efforts to initiate and stimulate a dialogue on these issues at a national and international level are greatly appreciated. I hope that there will be many future discussions on what we can do to restore lost human uses of the environment.

Overview of Conference Objectives: Restoration Based on Cost-Effective, Cost-Reasonable Reinstatement of Impaired Public Resource Uses

*Richard B. Stewart**

This conference has 2 main stated objectives: to identify projects that can replace/restore interim lost human uses and to determine how much restoration is needed. Both of these objectives can be resolved through a single cluster of principles:

> Restoration should reinstate, on a going-forward basis, committed public resource uses impaired as a result of a spill or release by providing the public with resource uses equivalent in value to those impaired. Restoration projects should be cost-effective and cost-reasonable and should reinstate impaired uses as promptly as is feasible consistent with these requirements.

These principles resolve both conference issues. They define the basic objective of restoration projects: reinstatement on a going-forward basis of committed public uses impaired as a result of a spill or a release.[1] Resource injury consists of changes caused by a spill or release that impairs the services and uses that a resource provides to the public. Where a spill or release does not cause significant measurable impairment of public uses, there is no resource injury for purposes of natural resource damages (NRDs).[2] Where public uses are impaired, the objective of restoration is promptly to reinstate equivalent uses. These principles also provide the appropriate criteria for determining the needed level of restoration and for selecting among restoration alternatives. The restoration projects selected should provide public services and uses equivalent in value to those impaired. Restoration measures should be cost-effective and cost-reasonable and should reinstate public uses as promptly as is feasibly consistent with these requirements.

In accordance with this framework, reinstatement of public uses should not be a separate "add-on" element of NRD programs, over and above restoration, nor should restoration be divided into "primary" and "compensatory" components. Instead, there should be a single, integrated approach to restoration focused on prompt reinstatement of committed public resource uses. In appropriate cases, this approach calls for the use of temporary restoration measures to reinstate public uses in the interim while permanent restoration is being achieved. Trustees should evaluate various temporary

---

*New York University School of Law and Sidley & Austin

[1]I use the term "impaired" rather than "lost" human uses in order to underscore the focus of restoration on reinstating uses prospectively rather than seeking direct or indirect compensation for uses lost in the past.

[2]Similarly, the extent of any injury is defined by the extent of the diminution in public uses. Since restoration generally takes place following cleanup, the determination of whether there is any injury and the extent of any such injury should be based on the post-cleanup condition of the resource.

and/or permanent restoration options (including natural recovery, on-site rehabilitation, replacement, and acquisition of equivalent resources) in terms of their ability to reinstate public uses in as timely a manner as is feasible and select the option that will achieve this goal at least cost. Restoration measures should also be cost-reasonable, i.e., their costs should not, at the margin, exceed the benefits that they provide to the public.

Natural resource damage should be limited to the costs of reinstating impaired public uses and reasonable assessment costs. It should not include additional recoveries—whether denoted "compensable value" or "compensatory restoration"—or restoration measures based on past lost uses prior to the initiation of restoration or on nonuse claims. Imposing additional NRD liabilities on PRPs beyond going-forward restoration costs and reasonable assessment costs is unfair and unjustified.

The restoration principles summarized above reflect sound legal principles and public policy. They will ensure timely restoration consistent with the need to avoid waste of scarce societal resources and ensure fairness to responsible parties. In cases where trustees have followed these principles, they have fostered cooperative and constructive trustee/PRP information-gathering and evaluation and selection of restoration options, resulting in timely restoration. In other cases, trustees have ignored these principles by seeking restoration costs based on measures that go far beyond what is needed to reinstate impaired public uses and instead attempt to replicate the exact condition that a resource would have in the absence of a spill or release and by seeking additional recoveries based on past lost use and nonuse. Such claims have provoked controversy, mistrust, legal and factual uncertainty, litigation, and delay. Following the restoration principles set forth herein will avoid these problems and further the NRD programs' overriding objective of prompt restoration.

A number of issues must be addressed in order to operationalize the restoration principles set forth above. There must be methods for identifying any reductions in public resource services and uses that have been caused by a spill or release. This will require methods for determining changes in resource conditions caused by a spill or release, for linking such changes to changes in public services and uses, and for determining the character and amount of any reductions in those services and uses.[3] There must be similar methods for determining the means by which various restoration alternatives will enhance public services and uses and for determining the character and amount of such enhancements. There must also be methods for valuing the public uses impaired as a result of a spill or release and the uses provided by restoration measures in order to ensure that they are equivalent.

Economic welfare is the primary criterion for determining whether restoration projects are adequate: the resource uses provided by restoration should be equivalent

---

[3]This assessment should be based on the condition of the resource following cleanup and should assess the extent of any reductions in committed uses that will occur in the future following cleanup.

in public welfare or utility to any future post-cleanup decrement in uses caused by a spill or release.[4] Economic methodologies for making such determinations will be discussed during this conference. In specific cases, however, noneconomic techniques for scaling the public uses provided by resources and by restoration measures may serve as a practical "shortcut" tool for cooperative identification and selection of appropriate restoration measures without the need for detailed economic studies. These techniques will also be discussed at this conference. Both types of techniques can play an important and useful role in implementing the restoration principles set forth herein. But methods for scaling resource services that are not based on public uses and their reinstatement are not an appropriate basis for restoration decision-making. Such methods, including scaling of resource-to-resource services as authorized by NOAA, are incapable of providing an objective or workable basis for restoration decisions and give trustees excessive and potentially arbitrary discretion.

Restoration should be based on reinstatement of committed public uses

Remediation removes or contains contaminants to levels necessary to protect both the public health and ecological systems against significant risks of harm. Cleanups that meet these goals will, in almost all cases, allow natural processes of recovery to operate and reinstate a fully functioning ecosystem at the site affected by a spill or release. In some cases, however, it may take a number of years for completion of natural recovery. In these cases, restoration measures (i.e., measures other than a second, additional cleanup) may be needed and appropriate in cases where public uses will be significantly impaired during the period required for full natural recovery. The potential options include permanent restoration measures to reinstate public uses for the long term by accelerating natural recovery or by other means.[5] They also include temporary restoration measures, such as temporary acquisition of replacement or equivalent resources, to reinstate public uses in the interim pending completion of permanent restoration. For example, where a public fishery has been impaired by a spill and is in the process of recovering following cleanup, one might lease an equivalent privately owned fishery for public use in the interim before full recovery of the public fishery is accomplished. The measure or combination of measures chosen should aim to reinstate the impaired public uses in as timely a fashion as possible, consistent with requirements of cost-effectiveness and cost-reasonableness.[6]

---

[4]Restoration measures should satisfy requirements of timeliness, cost-effectiveness, and cost-reasonableness.

[5]For example, in the infrequent case where natural recovery may not be sufficient fully to reinstate impaired public uses, it may be appropriate to acquire, on a permanent basis, similar resources that will provide sufficient additional public uses to make up the shortfall and ensure full reinstatement of public uses.

[6]The requirement of prompt restoration, including use in appropriate cases of temporary measures to reinstate public uses in the interim pending completion of permanent restoration, eliminates the asserted need to award damages for lost use in order to prevent PRPs from dragging out permanent restoration.

Contrary to the position taken by some trustees and by NOAA and DOI in their NRD assessment regulations, restoration should not be based on replicating or approximating the precise physical, chemical, and biological conditions that an injured resource would possess had a spill or release not occurred. For example, NOAA's NRD assessment regulations define resource "injury" to include an "observable or measurable adverse change in a natural resource."[7] This definition authorizes trustees to equate the presence of residual contamination following cleanup with resource "injury" and to seek NRD for the costs of additional cleanup measures to remove the residual contamination in the guise of restoration.[8] The NRD programs, however, were not intended and should not function as a second round of cleanup measures. A cleanup remedy protective of health and the environment will already have ensured that a viable functioning ecosystem will be reestablished. The objective of restoration is necessarily different: to reinstate impaired public uses of a resource in cases where natural recovery following cleanup will take substantial time and interim impairment of committed public uses will be significant.

It follows that the goal of restoration should not be to replicate the physical, chemical, and biological baseline condition of a resource, i.e., the precise condition that the resource would be in if a spill or release had never occurred. It is impossible to replicate every feature of such a hypothetical ecosystem.[9] Rather, the appropriate benchmark is public resource use: restoration should be based on providing public uses equivalent in value to the committed resource uses that the public would enjoy in the future, post-cleanup, had the spill or release not occurred. Consider, for example, a fishery that historically afforded members of the public the opportunity to catch an average of 200 fish/day and would continue to provide the same level of fishing had a spill or release that impaired the fishery not occurred. Following cleanup, the fishery will provide an opportunity to catch only 100 fish/day until full natural recovery is accomplished. The objective of restoration is to provide the public, through temporary and/or permanent measures either on-site or off-site, a similar opportunity to catch an additional 100 fish/day or its equivalent in value, in order to reinstate public fishing opportunities to the 200 fish/day level or its equivalent in value.

There are several reasons why public services and uses rather than physical, chemical, and biological replication should be the benchmark for restoration. First, trustees sue on behalf of and as representatives of the members of the public, who value resources on account of the human services they provide and the public uses that those services

---

[7]15 C.F.R. §990.30.

[8]Under CERCLA, trustees have sought NRDs for additional post-cleanup removal of residual contamination at sites including the Butte/Silver Bow Creek NPL Site and the Berks, Pennsylvania Superfund Site.

[9]While cleanup will ensure reestablishment of a viable functioning ecosystem, that ecosystem will inevitably be different in some respects than the hypothetical ecosystem that would exist had the spill or release and the ensuing cleanup never occurred. It will be impossible to transform the post-cleanup ecosystem into an exact replica of the hypothetical ecosystem.

support. For example, members of the public may value a wetlands because it provides habitat for birds that they enjoy viewing. Restoration should accordingly focus on reinstatement of the public uses impaired as a result of a spill or release, including both non-consumptive and consumptive uses. Second, damages, including NRD, are an economic concept. From an economic perspective, resources are properly understood and valued in terms of the utility of the services that they provide to humans. Third, a focus on public services and uses is the only approach consistent with the broad array of restoration options provided under the NRD statutes, including on-site rehabilitation, replacement, and acquisition of equivalent resources as well as natural recovery. A replication approach would almost inevitably mandate on-site rehabilitation, disregarding the other restoration options that Congress provided. By contrast, basing restoration on public uses and services allows equal consideration and appropriate use of all of the statutory options.[10] Fourth, attempts at replication through intensive on-site rehabilitation will in many cases be extremely and unreasonably costly. A services-based approach allows use of less costly options for reinstating public uses, including temporary or permanent replacement and acquisition of equivalent resources and less intensive on-site rehabilitation.

Finally, reinstatement of committed public uses provides an objective and workable restoration benchmark that trustees and PRPs can agree upon and implement in order to achieve prompt restoration on a cooperative basis. Literal replication, by contrast, is impossible, for reasons already noted. Attempts at replication can succeed in only approximating, to varying degrees, baseline physical, chemical, and biological conditions. There are, however, no objective scientific principles for determining which of the many different elements and aspects of a natural resource are most relevant or important for restoration and how far the effort to replicate them should be taken. As explained more fully below, scaling based on resource-to-resource services, as authorized by NOAA, fails to resolve this problem and instead perpetuates it. Trustees, including NOAA, have sought to dodge this difficulty by asserting that they should enjoy broad case-by-case discretion to determine the extent and cost of replication-oriented restoration—in other words, "trust us." Many in the PRP community, however, are unwilling to accept a system of largely standardless administration discretion that can by used by financially self-interested trustees to claim arbitrary and excessive recoveries.

For all of these reasons, restoration should be based on reinstating the services and uses that natural resources provide to the public. Moreover, following the principle established in DOI's NRD assessment regulations, which authorize restoration of a water body as a drinking water source only if it was previously committed to public

[10]In *Kennecott Utah Copper Co. v. DOI*, 88 F. 3d. 1191 (D.C. Cir. 1996), the Court rejected Montana's claim that CERCLA's NRD provisions establish a presumption in favor of on-site rehabilitation over other types of restoration measures.

use as a drinking water source,[11] the resource in question should have been committed to the relevant public use at the time of spill or release causing the injury. Otherwise, trustees could require a PRP to finance a plethora of extensive and costly restoration measures in order to upgrade prior resource uses or accommodate wholly speculative future uses.

Trustees should select restoration measures that will reinstate equivalent public uses in a prompt, cost-effective, and cost-reasonable manner

Resources generally recover naturally following cleanup to levels that will be protective of human health and the environment. In cases where natural recovery will occur relatively rapidly—as is often the case, for example, with accidental spills or releases—or in cases in which it will take a longer time but where no significant public uses are affected or where substitute resources are readily available in the vicinity to support public uses,[12] no measures beyond cleanup may be needed or justified. But in cases in which natural recovery will take substantial time and there is a significant net impairment of the level or quality of public uses, it may be appropriate to undertake restoration measures to reinstate the impaired public uses on a going-forward basis through use of temporary as well as permanent restoration options.

In evaluating restoration options, one must be able to scale the impairment of public uses caused by a spill or release and the uses provided by restoration measures in order to determine whether the restoration measures are appropriate and adequate to reinstate public uses. As already explained, resource injury and the adequacy of restoration should be understood in economic terms. Thus, the ultimate question is whether the uses provided by proposed restoration measures are equivalent in public welfare or utility to any future, post-cleanup decrement in uses due to a spill or release. This implies use of economic methods to determine the values of consumptive and non-consumptive resource uses on both sides of the equation. Such methods, including travel cost methods, are relatively well-developed and reliable. As discussed below, however, in given cases there may be alternative practical "shortcut" means of determining whether restoration measures are adequate. The evaluation must, however, focus on reinstating equivalent public uses. Accordingly, NOAA's resource-to-resource scaling, which is not focused on public uses and their reinstatement, is not a valid tool for restoration decision-making.

In assessing potential restoration measures to reinstate public resource uses, one should consider the full array of statutory restoration options, including on-site rehabilitation and temporary and/or permanent replacement or acquisition of

[11]See 43 C.F.R. §§ 11.14(h), 11.62(b)(ii).

[12]In their paper for this conference, Thomas Birdsall, Ralph d'Arge, and Edward McGrath emphasize the importance of taking into account currently available substitute resources in determining whether a spill or release at a given site has impaired public uses. As they point out, contamination of the Ridgeway Reservoir did not impair public fishing opportunities because ample alternative fishing sites were available in the vicinity.

equivalent resources. They should evaluate the costs of these options, the benefits that they will provide to the public in terms of enhanced public uses, and the timing of those benefits. The costs of restoration measures not only include the direct financial outlays to implement them but also any adverse environmental impacts that may be associated with measures such as dredging of sediments or conversion of uplands to wetlands. One should then select the restoration measure or combination of measures that will reinstate, as promptly as is feasible, on a temporary as well as a permanent basis, impaired public uses.[13] The costs of various measures to accelerate permanent reinstatement of impaired public uses, by hastening natural recovery through on-site rehabilitation or by other means such as permanent acquisition of equivalent resources, must be balanced against the costs of temporary measures to reinstate such uses on an interim basis pending completion of permanent restoration. These various alternatives must be weighed in order to determine the measure or combination of measures that will promptly reinstate public uses at least cost.

The application of the cost-effectiveness requirement in cases where both temporary and permanent restoration options are available may be illustrated by the following example: Consider a stream on public lands that supported a trout fishery. A release into the stream has impaired the fishery. Following cleanup, it will take 15 years for the fishery to recover naturally. In the interim, fishing opportunities for the public will be 100 fish/day, versus 200 fish/day had the spill or release not occurred. There is a similar trout stream nearby where streamside land is privately owned that could provide the public with comparable opportunities to catch 100 fish/day. The land can be leased in order to provide public access to the stream at a cost of $15,000 per year. Suppose that intensive on-site rehabilitation could reinstate the baseline level (200 fish/day) of trout fishing at the public stream in 2 years at a cost of $100,000. In that case, the cost-effective restoration option is to proceed with on-site rehabilitation while leasing the private streamside land during the 2-year period that it will take to achieve permanent restoration on an accelerated basis. Impaired public uses will be reinstated on both a temporary and a permanent basis at a total cost of $130,000, which is significantly less than the $225,000 cost of relying on natural recovery to achieve permanent restoration and leasing the private streamside land for the 15-year period of natural recovery.[14] But if intensive on-site rehabilitation of the public stream instead costs $500,000, the cost-effective measure for reinstating impaired public uses is to lease the private streamside land for the entire 15-year period that it will take natural recovery to occur, at a cost of 225,000, versus $530,000 for on-site rehabilita-

---

[13]In addition, the measure selected must be cost-reasonable.

[14]The example ignores discounting issues that must be addressed in actual cases in order to make an appropriate evaluation of restoration options that incur costs and provide benefits over different time periods. Further, the example assumes that the value to the public of the fishery equals or exceeds the costs of the temporary and permanent restoration measures and that the measures are therefore cost-reasonable. The issue of cost-reasonableness is discussed further below.

tion and leasing the private streamside land for 2 years.[15] These examples illustrate the way in which restoration decision-making should focus on promptly reinstating impaired public uses in a cost-effective manner.

In addition to being cost-effective, restoration measures should also be cost-reasonable (i.e., the financial and environmental costs of measures to reinstate impaired public uses pending natural recovery should not exceed the benefits provided to the public). Otherwise, society would be wasting scarce resources by spending more to reinstate uses than those uses are worth to the public. The operation of the cost-reasonableness requirement may be illustrated by the following example. Assume that a variety of on-site rehabilitation measures to accelerate natural recovery of a resource can be taken. Natural recovery would take 15 years. Various on-site rehabilitation measures can accelerate natural recovery and reinstate impaired public uses in 8 years at a cost of $4 million, 5 years at a cost of $6 million, 3 years at a cost of $25 million, and 1 year at a cost of $40 million.[16] The annual value of impaired public uses is $1 million.[17] The rising incremental costs of accelerated on-site restoration must be balanced against the incremental benefits of earlier reinstatement of impaired uses in order to determine which option will reinstate impaired uses as promptly as possible consistent with the cost-reasonableness requirement that the incremental benefits of a restoration measure exceed its incremental costs. The 8-year measure would reinstate resource services 7 years earlier than natural recovery, thereby generating benefits of $7 million at a cost of $4 million, producing net benefits of $3 million. By the same logic, the 5-year program would produce net benefits of $4 million, the 3-year program would produce net benefits of $13 million, and the 1-year program would produce net benefits of $26 million. The 5-year restoration option should therefore be chosen; efforts to further accelerate recovery would cost more than the benefits that they provide to the public.[18] In cases where none of the available restoration measures is cost reasonable, the scope and timing of restoration should be scaled back to the point where the cost-reasonableness requirement is satisfied, in order to ensure that society does not spend more to reinstate impaired uses than the value of those uses to the public.

---

[15]In actual cases, of course, the array of restoration options is often more extensive than the 2 alternatives in the example. The example also assumes that the 15-year lease option is cost-reasonable.

[16]For simplicity of exposition, it is assumed that alternative means of reinstating public uses, including temporary or permanent replacement or acquisition of equivalent resources, are not available. As reflected in the previous example of the trout fishery, such alternatives are often available.

[17]Again, the example ignores discounting.

[18]It would make no sense to impose "compensatory restoration" damages based on the impaired uses during the 5 years that it will take to achieve full restoration of the resource. Such recoveries would supposedly be spent to compensate the public for the interim impairment of use. But, by hypothesis, there is no restoration measure available to reinstate impaired uses in the interim that does not cost more than the value of the uses provided to the public.

Accordingly, the restoration decision-making process may be summarized as follows: one should identify a variety of available restoration options that will reinstate impaired public resource uses on both a temporary and permanent basis. One should select the least costly option for reinstating equivalent public uses as promptly as possible, provided that it also satisfies the requirement of cost-reasonableness.

NRD should not include surplus recoveries, over and above restoration costs, based on past lost use or nonuse

Injury to human uses of a natural resource caused by a spill or release is fully and appropriately redressed by the approach to restoration presented herein, which focuses on prompt reinstatement of impaired public uses on a going-forward basis. There are several reasons that trustees should not seek or obtain separate recoveries—over and above the costs of restoration measures to reinstate prospectively impaired public uses—based on past lost uses under labels such as "compensable valuation" or "compensatory restoration." First, surplus trustee recoveries based on past lost uses by others would be inconsistent with the Congressional design of the NRD programs. In the case of CERCLA, Congress in 1980 rejected legislative provisions that would have provided a federal cause of action for private economic losses resulting from resource injury. OPA provides for recoveries based on lost uses by private persons, but only by a property owner suffering a loss, not by trustees.[19] Other potential claims by private persons for lost use are properly addressed by state law. Second, any "compensable value" or "compensatory restoration" recoveries based on past lost use would be paid to trustee agencies, not to the individuals who may have suffered a loss of use. There is also no requirement or consistent trustee practice that ensures that the benefits from trustees' expenditures of past lost use recoveries accrue to the individuals who may have suffered a loss, an objective that is in any event impossible to achieve in the cases of losses suffered in the distant past. Accordingly, it is false and misleading to characterize surplus recoveries based on past lost use through labels—such as "compensatory restoration" or "compensable value"—that imply compensation of those injured. The use of the "compensatory restoration" label is especially misleading when restoration is aimed at replicating resource conditions that bear no relation to reinstating committed public uses. Third, recovery under the federal NRD statutes for past lost use is unfair and would not be justified by principles of corrective justice even if recoveries were to accrue to the individuals who suffered a loss. NRD liabilities are near-absolute and bear no relation to fault.[20] Retroactive liability under CERCLA based

[19]OPA Section 1006(d)(1)(B) authorizes trustees to recover for "diminution in value of [injured] natural resources pending restoration;" under the restoration principles stated herein, this provision should be interpreted as including the costs of temporary restoration measures to reinstate public uses pending completion of permanent restoration. Moreover, OPA Section 1006(f) provides that NRD recoveries in excess of the costs of restoration and damage assessment must be paid by trustees into the Oil Spill Restoration Trust Fund.

[20]In order for a trustee to recover NRDs from a party, however, the trustee must prove that the party's spill or release caused resource injury.

on pre-1980 lost uses, stretching back in some cases to the early 19th century, is especially offensive to corrective justice principles as well as contrary to the limitation on retroactive liability adopted by Congress in CERCLA in 1980. Fourth, trustee efforts to obtain surplus recoveries based on lost use unnecessarily provoke conflict and controversy, generate delay, uncertainty, and high transactions costs, and impede prompt restoration.

Like remediation, restoration is a prospective enterprise based on providing future protection or reinstatement, not a mechanism for attempting to provide compensation for past resource impairments. Thus, remediation authorities have properly refrained from seeking additional recoveries, over and above the costs of ensuring future protection of public health and the environment, to finance still further cleanup as "compensatory remediation" for the presence of pollution during the period between the spill or release and the implementation of cleanup. Similarly there is no justification for imposing additional NRDs to finance further restoration measures, beyond those needed to reinstate prospectively impaired public uses, as "compensation" for past impairments. Thus, in the fishery example presented earlier, where a spill or release causes public fishing opportunities at a site to be reduced from 200 fish/day to 100 fish/day, restoration measures should be selected with the aim of providing the public with comparable opportunities to catch an additional 100 fish/day or its equivalent in value, not some higher level (such as 150 fish/day) to "compensate" for impaired fishing opportunities in the past.

For several reasons, there should also be no additional NRD recoveries, over and above restoration costs, based on nonuse losses. First, while the public undoubtedly places a high value on the preservation of certain natural resources, this value is fully served by protective government regulatory and resource management programs and, in cases where injury occurs, by prompt restoration. Any possible nonuse losses associated with temporary resource injury in the interim before restoration is accomplished are too evanescent and fleeting to serve as an appropriate basis for recovery of additional damages beyond the costs of restoration. Second, any such recoveries could not in any event compensate for nonuse losses. Because they are surplus to the cost of restoration, such recoveries will necessarily be spent on other measures that bear little or no relation to any nonuse value of the injured resource, which is already being addressed through restoration. Further, as with NRD recovery for past lost use, nonuse recoveries are not paid to the individuals who may have suffered a loss, and there is no assurance that such individuals will obtain commensurate benefits from trustee expenditure of the surplus recoveries. Third, as environmentalists often point out, the value to the public of preserving significant natural resources is primarily noneconomic in character. Seeking to impose monetary damages based on nonuse values ignores this basic moral reality and improperly seeks to place a price on values that are noneconomic in character. Fourth, there is at present valid and reliable methodology available for quantifying nonuse losses in monetary terms; CVM and conjoint analysis have yet to prove themselves reliable in the nonuse context. Fifth, as with NRD claims based on past lost use, trustee efforts to obtain enormous additional recoveries based on nonuse claims inevitably provoke intense controversy, litigation, high transaction costs, and delay.

Appropriate methods should be used to scale resource injury and restoration projects to ensure reinstatement of impaired public uses

In order to ensure that restoration projects adequately and appropriately reinstate impaired public uses, one must scale the diminution in public uses resulting from a spill or release and the enhancement of public uses provided by restoration projects in order to determine whether the enhanced uses provided through restoration are equivalent to the impairment. As previously explained, damages is an economic concept; scaling should accordingly be based on the economic welfare of the members of the public. Restoration measures should provide the public, on a going-forward basis, resource uses equivalent in public welfare or utility to the decrement in uses due to a spill or release. The relevant decreases and increases in the public's economic welfare can be measured by techniques such as travel cost methodology or by other methods, such as those discussed by Mathews et al. (this volume), to scale the utility provided to resource users by different resource use opportunities.

It does not necessarily follow, however, that any measure that provides the public as a whole with increased economic welfare equal to the impairment caused by a spill or release qualifies as appropriate restoration. Certain distributional considerations should also be taken into account in determining whether the requirement of equivalency is satisfied. First, the video arcade cannot qualify as a restoration measure. Second, the restoration measure must be located at or in the vicinity of the resource injured; a restoration measure in one part of the country cannot appropriately compensate for impairment of uses in another part of the country. Third, there must be an appropriate relation between the type of uses impaired and those provided by the restoration measures. The uses need not and often cannot be identical, but should be similar. The flexibility afforded by the concept of equivalency enables trustees and PRPs to agree on workable and practicable restoration alternatives. This flexibility is illustrated by the Cantara Loop example discussed by Birdsall et al. (this volume). The PRP and trustee authorities agreed to development of publicly available put-and-take stocked trout fishing ponds to provide a temporary substitute for catch-and-release fishing in the river while the river fishery was recovering. The 2 fishing experiences were not identical; some members of the public placed a higher value on the original uses while others preferred the uses provided through the ponds. The parties reasonably concluded, however, that the substitute provided reasonably equivalent resource uses to the public. Developing appropriate criteria for restoration equivalency is likely to be an important research task for the future.

While the NOAA NRD assessment regulations provide for scaling based on economic valuation in some cases, they afford primacy to scaling based on resource services, including resource-to-resource services, without reference to public uses or economic welfare. There are a number of fundamental flaws involved in making this type scaling the basis for restoration decisions. Basing restoration solely on resource-to-resource services in the abstract severs the essential link to committed public uses and public welfare. It allows trustees to pursue very costly replication-based approaches to restoration even in cases where there has been no significant impairment of public uses or where alternative, far less costly means of reinstating those uses are available. Moreover, as noted previously, replication of all baseline resource-to-resource services, either through on-site rehabilitation or through other alternatives, is literally impossible. One cannot create the exact physical, chemical, and biological conditions of the hypothetical ecosystem that would exist if a spill or release, and the ensuing cleanup, had never occurred. Nor can science tell us which of the myriad resource-to-resource services that a resource would have provided in the absence of a spill or release should be selected for reinstatement over others or the proper extent of reinstatement of any particular service, especially when reinstatement of one service may impair reinstatement or maintenance of other services. An example of such a trade-off is provided by the Fields Brooks NRD site in Ohio where trustee authorities have called for extensive conversion of uplands into wetlands as a restoration measure for dealing with injury to existing wetlands. There is no objective, scientific basis for determining whether the increased resource-to-resource services provided by the newly created wetlands outweigh the losses in entirely different resource-to-resource services resulting from converting the uplands. Unless committed public uses and the economic value of such uses are brought into play in order to evaluate the losses caused by a spill or release and the gains provided by restoration, the restoration decision process is rudderless. In lieu of an objective criterion that can be implemented in workable fashion—reinstatement of public uses of equivalent value—NOAA's approach gives trustees essentially arbitrary power to pick and choose among restoration objectives and measures and to generate enormously and excessively costly restoration projects. Such a decisional approach is unsound in principle and creates an unacceptable risk of arbitrary decisions.

A form of public-use-based resource scaling may, however, serve as a practical guide to cooperative trustee/PRP restoration decisions in certain cases without the need for full-fledged economic valuation of impaired uses and the enhanced uses provided by a restoration measure. To invoke an earlier example, if a trout stream with privately owned access available for lease is near a public trout stream that incurred a spill and is in the process of recovering, and if the 2 streams provide similar fishing opportunities and scenic amenities and are similarly accessible to the public, interested parties may agree that the uses that would be provided to the public by the privately accessed stream are equivalent in value to those provided by the public stream without the need to resort to full-fledged economic studies to quantify the values of the 2 sets of uses. But recognizing the potential utility of public-use-based resource scaling as a guide in particular restoration decisions is a far cry from NOAA's approach, which authorizes trustees to divorce resource scaling and restoration decision-making from public uses and abandons requirements of cost-effectiveness and cost-reasonableness.

A focus on reinstatement of public uses will promote cooperative approaches to prompt restoration

Basing restoration on reinstatement of impaired public uses provides an objective, practical focus for restoration decision-making that promotes cooperation between trustees and PRPs and fosters prompt restoration. This is the lesson of experiences at sites such as Cantara Loop and Lavaca Bay. In other cases, however, trustees have declined to make reinstatement of impaired public uses the focus of restoration. Instead, they have sought far more costly restoration measures based on approximating the physical, chemical, and biological conditions that a resource would have had, had a release not occurred. They have also sought additional recoveries, over and above the costs of restoration, based on past lost use and nonuse claims. As experience at sites such as Berks, Clark Fork, and Los Angeles Harbor reflects, such an approach almost inevitably provokes controversy and mistrust, uncertainty, litigation, delay, and high transaction costs. As NOAA and DOI, along with other trustees, prepare to assert large numbers of additional NRD claims, the choice between these 2 approaches has important implications for the future of the NRD programs. If an approach focused on reinstatement of impaired public uses is chosen, it will be possible to achieve prompt restoration at reasonable cost to all concerned. If that approach is rejected, the NRD programs will be plagued by antagonism, high costs for all parties, and failure to achieve timely restoration.

Conclusion

The approach to restoration decision-making developed herein makes reinstatement of impaired human uses on a going-forward basis the focal point of restoration. It reflects sound law and public policy and will promote constructive solutions to restoration. This approach enables decision-makers to resolve appropriately the 2 issues posed by the conference. Restoration projects should be selected in order to reinstate committed public resource uses in a cost-effective, cost-reasonable, and timely manner. The level of restoration selected should provide the public with resource uses equivalent in value to uses impaired as the result of a spill or release.

Overview of Conference Objectives

*Martin J. McHugh**

Natural resource trustees and the regulated community are making progress in the task of restoring natural resources injured by oil spills and releases from contaminated sites. Many public and private stakeholders are working to avoid the expensive and time-consuming path of litigating formal natural resource damage (NRD) claims and have made concerted efforts to achieve restoration by more cooperative means. The desire by parties to find more effective and timely ways to address NRDs and restoration is reflected in recent initiatives such as the provisions for cooperative damage assessment within the rules promulgated by the National Oceanic and Atmospheric Administration (NOAA), the efforts to integrate assessment and restoration into the cleanup process, and the sponsorship of this conference, which will aid in the development of restoration strategies for lost human uses of the environment.

The challenge of recreating or replacing what natural processes have created over many years has not daunted those who have pursued new, creative, and constructive approaches to restoration. However, the participants active in facing this challenge have identified important issues that need to be addressed in order to promote the shared goal: more timely, effective, and efficient restoration. The purpose of this conference is to benefit from past experience and to explore these issues by focusing on one component of the overall restoration goal: the restoration of interim loss of human uses of natural resources due to releases of hazardous substances and oil. The 2 primary objectives of the conference are to 1) identify projects that can replace/restore interim lost human uses and 2) determine how much restoration is required. The collective experiences of state and federal natural resource trustees as well as the regulated, consulting, and environmental communities will be drawn upon to meet these objectives. To further these objectives, the following observations and issues are offered from the perspective of New Jersey's natural resource damage assessment and restoration program. While restoration has been pursued in New Jersey for a number of years, the formal program, in existence for nearly 4 years, draws on an experience of response to over 50 oil spills and hazardous sites, a dozen of which are currently in various stages of restoration or restoration planning.

Background

When Congress established the provisions for natural resource damage assessment (NRDA) and restoration in the Superfund program, it acknowledged that efforts to clean up contaminated sites and oil spills may not address the harm to natural resources and the losses associated with their impact to fisheries, wildlife, and public lands and waters. The Superfund cleanup program would strive for successful cleanups to eliminate or isolate the contamination, reduce the threat to human health, and,

*The views and opinions expressed in this paper are solely those of the author and do not necessarily represent the position of the New Jersey Department of Environmental Protection or the State of New Jersey.

possibly, the risk to natural resources. However, Congress anticipated that in many cases successful cleanups might not result in any restoration of natural resources or restoration to a level that would make the environment and public "whole." Historically, releases from contaminated sites and oil spills have injured fish and wildlife, have closed public parks and swimming areas, and have restricted the use of lakes, river, and streams. These impacts can linger for years after the cleanup, and the persistent nature of many of the substances contaminating natural resources can result in permanent impacts that may prevent any natural recovery. Congress therefore acknowledged the need to authorize a program pursuant to the Comprehensive Environmental Response, Compensation, and Liability Act (CERCLA) that would provide for the identification of natural resource injuries and the means to accomplish restoration.

Restoration as compensation for natural resource injuries is derived from the government's legal responsibility to administer and protect natural resources that are held in trust for the benefit of the public. This stewardship responsibility was initially codified in federal law, in CERCLA, and in the Clean Water Act, and then reaffirmed by Congress with the passage of the Oil Pollution Act of 1990 (OPA). While some states followed this federal lead by enacting separate NRD statutes, many states had preexisting authority within general environmental statutes. The legal "trustee" responsibility set forth in federal and state law advances common law principles arising from the Public Trust Doctrine. The legal rationale for restoration of natural resources is clear from a number of standpoints. From a public-health, quality-of-life, and conservation standpoint, the public attributes an intrinsic value to fisheries, wildlife, lands, and water. In addition, the active use of natural resources is identified with a vast array of both consumptive (fishing and hunting, etc.) and non-consumptive uses (hiking, boating, camping, wildlife viewing, etc.). Thus, one specific resource can provide a range of values. For instance, use values associated with waterfowl can range from bird watching to bird hunting. In both cases, a complete and fulfilling experience can be dependent on the ability of participants to enjoy all of the resources in the marsh habitat of waterfowl, even if they do not spot a single bird. It is important to note that together, the intrinsic and use values attributed to natural resources are also reflected prominently in the health of numerous local and regional economies. From this economic standpoint, the restoration of fisheries, wildlife, lands, waters, and other resources takes on additional import for the government and the public.

In general, the restoration of lost human uses in almost all cases entails the restoration of the biological resources that provide the services upon which all uses are based. In order to pursue a full claim for restoration, it is necessary to undertake a preliminary identification of the baseline natural resources and the services provided by such resources prior to the release. The next steps include an assessment of the injury caused by the release and quantification of the injury from the time of the release and into the future prior to restoration. Furthermore, the quantification of lost services associated with the injured natural resources is a necessary component of a restoration process that will make the environment and public whole.

Full restoration may also require the assessment of possible lost intrinsic or passive-use values discussed above, in addition to consumptive and non-consumptive use values. While the damage assessment rules describing the above process have generated much debate, the passive use or "nonuse" aspect has created the most controversy. It is not necessary to reach this issue in order to meet the objectives of this conference. Similarly, issues such as past losses, specific assessment methodologies, and others that may be the subject of current or pending litigation can be put aside in order to focus on restoration of interim lost human uses. It is possible that by narrowing the focus to the one facet of restoration involving lost human uses, conference participants may discover successful approaches, applicable elsewhere, that also may facilitate the resolution of related restoration issues.

Restoration of interim lost human uses

In many instances throughout the literature of NRDA, terms have been used interchangeably, e.g., "damages" and "injury." The restoration of interim lost human uses is a phrase that has been given another description in the damage assessment regulations promulgated by NOAA, i.e., "compensatory restoration." This aspect of restoration is directed at compensating the public for the "natural resource outage," the loss of a resource and the services it provides from the time of the release until the time it is restored. The need for compensatory restoration or restoration for interim losses in many situations is due to the realities of the cleanup process. Cleanups of releases from contaminated sites and even oil spills can take many years. Following a cleanup, residual contamination may remain in the environment, potentially impacting resources for more years to come. This may be temporary, until resources recover naturally, or there may be a lingering impairment in perpetuity. This of course will depend on the nature of the substance released, the physical characteristics of the ecosystem, and the resources impacted. It may be that a cleanup will restore the use of a resource. Some cleanups involve the restoration of the use of a resource (such as the remediation of groundwater). In such cases, the need for compensatory restoration will be dictated by the baseline of services provided prior to the release and the length of time for the completion of the cleanup. The degree of compensatory restoration then becomes a function time of impact or time of recovery, if recovery occurs. The complexity of determining the need for and degree of compensatory restoration will depend on the nature of the resources impacted and the relation of those resources to the services provided.

In the case of some oil spills along the coast, it has been the experience of state trustees that public beaches impacted by the deposition of tarballs may remained closed, either officially or de facto, for many weeks while the oil washes in and out with the tides, with cleanup crews working diligently. The lost human use aspect is heightened if such spills impact bathing or fishing areas during the traditional tourist season. The selection of restoration projects to compensate for interim lost use of the beaches may not require regard for ecological resources but will entail the enhancement of access to the affected area or comparable substitutes, in order to compensate for access lost or devalued by the spill. If the spill impacted wetlands that provided bird watching opportunities, the selection of interim restoration measures becomes complicated by the need to estimate the impact of oil residues on the wetlands, the time to natural recovery (since cleanup is usually precluded), and any associated loss of bird-watching opportunity. Interim restoration measures may then require the manipulation of ecological resources on site or within the watershed to increase bird habitat. This may be performed in combination with some level of increased public access to the restored area if it is feasible and does not threaten the integrity of the underlying ecological resources providing the human uses.

In New Jersey, there are 2 notable restoration projects underway that focus on the restoration of lost human uses due to the closure of public shorelines and waterways as a result of oil spills. The BT Nautilus grounding in June 1990 resulted in the injury of natural resources from the Port on New York/New Jersey down to Cape May, New Jersey. Injuries included the closure of Atlantic Coast bathing beaches at Island Beach State Park and the de facto closure of miles of other coastal beaches. In order to restore the lost access, use, and enjoyment of the beaches, an interpretive center will be developed at the park, which is centrally located in the spill impact zone and the state. The facility will increase access to coastal and estuarine resources in 2 ways. First, it will provide a year-round physical access point for aquatic, walking, and biking tours of the 10-mile shoreline park, which contains the state's most dynamic mix of coastal and estuarine resources. Second, the interpretive program, displays, and meeting area will increase visitors' access, use, and enjoyment of resources by enhancing their knowledge and understanding of the fish, wildlife, and habitat (many of which were also impacted by the spill) found in this unique coastal ecosystem. This restoration project is just part of the overall restoration for injuries to wildlife, wetlands, and other resources caused by the spill.

On the western side of the state, the *MT Presidente Rivera's* 1989 spill into the Delaware River had a similar effect on the public's use of the river and the shoreline during the extended cleanup. Among the injuries resulting from the spill was the loss of use of the river for fishing/boating and the loss of shoreline access. New Jersey's Fort Mott State Park was impacted by shoreline oiling, and because of its location, it was utilized as a staging area for cleanup operations. In partial restoration of these lost human uses, a portion of settlement funds was combined with other sources to restore a historic earthen pier at the impacted park. The project will increase access to natural resources by providing a physical access point to the river. In addition, the pier will enable an existing passenger ferry, which currently runs from Fort Dupont in Delaware to that state's Fort Delaware and nature area on Pea Patch Island, to complete the journey across the river to dock at the restored pier in Fort Mott State Park. This will enable New Jersey visitors at Fort Mott to experience the resources of the river and to visit the

State of Delaware's nature area and historical forts. Delaware visitors will now be able to travel to New Jersey's park, permanently connecting each of the states' official coastal heritage trails and opening a new venue for the enjoyment of the resources shared by the states bordering this river.

The above examples of human-use restoration are projects that would normally be associated with oil spills not requiring the manipulation of ecological resources. However, additional human-use restoration requiring specific ecological restoration (i.e., wetlands and wildlife restoration) is underway for both spills. Due to the nature of oil spills, the scientific knowledge of oil types, and extensive experience with oil impacts to ecosystems, it is possible to predict the weathering of oil and its effect on natural resources for the purpose of planning such ecological restoration. In contrast, contaminated sites can present a more involved process to access injuries, lost uses, and the appropriate degree of restoration for interim lost human uses. Contaminated sites present many variables not generally associated with oil spills, including 1) chronic releases of unknown volumes that are often not visible, 2) a mixture of hazardous substances, 3) sublethal or long-term impacts that are difficult to assess, and 4) the difficulty of obtaining historical data on lost human uses. The initial focus of cleanup programs on human-health risk generated remedial investigations that in most cases did not contain enough ecological data necessary to fully characterize injury. Fortunately, both the U.S. Environmental Protection Agency and the states have begun to broaden the scope of site investigations by increasing ecological evaluations and ecological risk assessments. These can be very useful tools for natural resource trustees because they contain substantially the information needed to "pre-assess" a site, to begin, and even to complete an assessment of natural resource injuries. What a typical remedial investigation does not contain, however, is information on past injuries that may have naturally recovered to some degree and human-use data to determine compensatory restoration. When natural resource trustees are integrated into the cleanup programs, this lost human-use information can be requested and obtained more easily than reconstructed later.

The human uses lost as the result of releases from contaminated sites typically derive from the ecological resources impacted by the releases. In such cases, natural resource services cannot exclusively be viewed as an abstract activity that may be restored independently of the injured ecological resources from which the service flows. This concept derives from information generated through the promulgation of the damage assessment rules.

In addition to the above complexities, the trustees and regulated community have had less experience with restoration associated with hazardous sites. This experience has shown, however, that when trustees are not involved in the investigation, feasibility study, and remedy selection process, the need for increased restoration may result. For example, a wetland that is dewatered by the extraction and treatment of groundwater may increase the need for restoration if the treated water is pumped out of the watershed. Trustee involvement can spur efforts to reduce the injury or avoid it by returning the treated water to the watershed (e.g., through sheet flow or reinjection). The involvement of natural resource trustees will help promote less destructive remedies that will aid in reducing the need for additional restoration.

Conclusion—restoration realities

Ultimately, the strategies to restore interim lost human uses associated with a spill or release must be guided by the general principles established under both CERCLA and OPA to restore, replace, or acquire the equivalent of resources that have been injured. Despite the complexities referenced above, the application of this hierarchy for the selection of appropriate restoration projects has produced successes for restoration of interim lost human uses and for restoration of other services as well. A trustee or responsible party with experience in applying this hierarchy has probably faced certain typical issues that arise in the course of proceeding through the process of selecting actual restoration projects. The following list highlights some of these issues for reference during this conference. However, the key restoration realities to remain apprised of are the inherent complexity of natural resources, their interrelation and function within differing ecosystems, the range of direct/indirect services they provide to humans, and the range of values placed on these services by humans. When releases of hazardous substances or oil are added to this equation, trustees will seek to apply current scientific information combined with past experience to make what is necessarily a case-by-case restoration determination. This reality is problematic for the regulated community, which necessarily seeks predictability in order to forecast liability. It will therefore benefit all stakeholders to work toward general strategies and guidance that can be applied to case-specific conditions to improve the process for trustees and the regulated community. The effort to achieve the objectives of this conference will help lay a foundation for this restoration goal.

Direct restoration

The restoration of the actual resources harmed by a release from a hazardous site or an oil spill presents the issue of availability of options on the actual site or in the vicinity. Restoration options can be limited by numerous on-site conditions (e.g., size, open space no affected by remedial structures, etc.). Options in the geographic vicinity may also be limited by other contamination. Due to the protracted nature of the cleanup of contaminated sites, it is not always certain when a cleanup will be completed in order to allow for on-site restoration.

Replacement

Replacement (which is equivalent to creation of new resources or enhancement of existing resources to achieve a net gain of services) has a successful track record limited to a few habitat types (e.g., wetlands, stream beds) and limited to a small number of species (e.g., waterfowl, piping plovers, salmon and trout fisheries). The time from injury until full restoration for some ecosystems can be substantial due to natural processes, which in turn increases interim losses (e.g., when replacing mature upland forests, it may not be feasible to plant 50-year-old trees).

Acquisition of equivalent

Equivalent resources are often not available for purchase or lease in the vicinity of the injured resources. In the case of purchasing habitat, in order to offset the fact that a net gain of services will not be accomplished, larger areas are sought. Again, the availability of large contiguous areas may be very limited. Evaluating the equivalency of resources that are of a different type is the most complex step of this restoration option. NOAA's guidance documents may prove instrumental in meeting this need.

General issues

- Trustees generally lack the financial resources to aid the responsible party in identifying restoration projects. Trustees do not have access to Superfund, and few state trustees have annual appropriations.
- Trustees require the means to better communicate with land preservation entities within and outside of state and federal government in order to become quickly apprised of restoration opportunities that can be conveyed to responsible parties and to form restoration partnerships.
- Trustees need the resources to refine the methods for community involvement in restoration planning in order that all parties benefit from the experience and knowledge of local experts and interested groups.
- Despite the data on certain fisheries and wetlands projects, consistent objective criteria for measuring restoration success is needed for trustees to be able to monitor restoration projects.
- A national database is necessary to compile information on restoration successes and failures as a reference for all stakeholders.
- An effort to expand the view of restoration to a landscape or watershed perspective would give more flexibility to the restoration process. This is consistent with the initiative to compile environmental information based on ecosystems (e.g., estuary programs) and the movement to base new environmental regulations on landscape or watershed approaches.
- Regional restoration plans developed by estuary programs and similar ecosystem advisory authorities can provide a source of readily identified restoration projects. Natural resource trustees should consider increased participation in such programs and the regulated community should become familiar with programs in their operations area.
- Trustees, cleanup programs, and the regulated community need to promote the integration of damage assessment as part of the investigation and remediation of contaminated sites in order to reduce transaction costs and overall NRD liability by 1) enabling the collection of NRD information during the remedial investigation, 2) promoting remedy selection that is more protective of re-

sources, and 3) creating opportunities for restoration to be "built into" the selected remedy.

- The trend toward restoration-based damage assessments should be continued as the alternative to monetary-based assessments, which promote litigation, delays in restoration, and less cooperation.

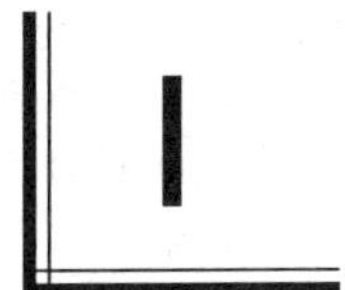

A Proposed Framework for Developing and Selecting Compensatory Restoration Projects under Federal Natural Resource Damage Assessment Statutes[1]

Robert E. Unsworth,[2] Mark D. Barash[3], Michael T. Huguenin[2]

Much of what has been written about the natural resource damage assessment (NRDA) process has centered on the manner in which monetary damages are estimated and recovered. Current approaches to NRDA, however, focus on effective and timely restoration of injured natural resources and the services they provide. This paper proposes a functional framework for the development and selection of restoration projects to compensate the public for interim losses in services. Specifically, it attempts to answer 3 commonly raised questions regarding the nature of appropriate compensatory restoration actions. In doing so, it clarifies and expands on the guidance currently available to trustees, responsible parties, and others involved in the restoration planning process.[4]

The category of restoration actions that aim to compensate the public for services lost from the time of an oil or hazardous substance release through restoration of the underlying resource to its baseline is referred to in the National Oceanic and Atmospheric Administration's (NOAA) regulations for damage assessment under the Oil Pollution Act (OPA) as "compensatory restoration" [15 C.F.R. §990.53]. While the Department of the Interior's (DOI) regulations for the conduct of damage assessments under the Comprehensive Environmental Response, Compensation, and Liability Act (CERCLA) [42 USC 9601-9675] and the Clean Water Act [33 USC 1251-1387] do not explicitly mention compensatory restoration, the conduct of restoration activities to compensate for interim losses in services is discussed in its regulations under use of compensable value awards [43 C.F.R. §11.84]. The common goal under these frame-

[1]The views and opinions expressed in this paper are solely those of the authors and do not necessarily represent the position of the United States Department of the Interior or of the United States government.

[2]Industrial Economics, Incorporated, Cambridge, MA.

[3]Office of the Solicitor, U.S. Department of the Interior, Boston, MA.

[4]While there are a number of challenging and interesting issues associated with the selection of primary restoration options, this paper focuses solely on the approaches used to identify and select compensatory options.

works is to use natural resource restoration as a means to make the public whole for its losses. Thus, without compensatory restoration, the public will be left uncompensated for actual losses incurred.[5]

In many cases the selection of appropriate compensatory restoration activities is noncontroversial. For example, the release of a contaminant might result in reduced catch rates for recreational anglers for a short period of time, but not in other significant short- or long-term changes to the affected natural resources or the services these resources provide. If options to address some other source of impairment to the fish population at the site can be quickly and easily adopted, thus enhancing future catch rates as compensation for past losses, such actions may be sufficient to achieve the objective of compensable restoration. The identification and selection of restoration actions in cases such as this generally do not represent much of a challenge for trustees or responsible parties.

In other cases, however, it may not be feasible, desirable, or sufficient to produce, as a means of compensatory restoration, additional use opportunities of the same type and quality as those that were lost. This may be due to resource capacity constraints, the continued presence of a hazardous material, a conflict with resource management goals (e.g., limitations on access to allow for resource recovery), or other factors that constrain the ability to provide compensatory restoration "on-site and in-kind" [61 *Federal Register* §448, 5 Jan 1996]. For example, a water body that has been closed to recreation for many years may have experienced thousands of present value lost-use opportunities. Even given full recovery to baseline, the resource might not be able to support the level of additional recreational use necessary to fully compensate the public. Similarly, actions to increase the use of a fishery that continues to pose a health threat even after primary restoration is complete might not be viewed as desirable by state or local health officials. In other cases, complex and fundamental changes in the services provided by the resource may have occurred, and these changes may not easily be described in terms of lost visitor days or other simple metrics. For example, contamination of a site may have led to a change in its aesthetic value.

We present 3 questions commonly raised by trustees, responsible parties, and members of the public involved in NRDA. We then address these questions through 3 fundamental principles regarding the selection of compensatory restoration projects. We provide support for these principles based on the legislative and public policy histories of CERCLA and OPA's damage assessment provisions and the resultant regulations and regulatory guidance issued by NOAA and DOI. Finally, we provide several hypothetical case studies that demonstrate the role these principles should play in the restoration planning process.

[5]It could also be argued that without the requirement of compensatory restoration, there would be no incentive to choose more aggressive primary restoration actions designed to speed natural recovery of the resource (i.e., failure to recognize the value of interim losses from the time of the release through full recovery will lead trustees and responsible parties to choose primary restoration options that restore resources more slowly than is appropriate).

A key term used in this paper, "human use," has been defined by various parties in different ways during discussions of the NRDA process. We define human use as the human derivation of value from a natural resource. Values may derive from a wide variety of consumptive (e.g., hunting), nonconsumptive (e.g., bird watching), and passive uses (e.g., a desire to protect an endangered species regardless of opportunities to see that species firsthand). Under this definition, changes in human use resulting from a release of a hazardous substance may be expressed in terms of direct human behavioral changes or changes in attitudes toward or perceptions of the resource.

This definition may be viewed by some as overly broad, especially in so far as it incorporates passive-use values. Passive-use values are commonly associated with the tool often used to measure them: contingent valuation. The purpose of this paper is not to reopen the discussion of whether contingent valuation accurately measures passive-use values or whether such values should be included in damage claims; these arguments are familiar to most in the NRDA community. We do believe, however, that it is difficult to draw a fixed line between the value the public holds for natural resources associated with their current direct use (e.g., fishing, swimming), and those associated with indirect or passive uses. For example, society may value the option to study an endangered freshwater mussel species even if it is not currently exercising this option in order to better understand why the species appears immune to certain cancers. Similarly, an individual might move to a region due in part to the region's reputation for a clean environment. In these cases, individuals derive value from natural resources without directly interacting with them. Changes in the quality of the environment due to a hazardous substance release, however, could clearly affect these individual's behaviors and attitudes. The principles presented in this paper should apply equally to active- and passive-use losses.

In addition to development and selection of compensatory restoration options, trustees must appropriately scale the selected projects to make the public whole for its losses. For example, the trustees may conclude that wetland construction is the best means to compensate the public for interim losses resulting from a release. A question that remains, however, is how many acres of wetland will be required to make the public whole. While important to the policy debate, this topic is not addressed directly in this paper, but we hope it will be addressed more fully by other papers given at this conference.

Commonly asked questions

Despite the guidance provided in NOAA's and DOI's regulations and associated documents, several questions regarding the identification and selection of appropriate compensatory restoration actions are commonly raised. These include the following:

- *Is it appropriate to provide compensatory services via projects that do not involve restoring the resource that originally provided those services?* For example, the release of a hazardous substance may have resulted in a reduction in the population of an important game fish. Because of this population effect, recreational catch rates may have been depressed from the time of the resource through recovery of the resource to baseline condition. In this case, would a stocking program designed to enhance catch rates in the future be sufficient to meet the goal of compensatory restoration?

- *What does the relationship need to be between the particular human uses, values, or resources that were lost and the resources and services gained through the selected restoration projects?* That is, how broad a suite of projects can be considered for compensatory restoration? For example, we are aware of a community that identified construction of a bike path as a means to compensate for lost use of a groundwater resource. A related but more specific question that has been raised is whether the provision of an equivalent level of consumer surplus (economic welfare) represents an acceptable linkage.
- *Do the selected projects need to be conducted near the site where the injury occurred?* That is, does restoration need to take place in the ecosystem or political entity that suffered the loss? For example, can a restoration alternative designed to compensate the public for a fisheries closure be undertaken in a different, but nearby, watershed?

Three principles for identification and selection of restoration alternatives

Available guidance on the identification and selection of compensatory restoration alternatives fails to address several important questions that are commonly raised in the course of damage assessments. As a result, compensatory restoration alternatives for many cases are being identified and selected using ad hoc processes and criteria. The absence of a clear set of goals and a standard framework makes it difficult for trustees to act consistently, especially as the number of cases brought by state and tribal trustees increases. Such inconsistency makes it equally difficult for responsible parties to understand their potential liabilities and to participate in the damage assessment and restoration planning process in an effective manner. In addition, this inconsistency could result in the development of claims that fail to meet the original intentions of Congress in establishing the damage assessment provisions of CERCLA and OPA.

The following are a set of principles to guide trustees and responsible parties in identifying and selecting from among restoration options. These principles are intended to expand on and clarify, not replace, the guidance already provided by DOI and NOAA. It will not, in all cases, be possible or even desirable to abide by all of these principles, but they should form a guide and act to clarify some significant questions raised during the course of restoration planning. Other principles may be identified; however, we view these as addressing the most fundamental issues commonly raised in the damage assessment process.

Principle 1:
Restoration of lost human uses should be based on restoration or enhancement of the natural resources that form the basis of those uses

All human uses of natural resources derive from some service provided by the resource (e.g., the opportunity to catch fish, the aesthetic value of a pristine river, the value of a wetland in supporting a bird migration). In many cases it is feasible to provide replacement services without actually enhancing a natural resource. For example, to compensate for a long-term reduction in fish catch by recreational anglers, it might be possible to simply stock the river with adult fish for some number of years into the future, thus increasing the catch rate of anglers using the resource. A preferred option, however, would be to undertake resource enhancement projects to allow the river to support a greater naturally sustainable population of native fish. While restoration of lost human uses without concomitant restoration of the resources that support these services may still be required in some cases, this should be viewed as a less preferred option for compensation for interim lost use.

In some cases trustees have considered options to "acquire the equivalent" [15 C.F.R. §990.25] of the resources and services lost as a result of a release. Since the purpose of the damage assessment process is to make the public whole for its losses through the restoration of natural resources, it is imperative that resources be acquired only in cases where those resources might otherwise be at risk of loss or degradation. For example, acquisition of wetland in an area with effective and consistent wetland development regulations might not provide the public with services beyond those which they already had.

Principle 2:
The link between the resources and services lost as a result of the release and the resources and services gained through the proposed compensatory restoration actions should be reasonable and explicit

A common issue encountered among practitioners of NRDA is how connected the proposed restoration action needs to be to an injured resource or lost human use. We believe that a strong bias should exist toward restoration options that can be reasonably and explicitly linked to the lost service (and thus, the users who suffered the loss) and the injured resource. In short, simply doing good things for the resource or the affected community is not a sufficient justification for a restoration alternative, nor is it consistent with the damage assessment provisions of CERCLA or OPA. As an extreme example, an option to use funds recovered as part of a compensable damage claim to offset a community's water and sewer bills would not fall within the spirit of the statutes under which these claims are made, despite the fact that arguments could be made that the public could be made as well off.

Welfare economics provides tools that can enable us to place economic values on natural resources and the services they provide. Given that these tools can be used to measure the value of both lost services and those proposed as part of a restoration program, the argument has been made that the public can be made whole through the provision of services of similar value, but not explicitly related to, the services that were lost. In these cases value is expressed in terms of economic welfare losses and gains (e.g., consumer surplus changes). For example, the lost use of a river for recreational fishing from the time of a release through full recovery to baseline might be estimated to be worth $1 million. A project to provide a bikeway near the site might be expected to yield a similar welfare gain, and thus might be offered as a means of making the public whole for its loss. The selection and scaling of restoration options may, in some cases, benefit from efforts to assess the associated economic welfare losses and gains. Principle 2, however, argues that such an approach should not form the sole basis of the restoration option selection process.

Principle 3:
The link between the resources and services lost as a result of the release and the resources and services gained through the proposed compensatory restoration actions can, if necessary, transcend physical and political boundaries

Another common question asked of NRDA practitioners is whether there are any limitations to the geographic scope of the projects that can be selected for compensable restoration. For example, does the restoration need to take place within the watershed in which the release and injury occurred? Can compensation for interim lost use be provided on a different stream from that which suffered the loss?

It is our belief that there can be no universal physical or political limitations imposed on the consideration of restoration options, but instead the scope should be determined by the nature of the injured resource and the human users of that resource. For example, the appropriate geographic scope for actions to restore lost fishing trips would be all of the substitutes that users of the injured resource might reasonably access. Information on reasonable substitutes is often available as a result of the damage assessment process or from regional resource managers. Alternatively, the appropriate scope for a restoration project for an endangered bird species affected by an oil spill might be defined as the full range of the species. As an extreme example, we can imagine situations in which a spill results in the death of several hundred endangered birds somewhere on the east coast of the U.S., but where the most cost-effective restoration alternative involves protection of the bird's wintering habitat in South America. Thus, the appropriate geographic scope for restoration actions might be defined differently for different categories of loss, even at the same site.

While this principle states that there are no predefined geographic bounds for restoration actions, it also implies that on-site restoration might be the most preferred option (i.e., given obvious ecological and economic linkages). Specifically, it can be argued that options that are more distant from the site in question, both geographically and ecologically or economically, are by definition, going to be less effective and efficient to implement. For example, the more distant a proposed substitute use opportunity, the less likely users of the injured resource will benefit from it. Similarly, while options to improve the habitat of a species at some distance from the site of injury may exist, the more distant these projects are from the site of the original injury, the more difficult it will be to demonstrate benefits to the injured population (i.e., the weaker the ecological link). There may be, however, obvious technical characteristics that limit the availability of such on-site options. For example, the continued presence of contamination may limit the trustees desire to encourage a recreational fishery at the site. Alternatively, a resource may have fully recovered, thus offering no opportunity for additional restoration. For example, a spill may have resulted in the death of a number of endangered birds. If everything reasonable is already being undertaken at the site to protect these birds, it may not be feasible to spend additional funds at the spill location. Thus, as with the other principles described in this paper, there may exist other factors that influence the process used to select restoration alternatives.

The NOAA regulations explicitly allow trustees to consider all or part of an existing regional restoration plan or other existing, planned, or proposed environmental restoration projects as one of a range of restoration alternatives [61 *Federal Register* 455, 5 Jan 1996]. While the regional restoration planning process envisioned in the NOAA rule is a relatively formal process (e.g., the requirement that public comment be received on the plan), in many cases trustees have considered alternatives that involve taking advantage of existing plans or combining the settlements from several cases into one restoration fund. In these cases the trustees hope to achieve economies in planning and implementation of the restoration option. Under this principle, restoration activities may be undertaken at the regional level if careful consideration is given to the human use or ecological linkage between the regional plan and the injury it is intended to compensate for. It is our opinion that the regional restoration planning option is not pursued as much as it should be by trustees. Such options hold the potential for substantive restoration activities while also reducing planning and implementation costs and facilitating quicker settlements of damage claims.

The legislative and policy basis of these principles

The concept of restoration, as a remedy, although similar to the doctrine of penance, or "putting right, things wrong," was never comfortably endorsed by the English common law. In the United States, while restoration has not been the general rule, its application to natural resource concerns predates current federal environmental legislation. In *Feather River Lumber Co. v. United States* [30 F. 2nd 642 (9th Cir. 1929), page 644], an action for damages to federal land arising from a negligently caused fire, the Court held that the proper measure of damages for injury to young timber includes the "cost of restoring the land to the condition in which it was before the fire." The Court noted that this measure of damages represented that which is required to make the government whole. Beyond the confines of the courtroom, this approach is enshrined on cardboard signs in souvenir shops throughout the country, which state "Pretty to look at, fun to hold, but if you break it, we mark it sold!" It is also a recurring theme within the modern American family, as in "Johnny, if you break anything with that ball you'll have to buy a new one with your own money."

Nonetheless, restoration as it presently relates to oil spills and hazardous material releases is a construct of statutory law. The primary relevant statutes, OPA [33 USC §§2710-2761, 104 Stat. 484], the Clean Water Act [33 USC 1251-1387], and CERCLA as amended [42 USC §§9601-9675] create causes of action for monetary damages for injures to, destruction of, or loss of natural resources. However, whether the result of the damage assessment process is expressed in terms of the biophysical change that must be compensated for (e.g., wetland services lost over some period of time), or in terms of the economic value of the loss (e.g., the economic value of some number of lost fishing days), the trustee will face the task of identifying and selecting restoration options to compensate the public for its loss. That is, while DOI defines compensable value to be "the amount of money required to compensate the public for the loss in services provided by the injured resources between the time of the discharge and release and the time the resources and the services those resources provided are fully returned to their baseline conditions" [43 C.F.R. §11.83(c)(1)], the statute requires that "[a]ll sums awarded as damages under CERCLA be used for the purposes of restoration," specifically, to "restore, replace, or acquire the equivalent of . . . natural resources." Oil Pollution Act is also clear on this issue, requiring that all sums recovered as damages be used to "implement a plan for the restoration, rehabilitation, replacement or acquisition of the equivalent of the natural resources." [OPA 1006(f)]

Although not directly defined in OPA or CERCLA, the term "restoration" as it applies to compensatory restoration is discussed in the regulations developed under each of these statutes. The OPA regulations, promulgated by NOAA, define restoration as "any action, or combination of actions, to restore, rehabilitate, replace, or acquire the equivalent of injured natural resources and services." [15 C.F.R. §990.30] These same regulations identify "compensatory restoration" as included within restoration generally and define it as "action(s) taken to make the environment and the public whole for services losses that occur from the date of the incident until recovery of the injured natural resource." [15 C.F.R. §990.30]

Department of the Interior's regulations define restoration in terms of activities undertaken to return an injured resource to baseline for physical, chemical and biological properties, or services [43 C.F.R. §11.14(ll)]. The regulations choose to discuss compensatory restoration in the context of restoration planning, stating that "[w]hen damages for compensable value have been awarded, the [restoration] plan shall also describe how monies will be used to address the services that are lost to the public until restoration, rehabilitation, replacement, and/or acquisition of equivalent resources is completed." [43 C.F.R. §11.93(a)]

Thus, the mandate of these laws, as expressed in the statute and implementing regulations, is to compensate public losses of resources and service use by restoring natural resources, where restoration is defined broadly to incorporate measures to enhance, replace, or otherwise put back resources or services. However, although the injured natural resources are, quite properly, the primary focus of all restoration efforts, the statute and regulations recognize that the specific nature of service losses may require that the trustees broaden the range of restoration approaches considered beyond the absolute confines of simply restoring the specific resources that were injured as a result of the release.

In pursuing claims under these statutes, the trustees are not without guidance in prioritizing among the alternatives of restoration, replacement, and acquisition. The legislative histories evince a clear preference for restoration over acquisition; "It is clear . . . that the primary purpose of the resource damage provisions of CERCLA is the restoration or replacement of natural resources damages by unlawful releases" [H.R. Rep. No. 99-253 (IV at 50)]; and "[t]hus. . .the legislation requires trustees to. . . prepare and implement a plan for repairing the injury due to the environment" [H. Conf. Rep. No. 101-653, page 108]. This view is restated by the court in *Ohio v. United States DOI* throughout its analysis of the proper statutory measure of damages [880 F.2d 432, 443 n.7, 446 (D.C. Cir. 1989].

These provisions do not simply reiterate the old maxim "if you broke it you have to fix or replace it," they also provide underpinnings for a framework to achieving these goals. First is the requirement that, except in emergency situations, all restoration be undertaken pursuant to an approved restoration plan. By regulation, the restoration planning process must involve the development of alternatives and their comparative analysis. Such a planning process achieves a number of results. The restoration plan clarifies the need to weigh the comparative merits of alternative actions before reaching decisions. In doing so, it recognizes that there is not necessarily a single correct restoration project or projects and that the decision process need not be easy. This planning process, applied to the hierarchy of restoration goals established by statute, constitutes the starting point for project selection. If one were to analogize restoration to a journey, although these elements fall short of telling someone exactly where to go, they do provide a conceptual goal (restoration of the injured natural resources), and a mechanism for finding the correct direction of travel (in the form of guidance on restoration plan development).

Second, the regulations issued by NOAA and DOI to support damage assessment under OPA and CERCLA provide guidance to trustees in the development and selection of alternatives for achieving compensatory restoration [15 C.F.R. §990.53-990.56 and 43 C.F.R. §11.82, respectively]. Department of the Interior's regulations call on trustees to develop a range of alternatives, from "intensive" through "natural recovery" [40 C.F.R. §11.82(c)], and to consider the services provided by the identified alternatives. Department of the Interior also provides 10 factors for trustees to consider in selecting among options [40 C.F.R. §11.82(d)].

NOAA's regulations also provide specific guidance to trustees for the process to be followed in developing and selecting restoration alternatives, including specific reference to compensatory restoration options. This includes detailed guidance on the approach to be used in scaling the selected restoration actions (i.e., establish the appropriate scale for the effort; e.g., the number of acres of wetland to be restored).

Like DOI, NOAA provides 6 evaluation criteria, as well as a separate cost-effectiveness criterion, against which each alternative should be considered.

Third, NOAA has issued a set of supplementary guidance documents that are intended to facilitate NRDAs under OPA [Guidance Documents ("Primary Restoration" and "Restoration Planning") for NRDA under OPA, August 1996]. Included in this series is a guide to the restoration planning process with a clear explanation of the need to identify compensatory restoration options that provide services of the same type and quality as those that were lost. The principles presented in this paper supplement the NOAA and DOI guidance, exploring in greater detail the issue of when services provided through compensatory restoration would (and would not) satisfy the "same type and quality" requirement [15 C.F.R. §990.53(d)(2)].

Our first principle is directly supported by the clear language of OPA and CERCLA. As previously noted, the statutory mandate in CERCLA and OPA is for monies recovered to be utilized for the restoration, replacement, or acquisition of natural resources [(OPA) 15 C.F.R. §990.53(d)(1)], with an express preference identified in the legislative histories for restoration of natural resources (CERCLA) and injuries to the environment (OPA) [15 C.F.R. §990.56(b)(1)(ii)].

The conference report for OPA and the associated debates clearly define restoration of injured resources as the preferred alternative. The acquisition of equivalent resources "should be chosen only when the other alternatives are not possible, or when the cost of those alternatives would, in the judgment of the trustee, be grossly disproportionate to the value of the resources involved" [H.R. Conf. Rep. No. 653, 101st Cong., 2nd Sess. 108 (1990)].

The preamble language to NOAA's regulations for the conduct of damage assessment under OPA clarify and generally support the principles defined in this paper. For example, NOAA states that "[w]hen developing the Draft Restoration Plan, trustees must establish restoration objectives that are specific to the injuries" [15 C.F.R. §990.55]. In addition, NOAA agreed with a commentator who noted that "the primary objective of the restoration process should be the timely restoration of the affected natural resources to levels that are adequate to support the services they normally provide to the biological community in general and humans in particular" [59 *Federal Register* 1136, 7 Jan 1994]. NOAA also appears to recognize in their preamble that simply increasing access or otherwise taking actions that will increase the use of a resource will not necessary be appropriate. The following is an example:

NOAA did not intend to suggest that increased use of an injured natural resource is a viable restoration alternative. NOAA suggests that one way of providing services for interim lost use pending recovery might be to provide public uses of a substitute site. The substitute site would have to be capable of sustaining such use without impairment. The suggestion of alternative services may also be a way to use those sums recovered representing diminution of use in a way to make the public whole for its loss. [59 *Federal Register* 1139, 7 Jan 1994]

There is additional support for our first principle in the preamble to NOAA's final rule. In general, both primary and compensatory restoration of services must be accomplished through actions to restore natural resources or to preserve or enhance the amount, quality, and/or availability of natural resources that provide the same or similar services. This may include actions to improve access to natural resources, although in selecting such actions, the trustees must carefully evaluate the direct and indirect impacts of the improved access on natural resource quality and productivity. In the natural resource damage context, a service may not be viewed as an abstract economic unit or activity that may be restored independently of the natural resources from which the service flows. [61 *Federal Register* p. 452, 5 Jan 1996].

Similarly, OPA provides that the measure of damages includes recovery of the cost of restoring natural resources and services to baseline plus compensation for interim losses (and for assessment costs). These recoveries are not to be distributed to affected groups or individuals, rather OPA requires that they be used to restore, rehabilitate, replace, or acquire the equivalent of the injured natural resources. The recoveries are to be collected and spent on natural resource restoration actions by the public agencies managing the natural resources in trust for the public. [61 *Federal Register* p. 484, 5 Jan 1996].

NOAA in its final regulations, under "Restoration Selection—developing restoration alternatives" acknowledges the linkage of service losses to the underlying natural resources when it states in regard to compensatory restoration that "[f]or each alternative, trustees must also consider compensatory restoration actions to compensate for the interim loss of *natural resources and service* pending recovery." (emphasis added) [15 C.F.R. §990.53(c)(1)]

The statutory support for a strong linkage between the restoration and the natural resources that were injured (Principle 2) arises in the explicit language of CERCLA, which mandates that trustees use recovered funds to restore the very injured natural resources ("such resources") which gave rise to the damages recovered [42 USC §9607(f)(1)]. This principle is reflected in the NOAA regulations as part of the specific guidance on the identification and selection of compensable restoration alternatives, and their linkage to the resources and services that were lost, which provides the following:

To the extent practicable, when evaluating compensatory restoration actions, trustees must consider compensatory restoration actions that provide services of the same type and quality, and of comparable value as those injured. If, in the judgment of the trustees, compensatory actions of the same type and quality and comparable value cannot provide a reasonable range of alternatives, trustees should identify alternatives that provide *natural resources and services* of comparable type and quality as those provided by the injured natural resources. (emphasis added) [15 C.F.R. §990.53(c)(2)]

Thus, there is a clear linkage implied between what was injured and the restoration actions that are selected.

Additional support for our first principles is found throughout the preamble to DOI's final rule on the conduct of damage assessments:

The Department has always intended restoration, rehabilitation, replacement, and/or acquisition of the equivalent resources to involve actions taken to return a resource to baseline. Apparent inconsistencies in the rule arise because trustee officials need a means of measuring injury in order to determine when restoration, rehabilitation, replacement, and/or acquisition of the equivalent resources is complete, and the concept of services provides that means. As was stated in the 1 August 1986 preamble to the original type B rule:

Traditionally humans have valued natural resources in monetary terms on the basis of services provided by the resources. This method logically may be extended to valuing damages to an injured resource on the basis of changes in services. This rule establishes the link between measured adverse changes in the condition of the resource, the injury, and the damages through the measurement of changes in the services provided by the injured resource. [51 *Federal Register* 27686]

In other words, although it is the natural resources that trustee officials are restoring, rehabilitating, replacing, and/or acquiring the equivalent of, such actions cause an increase in services, and that increase in services is used to measure the level of restoration, rehabilitation, replacement, and/or acquisition of the equivalent resources. [51 *Federal Register* 25 March 1994 (page 14272)]

The DOI regulations do not provide separate guidance for the identification and selection of compensable restoration actions. However, the general guidance provided includes

The authorized official shall develop a reasonable number of possible alternatives for the restoration, rehabilitation, replacement, and/or acquisition of the equivalent of the injured natural resources and the services those resources provide. . . .The authorized official shall then select from among the possible alternatives the alternative that he determines to be the most appropriate based on the guidance provided [in this section of the Interior regulations]. [43 C.F.R. §11.82 (a)]

As already noted, the DOI's regulations also provide definitions of "restoration or rehabilitation," and "replacement or acquisition of the equivalent" [43 C.F.R. §11.14]. Both of these definitions focus on the restoration of the injured resource, where restoration and rehabilitation involves actions to restore *the resource*, measured in terms of the physical, chemical, or biological properties it would have exhibited, or services it would have provided but for the release, and where replacement or acquisition of the equivalent refers to the substitution for an injured resource with *resources* that provide the same or substantially similar services.

In the preamble to the draft rule, DOI also provides insight into the types of restoration actions that are not appropriate. For example:

> Finally, the Department did not intend to suggest . . .that trustee officials may not use manufactured devices to assist the restoration of injured resources. The Department simply meant that trustee officials should not replace injured natural resources with artificial resources. [51 *Federal Register* 14272 (25 March 1994)]

This comment provides support for our first principle, in calling for alternatives that restore the resource that was injured, not simply actions that will replace the services provided.

These provisions furnish a common context from which to approach compensatory restoration planning—namely, an acknowledgment that natural resources are, quite properly, the primary focus of all restoration efforts. This preferential focus is, however, constrained by practical factors which may limit available alternatives, including the criteria defined in both DOI's and NOAA's regulations [43 C.F.R. §11.82 and 15 C.F.R. §990.54(a), respectively]. As a result, the specific nature of the service losses may sometimes require that the trustees broaden the range of restoration approaches to be considered beyond the absolute confines of simply restoring the specific resources that were injured as a result of the release.

This tension—the mandate to restore natural resources, but the need to do so in an effective yet feasible manner—leads to the need for our third principle. In regard to this principle, no explicit guidance is provided in DOI's regulation or preamble. There is, however, some discussion in the committee reports on *where* restoration has to take place:

> The committee therefore intends [that] any excess funds recovered be used, in such an instance, for the third purpose spelled out in the language of the amendment, which is to 'acquire the equivalent of the damaged resource.'. . .The committee expects that any such acquisition would provide resources of an equivalent nature at *a location as near as reasonably possible to the site at which the damages occurred.* [emphasis added] [H.R. Rep. No. 253, 99th Congress, 1st Session, pt. 4 at 50 (1985)]

Similarly, the Conference Report for OPA addresses this principle. The Conference Report defines "equivalent resources" as those that "the trustee determines are comparable to the injured resources. Equivalent resources should be acquired to enhance the recovery, productivity, and survival of the ecosystem affected by a discharge, preferably in proximity to the affected area." [H.R. Conf. Rep. No. 653, 101st Cong., 2nd Sess. 109 (1990)]

Justification for our third principle can be drawn from the fields of ecology and economics. Ecologists recognize natural systems as being interrelated and recognize that many species are dependent on a broad range of habitats. For example, a pair of bald eagles may rely both on a nesting site in eastern Canada as well as a wintering location in southern New England. Similarly, an endangered salmon run may be threatened by both acid mine drainage as well as hydroelectric operations many hundreds of miles away. Commonly applied resource management units, such as the watershed, will in many cases provide a relevant starting point for the restoration selection. In some cases, however, it may be necessary to transcend these and other boundaries in identifying appropriate restoration options. In economics it is common to talk of substitutes for a good or service. For example, a substitute fishing location for a site closed as a result of an oil spill would be one that is considered by users of the injured resource as a good alternative to the injured site in terms of its quality attributes, accessibility, etc. Such substitutes may be unrelated, in any direct ecological or physical way, to the system that was injured, but may be quite appropriate as replacement sites. Thus, the appropriate measure of linkage between an injury and the proposed restoration option should not be defined based on arbitrary political or geographic boundaries, but based on patterns of user behavior or the ecological needs of the affected resources.

Case studies

In this section we present 3 hypothetical case studies, each involving a different restoration challenge facing the trustees. The cases presented all involve relatively complex situations. The identification and selection of restoration actions in cases that involve relatively simple losses generally does not represent much of a challenge for trustees or responsible parties. We have purposely developed complex hypothetical examples to demonstrate how the principles presented in this paper might be applied. These hypothetical examples focus the discussion on interim human-use losses (i.e., this discussion does not specifically address the means by which injured resources might be returned to baseline).

Contaminated river sediments

Releases of a toxic substance from an industrial facility and associated waste disposal operations have resulted in contamination of the sediments and floodplain of a small river in the southern U.S. The levels of contamination in the sediment and in resident fishes have been sufficient to prompt public health advisories (i.e., children should avoid contact with the sediments, and all residents should avoid eating fish from the river). Based on a variety of studies, the trustees estimate that 3,000 additional fishing trips per year would take place but for the contamination, and those trips that were taken despite the contamination have been significantly reduced in value. Other forms of recreation have also been affected by the contamination (e.g., picnicking, hiking, tubing). Surveys of the public indicate widespread concern regarding the contamination; for example, visitors to a state park frequently express concern over the perceived health risks to children picnicking and taking part in other recreation near the river. Use of this park has been reduced as a result of public perceptions of the risk posed by the contamination. Actions to cut off the source of the contamination and to remediate hot spots have been successfully implemented, and the level of contamination is expected to drop below that which poses a health concern within 10 years. Additional remediation of the river and floodplain sediments has been deemed infeasible.

Following completion of the injury assessment the trustees undertook efforts to identify a range of restoration options as called for in the regulations. This effort involved members of the state trustee agency and local advocacy groups, resource managers, regional planners, town government representatives, and other community leaders. The following options were identified as a result of this effort:

1) Provide funds for annual stocking of the affected river with adult fish to create a seasonal put-and-take fishery at the site. The site currently supports a catch-and-release native trout fishery, which is used primarily by fly fishermen.
2) Increase streamside access for anglers by purchasing a parcel along the river that is currently in private ownership, thus opening a segment of the river not currently available to anglers.
3) Provide funds to enhance recreational opportunities at the state park. Options include new picnic shelters, landscaping, a modernized playground, and an improved interpretive center.
4) Construct a 10-mile bike path near the river, utilizing an abandoned railroad right-of-way.
5) Undertake actions to improve general water quality in the river with the goal of enhancing the native fish population. Actions might include addressing the remaining CSOs, controlling sedimentation from local truck-farms, and reducing runoff from a highway which crosses the river at two points.
6) Provide funds for an additional environmental enforcement officer in the county to enforce waste disposal laws. The goal would be to reduce the illegal dumping of used oil and other wastes to the river.
7) Provide funds for abatement of lead-contaminated soils at regional schools to offset perceived health risks to children at the site.
8) Acquire uncontaminated land to provide substitute recreation opportunities.

We can consider each of these options, or categories of options, in light of the principles described above. Table 1-1 summarizes the characteristics of the options and how they rate against the proposed Principles.

Four of the options (Options 1, 2, 5, and 6) relate to improvements in the fishery, direct use of which has been substantially diminished as a result of the release. Options 1 and 2 do not involve restoration of the injured resource, but instead are intended as a means to replace lost-use opportunities with substitute opportunities (i.e., substitute fish and a substitute location). Under the principles described above, these would be viewed as less preferred than Options 5 and 6, which provide for enhancement of the native fishery. Option 2, however, if required to fully compensate the users of this resource, would be preferable to Option 1, since this latter option provides no direct restoration of, or replacement for, the injured resource (i.e., Option

Table 1-1 Hypothetical case: contaminated river sediments relationship between restoration options and proposed principles

		Consistent with:		
Restoration option	Role in restoring lost use	Principle 1	Principle 2	Principle 3
1. Provide for stocking of fish	Create a put-and-take fishery at the site to compensate for past lost fishing opportunities	no	yes	yes, on-site
2. Acquire streamside access	Create new fishing opportunities near the areas that experienced the injury to compensate for lost fishing opportunities	yes	yes	yes, if new opportunity reasonable substitute for injured site
3. Enhance recreational opportunities at the state park	Enhance the value of trips to the state park to compensate for diminished value in past	no	yes	yes, on-site
4. Construct bike path	Substitute biking opportunities for lost recreational opportunities associated with the river	no	no	yes, on-site
5. Improve general water quality	Improve water quality with goal of enhancing the native fishery, and thus catch rates	yes	yes	yes, on-site
6. Fund additional environmental enforcement	Increase compliance with waste disposal laws in order to reduce the frequency of fish kills associated with illegal disposal practices	yes	yes	yes, on-site
7. Fund abatement of lead from contaminated soils	Reduce health risks posed by lead to children at regional schools	no	no	no, no evidence option will benefit users of degraded resource
8. Acquire substitute recreation site	Acquire lands near injured river to serve as substitute recreational sites	yes	yes	depends on location chosen for substitute

2 provides access to a substitute resource, and thus it could be argued provides a natural resource that in turn provides a use opportunity).

Options 5 and 6 appear to meet the spirit of all 3 principles. Option 6, however, raises questions regarding the efficacy of spending recovered funds to enforce behaviors that are already required by law. While this option might be deemed appropriate, additional consideration of this issue would be required by the trustees.

Options 3 and 4 provide means of compensating for the general reduction in recreationalist's use of the river's environment. Neither, however, provide for direct restoration of the injured resources (Principle 1). In this case an alternative option that addresses the public's general attitude toward the resource through a direct resource improvement (e.g., actions to create areas that are completely free of contamination), or which involved the purchase of a substitute property free of contamination (Option 8) would be preferred.

Option 7 was raised as a means for offsetting the perceived health threat posed by the contamination. This option, however, fails to meet the spirit of Principle 2 (defining some sort of linkage to the injured resource and the services it provided), or Principle 3 (defining a human use or ecological linkage to the injured resource, in terms of the location at which the restoration takes place). An option to reduce the perceived health risks posed by the site, such as removal of contaminated soils in areas accessed by the public, might be a better alternative for replacing this category of lost service.

Thus, the process of considering these options in light of the 3 principles proposed in this paper provides a means to determine the appropriateness of the various options. In many cases such as this, a range of options will be required to compensate for a range of lost-use opportunities and to provide sufficient compensation alternatives to make the public whole. Once a set of options has been selected, the next steps would involve comparing these options against the factors listed in NOAA's or DOI's regulations and establishing the extent to which these options provide sufficient compensation (i.e., scaling).

Western river system contamination

Mineral mining and processing activities over the past 100 years have resulted in the ongoing release of hazardous materials to a western river system. As a result, natural resources in a 20-mile stretch of the river and in several tributaries have been injured. Reported injuries include: a reduction in fish populations in the watershed, including the total absence of fish from the tributaries; a reduction in the abundance and diversity of vegetation and wildlife along the river corridor; the death of several hundred birds per year due to metals poisoning; and public health warnings regarding the drinking of water and/or consumption of fish from the river. Public knowledge of these injuries is widespread; in addition to the posted public health warnings, several areas of contamination appear as "dead zones" on the local landscape and are visible from an important regional highway.

Remedial actions at the site were successful in cutting off all ongoing sources of contamination and in fencing off areas posing an acute health risk. However, the injuries described above remain and are expected to continue into the foreseeable future. The trustees have conducted interviews with various stakeholders in the affected area and have gathered restoration options from regional resource managers and other officials. The following represents examples of the types of projects being considered:

1) Purchase conservation easements throughout the watershed to cut down on sediment, chemical, and nutrient loadings from local cattle grazing and farming operations.
2) Undertake other actions to improve stream water quality, including efforts to enhance streamside vegetation (reducing water temperature), placement of boulders and logs to create habitat, and removal of sediment in some areas to improve the substrate for spawning.
3) Purchase land under threat of development in the watershed.
4) Fund classes at regional schools designed to enhance students' understanding of the regional environment.
5) Fund a regional bird recovery center. This center would not address birds with symptoms of metals poisoning, but would provide medical attention to, with the goal of releasing, birds injured through illegal hunting and encounters with powerlines.
6) Undertake actions to enhance and provide greater public access to a substitute fishing stream in a nearby watershed through the provision of additional parking and boat ramps.
7) Landscape unvegetated areas, and construct roadside hedgerows to obstruct views of the dead areas.

As in our first hypothetical case study, we can consider these proposed options in light of the principles presented in this paper. Table 1-2 presents a summary of this analysis, as discussed below.

The first 3 options all provide for general improvement in regional water quality or actions to protect water quality in the future. All 3 of these options meet all of the proposed principles. Option 5 and Option 7 address specific symptoms of the contaminant release. Option 5 meets the first 2 principles, in that 1) it provides use opportunities by directly restoring an injured resource, and 2) direct linkages to the injured resource can be established. Whether it satisfies the third principle would depend on the location from which the injured birds are collected. Option 7 might be determined to be consistent with our first 2 principles, if in fact the action does directly restore some degree of quality to the injured resource (as opposed to simply "hiding" the injury). For example, the act of vegetating barren areas may provide habitat for wildlife not currently using these areas.

Table 1-2 Hypothetical case: western river system relationship between restoration options and proposed principles

		Consistent with:		
Restoration option	Role in restoring lost use	Principle 1	Principle 2	Principle 3
1. Purchase conservation easement	Improve general water quality to offset the effects of contamination and enhance habitat for various fish species	yes	yes	yes, on-site
2. Improve water quality	Improve general water quality to offset the effects of contamination and enhance habitat for various fish species	yes	yes	yes, on-site
3. Purchase land under threat of development	Take actions to prevent development that would otherwise affect water quality	yes	yes	yes, on-site
4. Fund education	Increase students' appreciation for the regional environment	no	no	possibly
5. Fund bird recovery center	Increase the scope and success rate of a regional bird recovery program with goal of off-setting the impact the contamination has on bird species	yes	yes	possibly; relationship to bird population in injured areas needs to be established
6. Enhance public access	Provide a substitute fishing location for local anglers	no; simply provides for greater access to existing resource	yes	yes, if site used by anglers experiencing diminished use opportunities
7. Landscape injured areas	Reduce the visual impact of injured areas. Possibly provides for enhanced wildlife habitat in those areas	possibly, unless primarily aesthetic	no	yes, on-site

Finally, Options 4 and 6 fail to meet each of the proposed principles. Option 4, viewed by members of the planning committee as a means to enhance students' appreciation for the environment, fails to meet each of the proposed criteria. Option 6 may provide for additional use opportunities to compensate for past losses (thus meeting Principle 2), but fails to provide for improvement in the underlying resource that provides such opportunities.

Urban oil spill

An oil spill has resulted in closure of 5 miles of beach for a period of 2 weeks. The beach adjoins a major metropolitan area and is heavily used by both residents who walk and drive to the beach and by tourists staying in local hotels. Common beach activities include walking, nature viewing, swimming, sunbathing, and picnicking. There are also paved paths running along parts of the beach for jogging and cycling. The trustees estimate that approximately 200,000 beach visits were lost from the affected beaches during the closure. All signs of the oil were removed from the beaches before they were reopened, and beach usage quickly returned to normal. For this hypothetical case, we assume that no ongoing biological injury exists. Possible restoration options that have been identified by the trustees include:

1) Purchase a parcel of neglected beachfront property 10 miles away, clean it up, and open it for public recreational use.
2) Design and build engineered structures to prevent beach erosion near the affected area.
3) Provide money for additional lifeguards to increase safety and provide additional areas of supervised swimming near the affected area.
4) Repave and expand the width of paved paths in the general vicinity of the affected beach.
5) Install a reef to enhance fishing and provide recreational diving opportunities.
6) Construct a boardwalk and self-guided tour to enhance/create nature viewing experiences.
7) Pay for a shuttle bus to provide free transportation to and from the beach for residents of low income areas in the metropolitan area.
8) Pay for the installation of lights and security personnel to keep sections of the beach open for evening concerts, shows, and events.
9) Spend money on programs and equipment to enhance the beach-going experience at the affected beach. Examples may include construction of permanent restroom and changing area facilities, planting trees for shade and aesthetics, and installation of trash receptacles and frequent beach trash collection and removal.
10) Pay for the elimination of a combined sewer overflow whose discharges are largely responsible for fecal coliform violations that occasionally prohibit swimming activity at the beach.

These options can be divided into several categories: 1) options to replace lost beach days, through the provision of additional use opportunities in the future (Options 1, 7, 10, and, possibly, 3 and 8); 2) options to enhance the quality of use opportunities afforded by the injured resource, either now or in the future (Options 2, 4, and 9); and 3) options to provide replacement use opportunities (Options 5 and 6). Each of these options, and the degree to which they are consistent with the proposed principles, is described in Table 1-3.

As noted in Table 1-3, 5 of the options are intended to provide additional future use opportunities similar to those that were lost. Option 1 involves the direct acquisition and creation of a substitute use opportunity; if it can be determined that this site is a reasonable substitute for the injured resource, than it would meet all of the principles. Option 10 provides for additional future opportunities in a different manner—through the prevention of other sources of degradation of the resource. Options 3, 7, and 8 serve to expand the use opportunities associated with the beach as a means of replacing lost opportunities in the past; Option 3 expands the area of the beach over which users can safely bathe, Option 7 expands the user group for the site to include individuals previously unable to access the site, and Option 8 extends the time period during which the beach can be safely used as a recreational location. Each of these options, however, fail to meet one or more of the proposed principles.

Options 2, 4, 6, and 9 act to enhance the quality of future use of the beach, through the maintenance of the beach's physical dimensions (Option 2), provision of greater access and the opportunity to stroll along the beach (Option 4), provision of a boardwalk and interpretive trail (Option 6), and improvements in the amenities and aesthetics associated with the beach (Option 9). Options 4, 6, and 9 fail to meet one or more of the principles proposed in this paper, as shown in Table 1-3. While Option 2 appears to meet all of the principles, the extent to which the beach erosion prevention actions described under this option meet Principle 1 would depend on the extent to which such actions result in other environmental problems.

Finally, Option 5 proposes the development of an artificial reef off the coast from the spill area. While this action would serve to improve the quality of the injured resource (Principle 1), there is no direct linkage to the injuries experienced or lost-use opportunities (Principle 2). In addition, it is not clear that the potential users of this resource were affected by the spill (Principle 3).

Conclusions

In this paper we identify 3 questions commonly raised during the restoration planning process. To address these questions, we propose 3 principles that clarify and expand on the guidance provided in DOI's and NOAA's regulations and associated guidance. These principles are in keeping with a progressively greater focus on resource and service flow restoration as the ultimate goal of NRDA process. It will not, in all cases, be possible or even desirable to abide by all of these principles, but they should form a

Table 1-3 Hypothetical case: urban oil spill relationship between restoration options and proposed principles

Restoration option	Roles in restoring lost use	Principle 1	Principle 2	Principle 3
1. Purchase land to create substitute recreation opportunity	Provide new destination and thus additional recreational trips in future	partly, to extent it improves degraded resource	yes	yes, if it truly substitutes for injured reserves
2. Prevent beach erosion	Maintain existing beach site in order to reduce future congestion associated with beach loss	yes, to extent action does not cause other problems	partial; past loss of opportunities offset by future improvement in quality	yes, on-site
3. Fund additional lifeguards	Improve quality and extent of current beach use opportunities	no	yes	yes, on-site
4. Improve paved paths along beach	Encouraged use of paved paths along beach, thus providing offsetting use opportunity and greater access	no	weak	yes, on-site
5. Install artificial reef	Provide substitute recreational opportunity near spill location	yes	no, separate user group	no, separate user group
6. Construct boardwalk and interpretive trail	Provide substitute recreational opportunity near spill location in attempt to off-set the public's diminished view of beach's environment due to release	no	limited	yes, on-site
7. Fund shuttle bus site	Enhance opportunity for use of beach by a population currently unable to gain access to it	no	no	no, new user group
8. Increase evening security	Expand time period over which beach is used to provide for off-setting use opportunities	no	limited	yes, on-site
9. Enhance the quality of the beach experience	Enhance general appearance and amenities of beach in attempt to off-set the public's diminished view of beach's environment due to release	no	partial	yes, on-site
10. Upgrade local sewage system	Reduce number of beach closures due to fecal coliform expected in the future to off-set past losses in use opportunities	yes	yes	yes, on-site

guide and act to clarify some significant questions raised during the course of restoration planning.

We recognize, and expect, that these principles will act to narrow the range of restoration alternatives viewed as appropriate following a given release event. It is our hope, however, that the principles presented also will foster greater creativity on the part of trustees and others involved in the restoration planning process. For example, these criteria may imply a greater role for ecologists, economists, regional planners and landscape architects, and other experts at the restoration planning phase of the assessment.

1a

Discussion Paper 1 on A Proposed Framework for Developing and Selecting Compensatory Restoration Projects under Federal Natural Resource Damage Assessment Statutes

*Kenneth L. Dickson, Dwight Barry, Steven Windhager**

The Unsworth, Barash, and Huguenin paper addresses a very important and challenging issue in natural resource damage assessment: how do you choose, from among various alternatives, the most efficacious and appropriate means of compensating for resources and services lost during the time between injury and restoration? Three "Principles" are proposed to guide trustees and responsible parties in developing and selecting compensatory restoration projects. The paper provides a convincing discussion about the need for guidance. It offers a cogent discussion of the legislative and public policy histories of the Comprehensive Environmental Response, Compensation, and Liability Act (CERCLA) and the Oil Pollution Act's (OPA) damage assessment provisions, and regulations and regulatory guidance issued by the National Oceanic and Atmospheric Administration (NOAA) and U.S. Department of the Interior (DOI) for supporting the proposed principles.

The 3 principles are the following:

- Principle 1: Restoration of lost human uses should be based on restoration or enhancement of the natural resources that form the basis of those uses.

Translation: Restoration and enhancement projects at and/or around the damaged resource site are preferred over projects that do not restore or enhance the damaged site.

- Principle 2: The link between the resources and services lost as a result of the release and the resources and services gained through the proposed compensatory restoration actions should be reasonable and explicit.

Translation: The nature of the resources and services provided by a compensatory project should be as similar in nature as possible to those lost.

*Environmental Science Program, University of North Texas, Denton, Texas

• Principle 3: The link between the resources and services lost as a result of the release and the resources and services gained through the proposed compensatory restoration action can, if necessary, transcend physical and political boundaries.

Translation: Where possible, do projects near the site of damage and loss of services, but do not eliminate outright alternatives that may be geographically distant from the site, as exceptional opportunities may exist in a regional context.

The authors suggest that these principles for developing and selecting compensatory restoration projects could serve as an explicit framework replacing the often ad hoc processes and criteria used in many past cases. To illustrate how the proposed principles can be used to assist in evaluating alternatives 3 interesting case studies—Contaminated River Sediments, Western River System Contamination, and Urban Oil Spill—are presented and discussed by the authors. For the purposes of this commentary, we will utilize only the first of these examples.

Critique

The authors are to be commended for developing a well-reasoned and professionally written manuscript. The inclusion of definitions and truisms greatly assisted these reviewers and compensated for the occasional lawyer language that obscured the authors' points or issues, including:

As already noted, the DOI regulations also provide definitions of "restoration or rehabilitation" and "replacement or acquisition of the equivalent" [43 C.F.R. -11.4]. Both of these definitions focus on the restoration of the injured resource, where restoration and rehabilitation involves actions to restore the resource measured in terms of the physical, chemical or biological properties it would have exhibited, or services it would have provided but for the release, and where replacement or acquisition of the equivalent refers to the substitution for an injured resource with resources that provide the same or substantially similar services.

What was that?

Putting these stylistic annoyances aside, the authors provide some very useful ideas on how to select between alternatives. However, it is my opinion that their principles should constitute the Second Tier of an assessment framework preceding by a First Tier consisting of evaluative criteria that address the ecological soundness, degree of certainty, and ecological sustainability of proposed alternative compensatory projects. We suggest the following preliminary First Tier Screening Principles:

Principle 1: Ecologically sound projects should be preferred over projects that provide services but are not as ecologically sound. This principle is designed to ensure that projects that are implemented to provide compensatory human services do not do so at an unacceptable ecological cost. For example, providing fisherman unlimited access to a stream can increase erosion along roads, paths and banks, trample vegetation, and destroy habitat.

Principle 2: The degree of certainty associated with a project's ability to provide the compensatory services should be evaluated and used in choosing projects to implement. Alternatives vary in the degree of certainty associated with their ability to provide the compensatory services. For example, stocking fish into a damaged stream to provide fisherman recreational opportunities (although ecologically unsound in many circumstances) may have less certainty to provide those services than purchasing another stream segment and providing access.

Principle 3: The probability that a project will provide sustainable services should be assessed and preference given to projects which provide services that are sustainable. Projects should be implemented which have a high probability to provide continuing services rather than simply providing services for a short period of time. Similarly, these services should be provided by projects requiring a minimum of maintenance and management. An example of the application of this principle would be preferring a stream habitat enhancement project to establishing a put-and-take recreational fishery.

We suggest that the Tier 1 Principles outlined above constitute the Screening Phase of the an Assessment Framework and that the principles developed by the authors constitute the Targeting Phase. In their manuscript, the authors used a table to illustrate how a series of hypothetical candidate alternative projects in 3 case studies met or failed their principles. A yes or no (all or none) relationship was noted between an alternative project and their principles. An alternative mode of presentation which may be more informative is to ordinate the principles and determine the degree to which a candidate project meets each of the criteria producing a resulting graph like Figures 1a-1 and 1a-2. The benefit of this presentation mode over the table format is that it keeps track of the degree of applicability of each principle to each candidate project. Figures 1a-1 and 1a-2 conceptually illustrate how candidate alternative projects could be evaluated relative to the Tier 1 and Tier 2 Principles. In this approach each principle is given equal weight; if users desire to give some principles higher or lower weights the approach would have to be modified. Projects that fall in the quadrant B are clearly preferable to those in quadrant C. Projects in quadrant C should be eliminated for further consideration. Projects in quadrant B should proceed to the Targeting Phase (Tier 2). Projects which fall in quadrants A and D should be examined carefully for the reasons of their occurrence in these quadrants. Note that it is possible to determine how each Principle affects the final location of an alternative. Perhaps those falling in the upper half of quadrants A and D should proceed to Tier 2 analysis. However, rule-based decision criteria should not substitute for professional judgements to take a candidate project to the next tier.

In Tier 2 the principles developed by the authors can be used to screen and ultimately select a project to implement that provides appropriate compensatory services in a ecologically responsible manner.

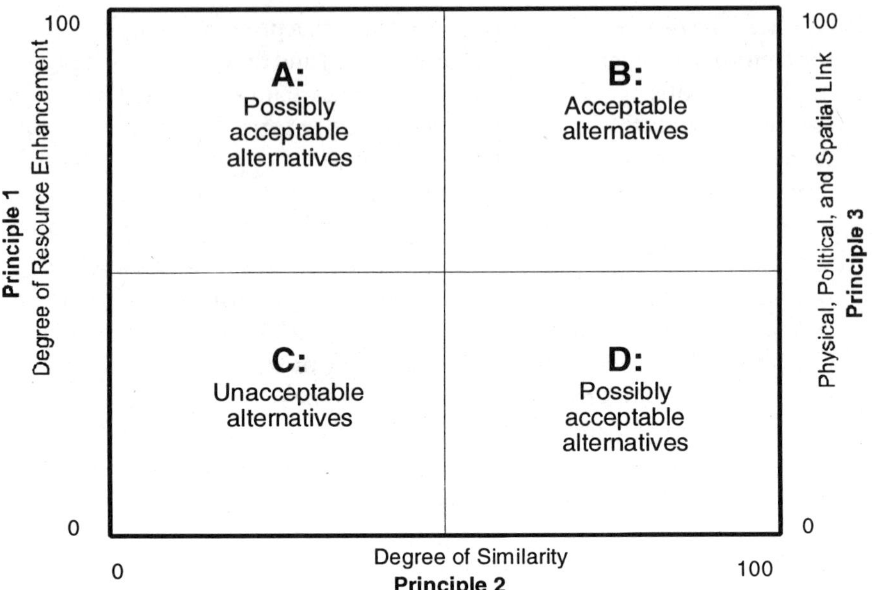

Figure 1a-1 The First Tier of evaluation for a proposed restoration project designed to screen ecologically unacceptable alternatives from consideration in the Second Tier of evaluation.

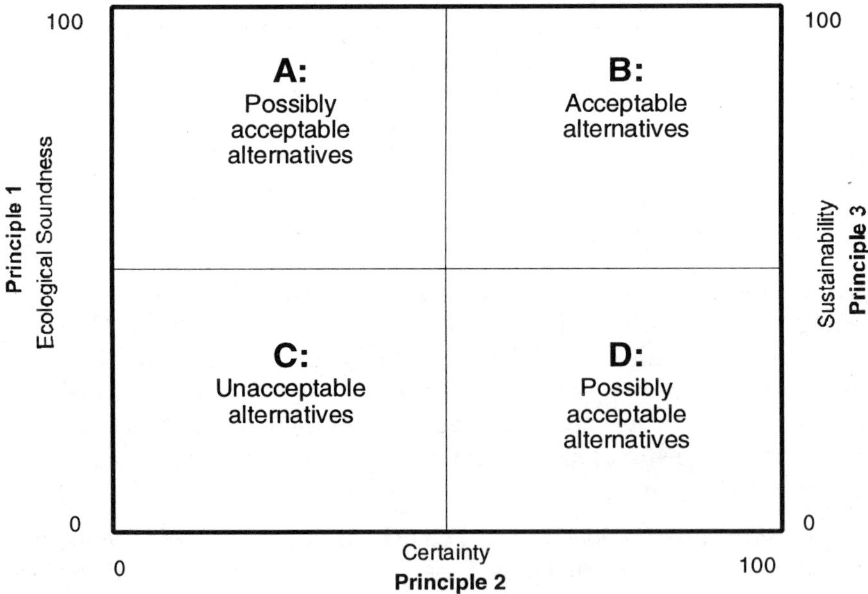

Figure 1a-2 The Second Tier of evaluation for a proposed restoration project designed to select a project from ecologically acceptable alternatives.

To illustrate the application of the Tier 1 Principles and Tier 2 Principles, Figures 1a-3 and 1a-4 have been developed to apply to the authors' sediment contamination case study.

Synopsis of case study

For a detailed description of the sediment contamination case study, see the authors' paper. In summary, a toxic substance release to a southern stream has contaminated sediments and resident fish, prompting public health advisories against consumption of fish and contact with sediments. Three thousand additional fishing trips per year would have occurred but for the contamination, and the value of trips taken has been therefore reduced. Picnicking, hiking, and tubing have also been affected. In addition, the public is concerned about possible adverse effects on children and their own health due to soil contamination in the floodplain. Remediation is underway and contamination levels are expected to be below health risk levels in 10 years. A variety of candidate alternative projects were identified by stakeholders to provide compensate for the lost services.

Each of the alternatives or candidate projects were evaluated using the Tier 1 and Tier 2 Principles discussed above and the results summarized in Figures 1a-2 and 1a-3. Figure 1a-2 illustrates how each of the projects meet or fail to meet the principles of ecological soundness, uncertainty, and sustainability. Figure 1a-2 shows application of the 8 candidate projects to the principles developed by the authors. In a real world application, decisions about the degree of compliance of a project with a principle would be made by a panel of stakeholders and persons knowledgeable about the environment and details of the proposed alternative. In Figures 1a-2 and 1a-3, I have made a judgement about the degree to which a project meets the principles.

Examination of Figure 1a-3 shows that alternatives 5 and 8 both fall in quadrant B and thus received high scores on all 3 Tier 1 Principles. Alternatives 2, 3, and 4 have attributes which make them worthy of further consideration. However, alternatives 1, 6, and 7 can be eliminated form further consideration to advance to Tier 2.

Figure 1a-4 illustrates application of the authors' principles to the 8 candidate projects. Alternative projects 1, 2, and 5 receive high rankings on all 3 of the principles and appear in quadrant B of the diagram, indicating that they should be finalists for consideration and implementation. However, the Tier 1 analysis shows that alternative 1—stocking of adult fish is neither ecological sound nor sustainable and thus should not be a candidate for further consideration or implementation. Note that alternative 8—purchase uncontaminated lands— ranked high in the Tier 1 screening analysis, but gets lower marks using the Tier 2 Principles. This is because it scores low on the principle of similarity to the damaged site.

By using a 2-tiered approach, one is able to eliminate alternatives which fail to meet the common sense ecologically based criteria embodied in Tier 1, and focus attention on the policy and regulatory based criteria or principles advanced by the authors.

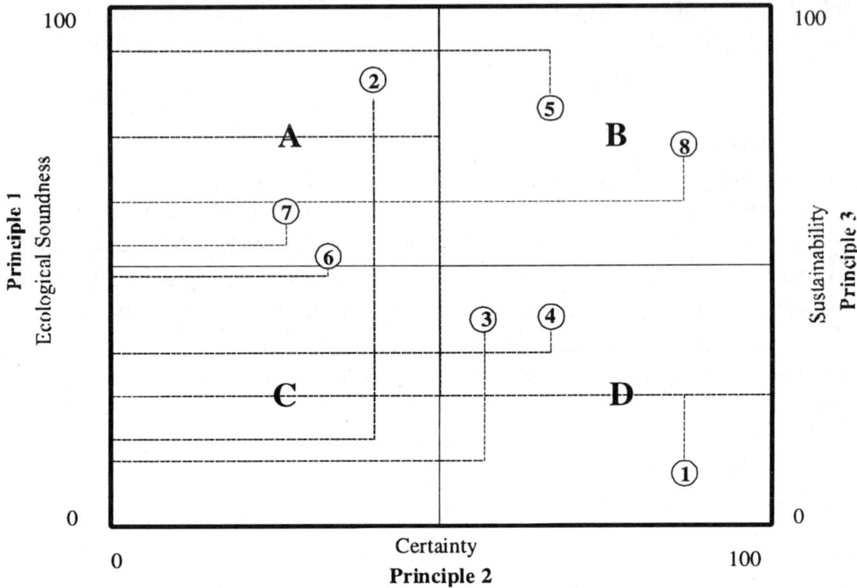

Figure 1a-3 The use of a Tier 1 evaluation in the authors' Sediment Contaminant Study

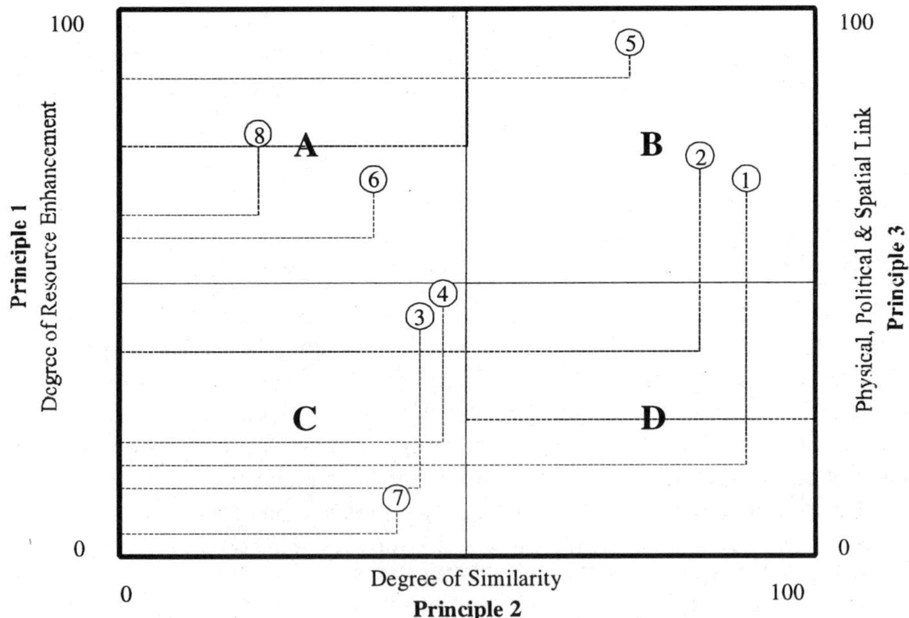

Figure 1a-4 The use of the authors' principles for an evaluation of the Sediment Contamination Case Study

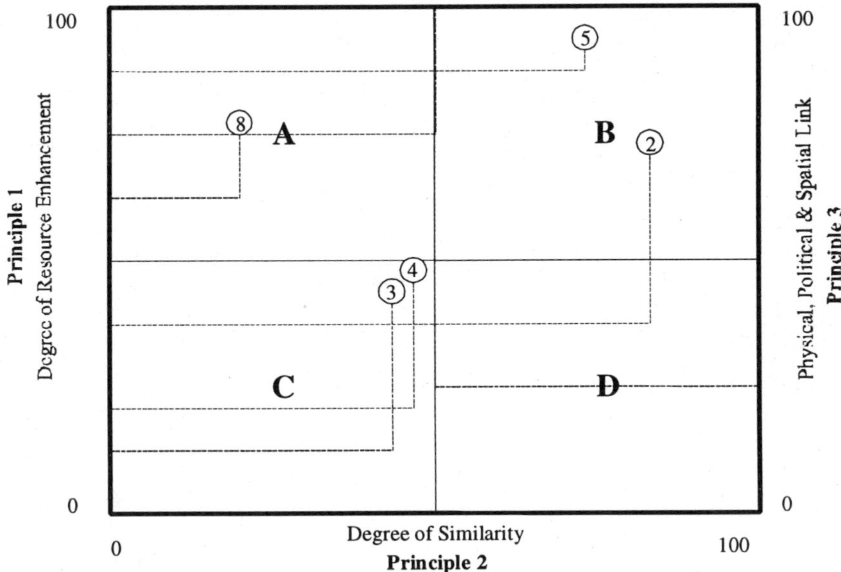

Figure 1a-5 The results of a 2-tiered evaluation of the authors' Sediment Contamination Case study

Additionally, the use of the ordination technique illustrated in Figures 1a-1 through 1a-5, provides an explicit explanation of how alternatives rank in regards to the Tier 1 and Tier 2 Principles. This should assist in communicating to the public, responsible parties, and trustees how decisions are made on which compensatory project to implement.

Conclusions

The Unsworth, Barash, Huguenin paper has developed a set of principles that appear to be solidly founded on the public policy and legislative histories of CERCLA's, OPA's, NOAA's and DOI's damage assessment provisions, regulations, and guidance. However, we suggest that the utility of their principles would be enhanced if they were used as a second tier evaluative tool, proceeded by an evaluation of candidate projects ability to meet common sense principles related to ecological soundness, certainty, and sustainability.

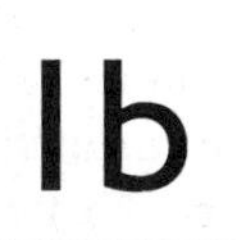

Discussion Paper 2 on A Proposed Framework for Developing and Selecting Compensatory Restoration Projects under Federal Natural Resource Damage Assessment Statutes

*John L. Duffy**

Although this paper was enjoyable to read, I do not agree with it. At the outset, I want to define 3 terms: 1) "primary restoration," which is the restoration of the injured resource to its baseline condition (no permanent injury); 2) "alternative restoration," which encompasses projects that are made necessary by an inability, because of physical or economic reasons, to return the injured resource to its baseline condition (permanent injury), and that "compensate" for the permanent injury to the resource; and 3) "compensatory restoration," which the authors define as "restoration actions that aim to compensate the public for services lost from the time of an oil or hazardous substance release to the restoration of the underlying resource to its baseline." Of the authors' 3 hypothetical case studies, for example, only the last involves a true issue of "compensatory restoration." Both the first and second examples involve situations in which complete restoration to the baseline, or pre-injury, condition is impossible. The authors repeatedly intermix the circumstances defined above as primary or alternative restoration when discussing compensatory restoration, particularly in drawing support for their framework from legislative and regulatory history.

Their 3 principles would complicate unnecessarily the trustee decisions for spending for lost use between the date of the injury and the date of the return to baseline conditions. Compensation for such a loss of services encompasses injury to such a wide variety of human uses, especially if you include, as do the authors, the often ridiculed passive uses that trying to match the replacement services during the interim period with the services lost and the persons who lost those services does not seem possible, or at least not possible without more effort than would make it sensible in light of the benefit produced. Moreover, by definition, such compensation is in addition to: 1) the cost of restoring the resource to its baseline condition, or 2) if impossible, the cost of the maximum feasible restoration, plus compensation for permanent injury to the resource. It is therefore unnecessary to consider restoration of

*Steptoe & Johnson, Washington, DC

the maximum feasible restoration, plus compensation for permanent injury to the resource. It is therefore unnecessary to consider restoration of the injured resource in our calculation of how to spend compensation for the loss of services during the period between injury and achievable repair.

Instead, we should spend the money on the best project, to be defined by the trustees in the exercise of their sole discretion. Any other approach risks the expenditure of the public's damages award on a less than best project. And what is the gain that justifies that risk?

Finally, I strongly disagree with the authors' discussion of restoration in which they make a number of unsupported, and in my opinion unsupportable, generalizations about the doctrine of penance and English common law. (If restoration were a big part of the doctrine of penance, Martin Luther would have had no reason to attack the Church's sale of indulgences.)

Restoration implies repair, often of something irreplaceable. If Johnny's ball had broken a vase brought over from Ireland by his sainted grandmother, an effort to glue it together would have been a restoration. If Johnny runs down to the local knickknack shop to acquire another vase as a replacement of an apparently fungible item, and an in-kind compensation for the damage done, it is not essentially different than giving his parents monetary damages.

The authors' souvenir shop example is, likewise, not a restoration but a forced sale, the consumer equivalent of a local speed trap. Compensation for damages should not exceed replacement value, which in the case of the souvenir shop means its wholesale cost, which is probably no more than one-fifth of the retail price.

I make these points not to be picky but because clear language leads to clear thought, and, if we think clearly about what the authors call compensatory restoration, we will conclude, I submit, that their principles for the exercise of trustee discretion are unnecessary and possibly counterproductive.

2

Scaling and Selecting Compensatory Restoration Projects: An Economic Perspective

*William H. Desvousges, Erin E. Fries, Sara P. Hudson, Richard W. Dunford**

The Oil Pollution Act (OPA) of 1990 seeks to "make the environment and public whole for injuries to natural resources and natural resource services resulting from an incident involving a discharge or substantial threat of a discharge of oil" (61 *Federal Register* 440). In response, the National Oceanic and Atmospheric Administration (NOAA) developed regulations in 1996 that focus on restoring such resources and services. These regulations represent a departure from the natural resource damage assessment (NRDA) regulations promulgated by the Department of the Interior (DOI) in 1986 (43 C.F.R. §11).

The NOAA regulations present new challenges to economists, as well as biologists and ecologists, because they contain procedures that differ from those previously used by NOAA and DOI. Most importantly, the NOAA approach now requires economists to predict how people will alter their use of natural resources in response to possible restoration actions. This requirement changes significantly the direction and emphasis of economic analysis, which had previously focused on estimating the value of foregone services. Therefore, there is little experience with this new approach to guide assessments.

In addition, the new NOAA approach is not based on a consistent conceptual framework. It mixes resources, services, and valuation concepts without properly developing the relationships between these key NRDA components. A consistent conceptual framework is crucial for reliably assessing damages. Moreover, such a framework is necessary to evaluate the efficiency of various restoration alternatives.

We provide an economic perspective on the process for determining the magnitude of damages in an NRDA. Specifically, we provide a conceptual framework based on microeconomic theory through which to view the NOAA approach to damage assessment. Our framework provides the context for discussing the challenges in evaluating restoration projects and selecting the most economically efficient projects. We include examples relating to the framework for both oil spills and hazardous-substance releases.[1]

*Triangle Economic Research, Durham, NC

[1]Although the NOAA approach now applies only to oil spills, DOI has indicated that it is considering a similar approach (61 *Federal Register* 37031).

Regulatory setting

In the NRDA regulations initially proposed by NOAA in 1994, natural resource damages had 3 components. The first component, restoration costs, was the cost of restoring the injured natural resource or its services to its without-injury (or baseline) state. The second component, compensable value losses, was the value of the services lost during the time between the occurrence of the injury and the return to baseline. Finally, assessment costs, the costs of performing the damage assessment, were the third component. This framework was consistent with the DOI regulations (43 C.F.R. §11).[2]

However, in August of 1995, NOAA proposed an alternative approach, later adopted in January of 1996 (61 *Federal Register* 439). Although it is difficult to know all the reasons for NOAA's change in direction, the controversy over the use of contingent valuation (CV) to measure so-called "nonuse losses" was a significant contributing factor. Comments regarding the reliability of CV accounted for a significant portion of the public comments on the initial NOAA proposal.

In the original NOAA proposal, nonuse losses and use losses comprised compensable value. Under the new rule, however, compensable value losses are replaced by compensatory restoration costs. Now, instead of calculating the value of the interim service losses, a compensatory restoration plan must be devised to replace forgone services with equivalent service gains. The responsible party is liable for the cost of that compensatory restoration, rather than the value of the interim service losses.[3]

A conceptual framework

Although NOAA's final rule provides a new NRDA framework that equates service losses and gains, it lacks the proper economic foundation for evaluating these service losses and gains. This section provides an economic perspective on assessing natural resource damages under the NOAA rule. This economic context provides a consistent way to evaluate all service losses and service gains.

Role of services in NRDAs

The NOAA rule places compensation within a framework of services lost as a result of injury and services gained from compensatory restoration actions. This focus is derived from the basic economic concept that people's value for a good is based on the

---

[2]Initially, the DOI regulations defined damages as the sum of assessment costs and the "lesser of" restoration costs and the compensable value that would be forgone if the restoration were not undertaken. Subsequently, DOI modified the regulations to define damages as the sum of all 3 components.

[3]However, if the trustees determine that "valuation of the replacement natural resources and/or services cannot be performed within a reasonable time frame or at a reasonable cost . . . trustees may estimate the dollar value of lost services and select the scale of the restoration action that has a cost equivalent to the lost value" (61 *Federal Register* 507). Therefore, NOAA allows for monetary compensation equal to the value of interim lost services as a fallback position. It remains to be seen how much the new framework, as opposed to the "fallback" position, will be used.

services provided by that good. This principle applies to any type of good, whether it is a marketed commodity or a natural resource (Kopp and Smith 1993). For example, people value a house, in part, because it provides the service of shelter. Likewise, people value the flow of services that come from wetlands, such as hunting, wildlife viewing, or the habitat provided for various species.[4]

With public services such as recreation uses, people directly experience the natural resource services on-site. Other services, such as habitat for birds or nursery areas for fish, must be perceived as meaningful to people in order to have value. Although benthic organisms provide a service because they are an integral part of the food chain for fish, birds, and other animals, they have value to people only if they provide perceptible direct or indirect human-use services.[5]

Under the NOAA regulations, the essential economic tasks in NRDAs are to measure the service losses resulting from the release of oil or hazardous substances and the potential gains that would result from restoration actions. To illustrate these tasks, it is useful to consider an example of service losses and gains. In Figure 2-1, service losses are shown as Area A. This stylized example shows a reduction from baseline and then a gradual recovery that occurs at the injured site. Time S represents the start of the spill or release, P represents the start of restoration, and R shows when recovery is completed. The dotted line extending to the baseline from P represents the path of natural recovery. Under the DOI regulations, damages are based on measuring the costs of the restoration actions that begin at P and the monetary value of the services that are shown in Area A.

The potential service gains from compensatory restoration actions are shown as Area B in Figure 2-1. As Figure 2-1 illustrates, compensatory restoration gains may come in one of two forms: restoration of services at the injured site *beyond* baseline, or generation of services at another site. As noted above, under the NOAA regulations, damages are based on the costs of primary restoration actions that begin at P and the costs of the compensatory restoration projects needed to achieve Area B. Clearly, if the costs of providing compensatory projects are less than the value of the services, the damages are lower under the NOAA rule than the DOI rule.

Conversely, if the costs of compensatory projects are higher, then the damages are higher.

To properly evaluate compensatory restoration actions, it is critical to establish the correct level of baseline services. NOAA's final NRDA rule defines baseline as "the

[4]In the NOAA final rule, services are defined as "the functions performed by a natural resource for the benefit of another natural resource and/or the public" (15 C.F.R. §990.30). These services include ecological services and public services. DOI's 1994 final rule for hazardous-substance releases describes services as "the physical and biological functions performed by the resources including the human use of those functions" (13 C.F.R. §11.14).

[5]Although the notion of economic value is based on human welfare, this anthropocentric focus does not mean that individuals do not value species' survival, habitat, or other ecological services.

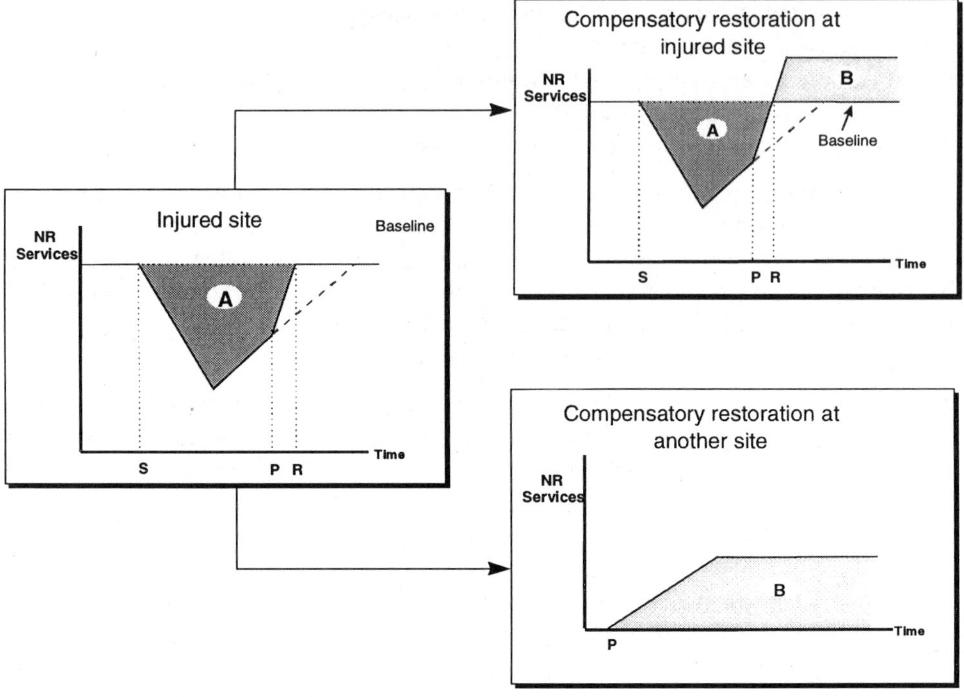

Figure 2-1 Example of service losses and gains

condition of natural resources and services that would have existed had the incident not occurred" (61 *Federal Register* 447). Therefore, its determination affects all subsequent analysis. For example, if the baseline is set too high, service losses will be overstated and the compensatory gains needed to offset these losses likewise will be overstated. This problem is especially pronounced if compensatory restoration is going to occur at the injured site in the form of service gains beyond baseline. In that case, compensatory restoration actions would have to generate services beyond an artificially high baseline.

In order to properly assess natural resource damages, baseline services must reflect the services that would have existed without the injury, rather than services before the injury. For example, suppose a release occurred in the 1940s in a rather pristine environment. However, the area became more industrialized over time, resulting in the building of highways and manufacturing facilities in the area. As a result, the baseline levels of ecological and public services in the area decline over time, completely independent of the release. Therefore, even though the resource was pristine before the release, we cannot assume that the relevant baseline condition is pristine. Because the baseline often is dynamic, its correct establishment must incorporate these types of intertemporal changes. Furthermore, this "without-injury" perspective complicates the establishment of baseline because often data are unavailable on the service levels in the absence of the injuries. Although the relevant temporal changes, such as the addition of highways, should be incorporated into the establishment of baseline, there may be no time period in the past for which the highways existed without the injury, making the determination of baseline services difficult.

The NOAA regulations call for the restoration of both natural resources and services. Clearly, such restoration does not have a valid economic rationale because, as discussed above, economics views the restoration of services as the relevant criteria because people value resources for the services they provide.

Finally, an important economic consideration is to measure people's value for the services in Area B such that it offsets the value of the services lost (Area A). The remainder of this framework addresses the economic concepts of value that can serve as the basis for this determination. NOAA's rule obscures the basic task by describing the process as "scaling" and indicates that "service-to-service" approaches are the preferred methods. As discussed in more depth below, the service-to-service approach replaces the injured services with services of the same type and quality. In effect, these approaches are a special type of valuation that assumes that similar resource services have the same value. NOAA's rule does allow for valuation-based approaches to be used when resources are not of the same type and quality (61 *Federal Register* 453).

Role of utility in NRDAs

The economic value of services comes, directly or indirectly, from human uses of resources.[6] To measure the value associated with service gains and losses, it is essential to place services within a basic economic context. The economic concept of utility provides the necessary organizational construct.[7] Utility is defined as the satisfaction that people receive from using a commodity or engaging in an activity. The level of utility, or satisfaction, is dependent on individual preferences.[8] Service gains are associated with increases in utility, while service losses are associated with decreases in utility (i.e., disutility). Thus, compensatory restoration actions should seek to replace the lost utility associated with an injury.

In general, different combinations of services can provide the same level of utility. Figure 2-2 presents a simplified example that includes 2 ecological services, riverine habitat services and wetland habitat services, on the x and y axes, respectively. The curves labeled u_1 and u_2 are called indifference curves and represent 2 levels of utility from various combinations of the 2 services. Any combination of riverine habitat and

[6]The NOAA rule defines value as "the maximum amount of goods, services, or money an individual is willing to give up to obtain a specific good or service, or the minimum amount of goods, services, or money an individual is willing to accept to forgo a specific good or service" (61 *Federal Register* 505).

[7]It is important to note that utility, unlike money, does not provide a cardinal measure of social welfare.

[8]To convert individual utility into societal utility, we make the simplifying assumption that individuals have similar preferences that can be combined. In practice, however, preferences are not the same across individuals and should be modeled as a function of personal characteristics like age, income, and other variables.

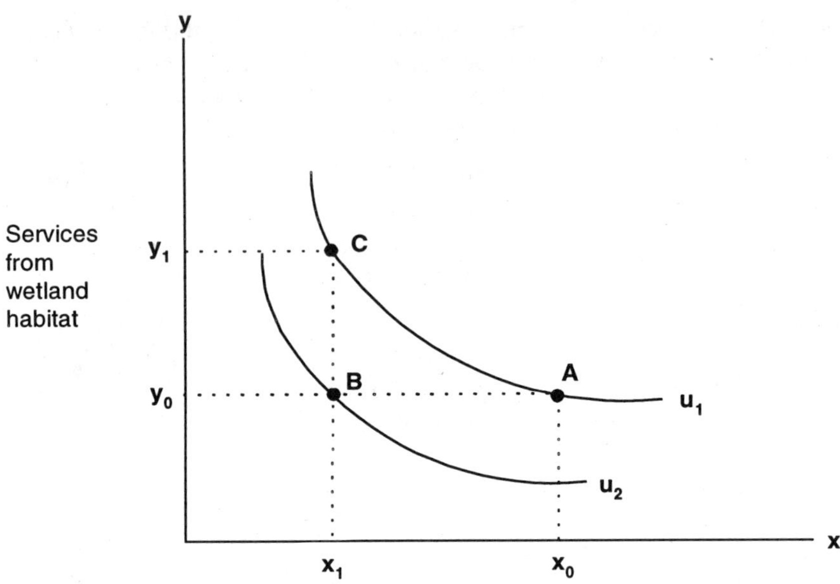

Figure 2-2 Indifference curves for habitat services

wetland habitat services along a single indifference curve represents the same level of utility.[9]

For example, Points A and C on Curve u_1 represent the same level of utility. Point A is a combination with a relatively high level of riverine habitat services and a relatively low level of wetland habitat services. Conversely, Point C indicates a combination with a relatively low level of riverine habitat services and a relatively high level of wetland habitat services. Because A and C provide the same level of utility, an individual is indifferent between Point A and Point C. The curvature of these indifference curves reflects the willingness to trade off one service for the other. For example, the slope at any point along Curve u_1 shows how much additional wetland service a person would require to give up a unit of riverine services and remain at the same level of utility. Any combination of services on u_1 has a higher utility than any combination of services on u_2 because u_1 represents a higher level of utility.

Now suppose that Curve u_1 represents the without-injury (i.e., baseline) level of utility and Point A is the baseline combination of services. Further suppose that u_2 represents the level of utility after a hazardous-substance release has occurred in riverine habitat. Given that the release affected only riverine habitat, riverine habitat services move

[9] Although Figure 2-2 shows standard indifference curves, these curves may have other shapes as well. For example, some individuals may derive utility only from riverine habitat, in which case their indifference curves would be vertical.

from x_0 to x_1 while wetland habitat services remain the same (see Point B in Figure 2-2). Point B is on a lower indifference curve, indicating a loss in utility. It is this loss in utility that should be compensated.

From an economic perspective, therefore, a hazardous-substance release or oil spill must result in a loss in utility in order for damages to occur. Thus, all effects from the release can be analyzed within this utility framework. Figure 2-3 illustrates the linkages. Following a release, a physical injury to a natural resource may occur. That injury may lead to a reduction in services provided by the natural resource. The reduction in services may cause a loss of utility, which results in damages. Thus, a clear link between release and injury, between the injury and a loss in services, and between the service loss and a loss in utility, is needed for damages to occur. The link between the release and injury usually is determined by biologists or ecologists. However, the link from injury through service loss to a loss in utility is made by economists, working with ecologists and biologists, through the observation of tangible behavioral effects of the injury.

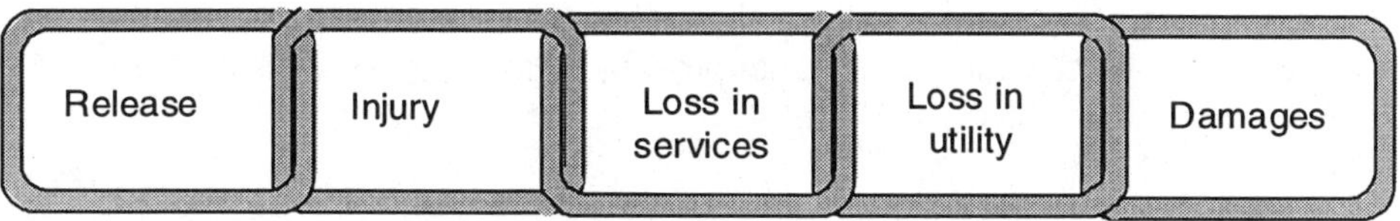

Figure 2-3 Necessary linkages for natural resource damages

The linkages that result in damages should not be assumed. Even in the presence of injury, it is possible that no losses in utility, and thus no damages, have occurred. For example, if a release injures an aquifer that is unsuitable for use because of hydrological limitations, the release may not result in a loss in services, thereby breaking the chain. Furthermore, an injury to sediments may result in such a small change in the service level that there is no resulting loss in utility, and thus no damages.

These same type of linkages also are important in the measurement of benefits from restoration. In other words, the chain works the same way for gains as it does for losses, as shown in Figure 2-4. In order to be effective, a compensatory restoration project enhances a resource, which in turn increases the resource services, which increases utility, resulting in benefits. Just as the linkages between an injury and damages cannot be assumed, the linkages from restoration actions and benefits must be evaluated. It is the evaluation of the chain shown in Figure 2-4 that represents the new challenge in damage assessment under the new NOAA approach.[10]

---

[10]The order in which the linkages for restoration benefits are made may differ in reality. Specifically, determining the desired utility and service gains is sometimes the first step in restoration. After the desired gains are determined, possible restoration actions are identified.

Restoration action
Resource enhancement
Gain in services
Gain in utility
Benefits

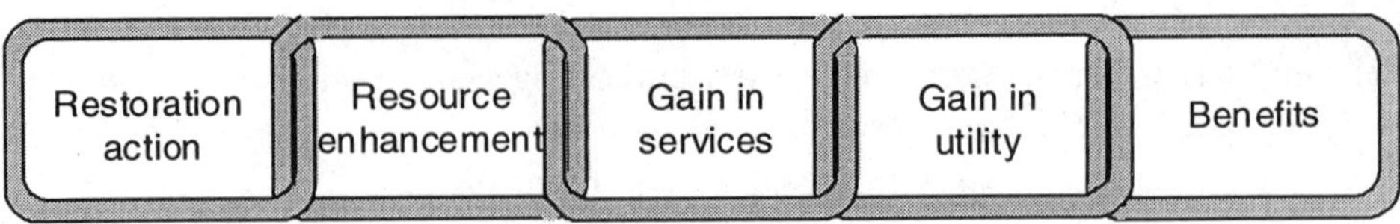

Figure 2-4 Necessary linkages for restoration benefits

After developing the link between injury and service losses or enhancement and service gains, economists measure changes in utility associated with the change in the quality of the resource. For example, a water-quality problem at a lake or river may decrease fishing days at that site or reduce the utility that anglers derive from fishing at that site. Similarly, the addition of boat launches at that same lake may increase total recreation at the lake or increase the utility for people who already use the site. If we understand how people's utility responds to various characteristics of a resource, such as the quality of access or the health risks of consuming injured fish, it is possible to construct an index of the utility associated with the change in quality. These examples illustrate gains and losses in public services. For ecological services, the conceptual basis is the same. However, empirically measuring the value of such services is far more problematic.

Utility's relationship to demand

For purposes of illustration, it is useful to examine utility in terms of its relationship to demand. Demand curves show the quantity of a service demanded at various prices. Given that demand curves represent trade-offs between consumption and dollars, this structure changes the metric of comparison from utility (as used in Figure 2-2) to dollars. Thus, demand curves represent a monetization of utility and allow economists to operationalize the concept of utility.

Figure 2-5 shows the demand for recreational fishing at a hypothetical site. At a given price, P_1, the quantity demanded is Q_1. The shape and slope of the demand curve for a given site is dependent on users' preferences and income as well as the quality and quantity of other substitute sites. Demand curves slope downward because of the inverse relationship between price and the quantity demanded. At higher prices, people will require a lower quantity, holding all other factors constant. The farther the demand curve is located from the origin, the more popular the site, because people demand more quantity at each price.

Demand curves are directly related to the indifference curves shown in Figure 2-2. Those indifference curves show a person's preferences and willingness to trade one service for another. The quantity of each service attainable by the individual is determined by adding a budget constraint reflecting the prices of the 2 services to Figure 2-2. The demand curve for one of the services reflects the quantity of that service desired at various prices for that service. Thus, demand curves show the willingness to trade dollars for consumption of a given good or service, subject to a

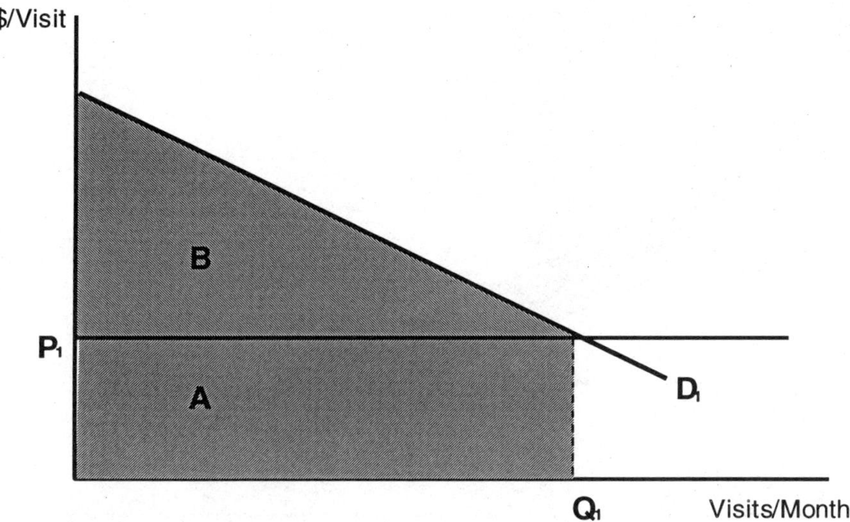

Figure 2-5 Demand for recreational fishing at a site

budget constraint. Demand curves represent the optimal trade-off people can make between dollars and consumption based on their preferences and the amount of money they have available.

Demand curves provide a way to derive a monetary estimate of the benefits gained from the consumption of the good or service. In Figure 2-5, Area A represents the cost of consuming that quantity (i.e., the per-unit price multiplied by the number of units consumed). The total area under the demand curve (Areas A and B) represents the total amount the person would be willing to pay for, and thus the total amount of benefit gained from, the consumption of Q_1 units. Thus, Area B represents the benefit in excess of the expenditures associated with that level of consumption. This area is known as consumer surplus, and it is the operational measure of utility used in damage assessments.

In addition, it is straightforward to illustrate the effects of a change in quality of the site, such as access limitation, water quality problems, or a restriction on fishing, using the demand curve. Figure 2-6 shows the possible recreational-fishing consequences from reducing the quality at a site. Demand for fishing services at this site decreases from D_1 to D_2. The potential loss in consumer surplus from the decrease would consist of 2 parts: the reduction in the number of fishing days as some people chose to forgo fishing (Area B) and the reduction in the quality of trips that continue to take place because people do not have the same fishing experience (Area A).

Conversely, shifts in recreation demand also may occur because of restoration actions. For example, suppose a new boat launch is built at the site. Assuming that D_2 represents the demand for fishing services at baseline, the enhancement to the site might

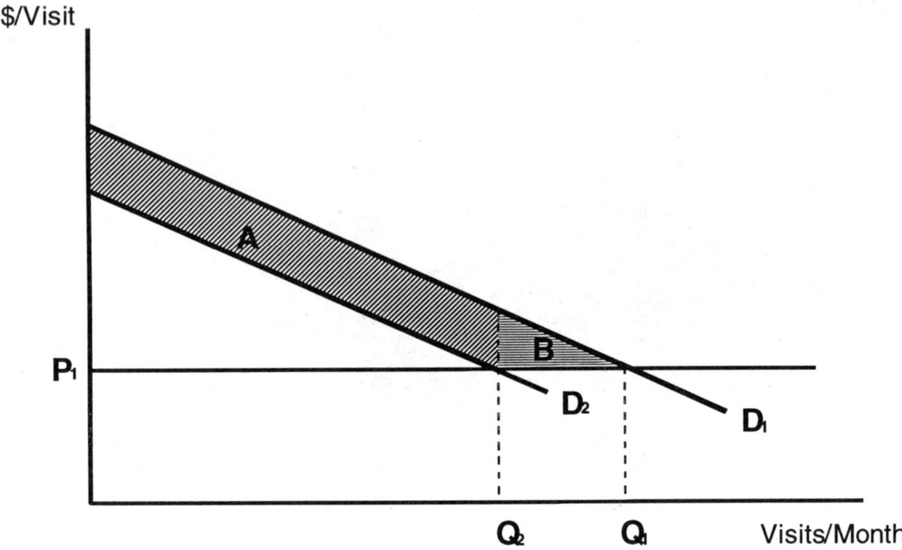

Figure 2-6 Shifting demand for fishing at a site

shift demand outward to D_1. In this case, the increase in consumer surplus includes Areas A and B, where A represents improved-quality fishing days for anglers who already visit the site and B represents additional fishing days at the site.

The measurement of utility trade-offs for service gains poses new challenges for economists. One of the most important challenges for use services will be the linkage of recreation choices to possible restoration actions. For ecological services, the challenges are even greater. It is not clear whether people can conceive of such trade-offs or whether they can perform the cognitive tasks that would be required. Whether such challenges can be met to provide measurements that are sufficiently reliable for damage assessment is an issue having little empirical evidence to date. Nonetheless, the concepts of preference trade-offs and consumer surplus provide a sound conceptual basis for evaluating service losses and gains.

Scaling methods

There are 3 basic approaches for quantifying utility losses and scaling potential restoration gains: behavioral models, stated-preference models, and service-equivalency models. Using the terminology of the NOAA regulations, these are called "scaling methods" because the objective is to determine the size or "scale" of compensatory restoration project that would offset the lost services. Table 2-1 provides an overview of each approach, focusing on its use for quantifying both losses and restoration gains. Many of the traditional economic approaches used to quantify losses are not likely to be well-suited for measuring gains.

Table 2-1 Comparison of scaling approaches

Method	Underlying premise	Services addressed	Data required	Statistical complexity	Ability to evaluate multiple compensatory-restoration alternatives
	Behavioral models				
Averting behavior	Value lost by a service reduction is estimated using costs people incur to avoid that reduction.	Drinking water, losses and gains	Survey data on actual averting behaviors taken and costs of those actions.	Low.	Past experience limited to losses. Gains have not been addressed.
Hedonic pricing	Value of environmental attributes is modeled as a component of the overall property value.	Recreation access losses and gains	Market transactions data on the total value of the property and the characteristics of that property including environmental quality.	Moderate to high. Based on strong assumptions that property markets are in equilibrium, change is costless, and all cost-contribution components can be identified and measured.	Limited to situations where the characteristics of the compensatory-restoration alternatives can be related to resource services. Must also avoid double-counting private losses.
Travel cost	Value of a site is derived from the travel cost expended to visit the site.	Recreation uses	Survey data on visitation to site by people living at varying distances; Limited site characteristic information.	Low to moderate for traditional, single-site models. Complexity increases with the introduction of multiple sites.	Very limited use because model estimates assume constant characteristics.
Random utility models	Value of a recreation site is a function of the value of each of its characteristics.	Recreation uses, losses and gains	Survey data on visitation and site characteristics for competing sites by people within the relevant geographic market.	High. The application of RUMs to recreation modeling is still evolving and these models are complex.	Well-suited for valuing different bundles of characteristics resulting from compensatory-restoration alternatives as long as those characteristics are included as site characteristics in the model.

Table 2-1 Continued

Method	Underlying premise	Services addressed	Data required	Statistical complexity	Ability to evaluate multiple compensatory-restoration alternatives
Stated-preference models					
Contingent valuation	Value of a good in hypothetical markets reflects the value that good would have in an actual market.	Public and possibly ecological services, losses and gains.	Survey data on willingness to pay for hypothetical good or program.	Low to High. Analysis ranges from very simple univariate statistics to highly complex models.	Only if the restoration alternatives are known in advance of the survey development and contingent market scenarios can be devised to represent them. Then, potentially, different versions for each alternative could be administered to separate samples. Unreliable when applied to non-use services.
Conjoint	Value of a good is determined by its attributes.	Pubic and possibly ecological services, losses and gains.	Survey data on trade-offs of hypothetical bundles of attributes.	Moderate. Complex statistical models are required to properly estimate the utility changes for changes in attributes.	Well-suited for valuing different bundles of characteristics resulting from compensatory-restoration alternatives as long as those characteristics are included as attributes in the model. Has not been applied to ecological services.
Service-equivalency models					
Habitat equivalency analysis	Lost resource services can be offset with replacement services without valuation.	Public and ecological services, losses and gains.	Services data only. No data on preferences. However, input parameters for assessing services may be expensive to measure if literature-based values are not available.	Low. If the strict assumptions are met, the analysis is straightforward.	If compensatory-restoration alternatives yielding services of the same type and quality as those lost can be identified, HEA can be useful for evaluating alternatives. Assumes people's preferences are such that they want the exact same services as compensation.

Behavioral models

All methods within this category use observed behavior to infer the value that people place on resource services. Although the use of actual behavior is a strength of these models, it can also be a limitation. For example, these models can only be used if sufficient data about relevant choices can be collected. Also, inferences from these models are limited to the set of choices upon which the models are based. Given that these models require data on actual choices, they are only useful for direct uses of natural resources. Finally, simplifying assumptions about behavior is required in some cases, which may bias the estimates.

Averting-behavior models

Averting-behavior models estimate the value of lost consumer surplus by calculating the costs of actions taken to avoid or mitigate some condition. For example, suppose that a release affects an aquifer, contaminating a community's water supply. The averting-behavior method could measure the willingness to pay for clean drinking water through individuals' expenditures on water filters and bottled water. To evaluate gains, averting-behavior models could be used in reverse. Instead of the costs of averting behavior being interpreted as a loss, the benefit of avoided averting-behavior costs would identify the scale or size of restoration actions. However, this model is limited to applications where such averting behaviors are quantifiable.

Hedonic pricing models

Hedonic pricing models are based on the idea that the value of a good (e.g., property) is a function of the value of each of its components. These models are used in NRDAs by including some measure of environmental quality as an attribute of the property and attempting to estimate the share of the value of the property that is attributable to that measure of environmental quality. These models can only be used for losses or gains if appropriate measures of environmental quality can be included in the model and if they are statistically significant. Then, by adjusting these measures, we could estimate gains and losses in consumer surplus. However, it can be difficult to find measures that reflect the actual injury and service losses and have explanatory power in the models. In addition, care must be taken not to double-count any private loss collected through tort claims.

Traditional travel-cost models

Traditional travel-cost models use the cost of traveling to a site as an implicit measure of the price of using that site. Based on this price and the observed trip behavior, these models estimate a demand curve for the site and calculate consumer surplus from that curve. These models have been used extensively in the past for determining the value of a day of recreation at a site. However, they have not been used for valuing quality changes. Traditional travel-cost analysis is not well equipped to calculate values when site attributes are changing, and it is likely to give biased results. Therefore, these models would be of limited use for scaling compensatory restoration alternatives.

Random utility models

Random utility models (RUMs) provide a significant improvement over the traditional travel-cost method. While they continue to use the cost of travel as an implicit price, the value of a site is modeled as a function of the values of its attributes. By taking this approach, RUMs can determine the relative importance of each site characteristic by evaluating the trade-offs among those characteristics made by users. By measuring value in terms of the sites' attributes, RUMs can be used to predict the quantity of additional recreation that would take place if the injury were not present or under different compensatory restoration scenarios, making it much more useful than traditional travel-cost models for scaling losses and gains.

Stated-preference models

Stated-preference models are based on information given by respondents in a survey setting, not on actual behavior. Thus, these models can provide more flexibility to value a broader range of services, both public and possibly ecological services. However, the hypothetical nature of the survey will generally reduce the reliability of the information collected from respondents.

Contingent valuation

Contingent valuation (CV) asks respondents directly about their willingness to pay (WTP) for a commodity. Instead of focusing on the services themselves, CV typically elicits WTP by focusing on an environmental program that restores services. Contingent valuation has many well-documented problems, especially when used to measure nonuse values that stem from its hypothetical nature.[11]

One of the challenges with CV is to design a hypothetical program that reflects the actual service losses at the site.[12] Even if this challenge is met, existing applications of CV typically value only one program and thus lack the flexibility of being able to estimate values for different compensatory restoration actions. Ideally, a technique should allow the valuation of different levels of an attribute or different combinations of attributes so that numerous restoration actions can be evaluated. This evaluation would only be possible if multiple CV scenarios were designed and administered. Even in this case, the compensatory restoration alternatives must be known in advance of the survey design and the number of respondents needed may be prohibitive. Combined with the reliability concerns for nonuse values, CV is of limited or no use for scaling gains.

---

[11]Nonuse values are defined as the values that individuals hold for resources that are independent of their use of that resource. See Hausman (1993) and the NOAA Panel Report (58 *Federal Register* 4601) for a full discussion.

[12]A variation on the conventional CV approach is the contingent-behavior technique. This technique describes a service loss or gain to respondents and asks about their behavior in the presence of the loss or gain (e.g., if a lake's water quality improved by 50%, how many fishing trips would you take to the lake?). See McConnell (1986), Duffield (1995), and Desvousges (1996) for more discussion.

Conjoint models

Conjoint analysis, like hedonic models and RUMs, is based on the premise that products are composed of various attributes, and the value of the composite good is a function of the value of its attributes. Conjoint models recover the utility for each attribute by asking respondents a series of questions, trading off pairs of products with varying attributes (in which respondents either choose one of the two products or rate one product relative to another). In a damage assessment setting, respondents are asked to evaluate service losses or gains through trading off environmental programs with different attributes. Then, using the observed trade-offs between attributes, the change in utility associated with either increases or decreases (i.e., gains or losses) for an attribute, such as fish-consumption advisory levels, can be estimated.

Conjoint analysis has several advantages over other techniques. One advantage is that its flexibility allows for the creation of attributes that may not exist currently. This flexibility can be crucial for measuring compensatory restoration gains. For example, a restoration program in a conjoint exercise may include recreation facilities that are not currently available in the area of the release. Despite the fact that they do not yet exist, conjoint analysis can recover individuals' utility for these attributes. Furthermore, because conjoint analysis values attributes separately, different combinations of attributes can be grouped together and the resulting compensatory restoration project can be valued. Contingent valuation typically only values one program, so it does not have this type of flexibility.[13]

Nonetheless, conjoint analysis has not been applied to ecological services, so it is difficult to know whether it can be reliably used to scale ecological losses and gains. It is possible that people's lack of familiarity with ecological services could hamper conjoint studies in the same way it does CV studies. Moreover, people may find it more difficult to trade off use services for ecological services because of the innate differences between these types of services.

Service-equivalency models

NOAA's final rule recommends the use of habitat equivalency analysis (HEA) for service-to-service scaling, especially when the lost services are primarily ecological services, such as species habitat or biological services (60 *Federal Register* 39816). HEA is based on the idea of compensating for lost services by replacing them with an equivalent flow of services.[14] Compensation may occur by creating new habitat or improving injured habitat beyond baseline (in cases where the habitat was not at its

[13]Stated-preference models can be used in conjunction with behavioral models to estimate changes in consumer surplus. Several studies have demonstrated the feasibility of jointly estimating these 2 approaches (Swaite et al. 1994; Adamowicz et al. 1994; Hensher and Bradley 1993).

[14]A basic tenet of economic theory holds that individuals can best determine how to maximize their own utility. Under this provision, replacing the lost service flows may be inferior to other possible uses of the money needed to replace those service flows.

maximum potential at baseline). Because all losses and gains are described in terms of service flows, a monetary metric is not explicitly included in HEA.

The HEA approach is based on the fundamental goal of equating the monetary value of service losses to the monetary value of service gains (Unsworth and Bishop 1994). Thus, the utility framework developed in this paper is applicable to HEA. However, HEA makes some very restrictive assumptions to eliminate monetary values from the calculations, avoiding the need to use economic valuation techniques to scale the compensatory restoration actions. In general, HEA requires the services lost from the injury and the services gained through compensatory restoration to be of the same type and quality and to face the same market conditions over the relevant time-frame (61 *Federal Register* 452). Under these assumptions, the per-unit value of lost services and gained services would be the same over time, which results in their elimination from the calculation. Therefore, we can compare the quantity of service flows and still be comparing the utility of those service flows, maintaining the conceptual framework underlying the behavioral models and stated-preference models.[15]

While the general requirements for using HEA may seem reasonable, the specific assumptions that must be met in order for HEA to accurately scale compensatory restoration include the following:

- The real unit value of the services of the injured habitat in its baseline condition is constant over time.
- The real unit value of the compensatory habitat prior to its transformation is constant over time.
- The real unit value of the transformed compensatory habitat at its maximum service level is constant over time.
- The relative reduction in the unit value of the injured habitat over time is equal to the relative reduction in the services of the injured habitat.
- The increase in the relative value of the transformed compensatory habitat over time is equal to the relative increase in services from the transformed compensatory habitat.

It is possible that one or more of these simplifying assumptions may be met in certain circumstances, but it is highly unlikely that all 5 assumptions would be met. Deviations from these simplifying assumptions will cause the estimated quantity of compensatory restoration to deviate from the quantity needed to make the public whole.

Habitat equivalency analysis was designed specifically to meet the new challenges posed by scaling compensatory restoration gains. However, in order to be effective, the strict assumptions discussed above must be met. Otherwise, comparing lost services

[15]A key component of HEA is the choice of a discount rate for putting both the lost and gained services in present value terms. Although we are discounting services operationally, we are actually discounting values. Therefore, a financial discount rate (3% in the NOAA regulations) is appropriate for HEA, as discussed in Desvousges et al. (1995).

and gained services without regard to their relative value will not yield the appropriate level of compensatory restoration. In addition, there may not be many feasible alternatives that will satisfy the strict criteria required by HEA. For large, complex ecosystems, replacement areas that provide services of the same type and quality under the same demand and supply conditions simply may not be available.

Habitat equivalency analysis has been used to provide a basis for settling some biological resource service losses in NRDAs. The approach has been used in lieu of trying to value such resource services with CV, which has demonstrated reliability problems and is expensive to implement.[16] However, these applications have been in situations where equivalent resources were located nearby and could be enhanced at reasonable costs. In some HEA applications, the parameters of the model are adjusted in such a way as to offset violations of its restrictive assumptions. Furthermore, uncertainties with respect to the HEA parameters are usually addressed by using "conservative" estimates of those parameters. This leads to estimates of compensatory restoration that overcompensate the public.

Integration of scaling methods

Despite the fact that the NOAA rule specifies 2 distinct services—ecological services and public services—it is important to avoid a simple summation of the value of the losses or gains when using different methods for different services. For example, suppose an HEA is used to determine a restoration action that results in the proper increase in fish-habitat services. Then, a RUM is used to estimate the value of lost fishing days resulting from the release and the value of gained fishing days from an enhancement. The cost of the fishing-days enhancement and the cost of the fish-habitat enhancement cannot be added simply because the fish-habitat restoration action scaled with HEA would be likely to result in an increase in angler days. Thus, the only angler days for which compensation is required are the days that would not be gained from the fish-habitat enhancement. Scaling compensatory restoration for these services in isolation, therefore, will likely lead to double-counting and an inefficiently high level of compensatory restoration action.[17]

Key factors affecting the magnitude of service losses and gains

Several factors affect the magnitude of both losses and restoration gains. These factors can be separated into those that affect the quantity of services and those that affect the value of services. Factors that affect the quantity of service losses include the following:

---

[16]In some cases, transaction costs for CV studies may be extremely large. For example, NOAA reportedly spent $5 million to $7 million to develop estimates of the value of the allegedly lost services for the *U.S. v. Montrose* case.

[17]The definitions of ecological and public services in the NOAA final rule are not mutually exclusive, which increases the likelihood of double-counting. Specifically, ecological services are defined as functions that one natural resource provides for another, and public services include functions of natural resources that provide value to the public (61 *Federal Register* 448). Thus, functions that one natural resource provides for another that are also valued by the public are included in both categories.

- the year when the service losses began,
- the magnitude of the initial service losses,
- the rate of natural recovery of services,
- the year when primary restoration actions begin,
- the rate of service recovery under primary restoration actions, and
- the year when services return to baseline under primary restoration actions.

As shown previously in Figure 2-1, these factors affect the size of Area A, which represents the quantity of service losses. For example, the year when the service losses begin is represented as "S" of the injured site. "P" shows the year when primary restoration begins. "R" is the year when services return to baseline under primary restoration actions. The rate of natural recovery of services is shown as the dotted line from P to the baseline.

The unit value of the forgone services is also an important determinant of the magnitude of the losses as a result of an oil spill or hazardous-substance release. The unit values are a function of the characteristics of the relevant services, individuals' preferences for those services, the price of those services, the characteristics and price of substitutes and complements for the relevant services, and income. Finally, the discount rate used to convert annual losses into their present value will affect the magnitude of the losses.

The factors that affect the quantity of service gains, which are similar to the factors affecting the quantity of service losses, include:

- the year when the service gains begin,
- the "growth" rate of service gains over time,
- the year when service gains reach their maximum,
- the useful life of service gains,
- the quantity of service gains each year between the time they reach their maximum and the end of their useful life, and
- the quantity of services lost as a result of the compensatory restoration actions, if any.[18]

These factors affect the size of Area B in the compensatory restoration scenarios in Figure 2-1. In addition to the quantity of service gains, the unit value of those services, the unit value of any forgone services as a result of compensatory restoration actions, and the discount rate will affect the aggregate, present value of the service gains.

[18]When a site other than the injured site is used for compensatory restoration, the services provided by the site prior to its transformation usually will be lost. For example, if a dry land area is converted to wetlands to replace wetland services injured by an oil spill, the services provided by the dry land area will be lost once the transformation to wetlands has begun. Both the quality and the quantity of lost services associated with the lost dry land should be included in the calculations.

In general, less severe injuries and quicker recovery from the injuries, either naturally or as a result of primary restoration actions, will reduce the required amount of compensatory restoration, other things being equal. Similarly, the sooner compensatory restoration actions begin and the faster the growth rate of the gain in services, the lower the cost of compensatory restoration actions will be. In addition, the longer the lifetime of the compensatory restoration actions, the less compensatory restoration will be needed, other things being equal. Finally, higher discount rates will increase the amount of required compensatory restoration because higher discount rates will increase the present value of losses and decrease the present value of gains.

Selection of restoration alternatives

After scaling compensatory restoration actions, it is necessary to select an alternative from the available possibilities. Because economics recognizes that society's resources are limited, the discipline can offer considerable insight into restoration-selection decisions. As discussed above, the concept of utility enables restoration outcomes to be expressed in a standard metric. In addition, economists have developed principles of economic efficiency that have been used in decision-making related to natural resources since the 1950s (Eckstein 1961). These principles also are well-suited to evaluating restoration selection because they provide an organizing framework.

The NOAA final rule lists several factors that trustees should consider in selecting restoration alternatives. In particular, the regulations state that the preferred plan should be selected from the feasible alternatives based on several criteria (61 *Federal Register* 442), as follows:

- cost to carry out the alternative,
- extent to which each alternative is expected to meet the trustees' goals and objectives in returning the injured natural resources and services to baseline and/or compensate for interim losses,
- likelihood of success of each alternative,
- extent to which each alternative will prevent future injury as a result of the incident, and avoid collateral injury as a result of implementing the alternative,
- extent to which each alternative benefits more than one natural resource and/or service, and
- effect of each alternative on public health and safety.

The final rule further specifies that trustees must select the most cost-effective restoration alternative when two or more alternatives are equally preferable based on these factors (61 *Federal Register* 442).

A complete evaluation of these criteria is beyond the scope of this paper (see Desvousges et al. 1995, for more discussion). However, we describe a few problems in these criteria below.

Cost-effectiveness and economic efficiency

Cost-effectiveness requires the selection of the lowest-cost alternative when two or more alternatives provide equivalent restoration benefits. In an NRDA context, the scaled restoration alternatives should provide the same level of utility because they all are scaled to make the public whole. Therefore, cost-effectiveness requires choosing the lowest-cost restoration alternative among the feasible alternatives.

While cost-effectiveness is an important criteria, it does not fully address economic efficiency, which requires that the selected alternative represents an optimal use of society's scarce resources. Thus, the cost of the selected alternative should be weighed against the benefits of the services it provides. An alternative whose costs greatly outweigh its benefits does not represent an efficient outcome. For example, if the most cost-effective alternative provides services valued at $100,000, but costs $2,000,000, then its costs greatly exceed its benefits. In this case, it would be inefficient to implement the selected alternative. Instead, it would be more efficient for the potentially responsible party to compensate directly the trustees acting on behalf of the public for the loss by paying $100,000 in damages, as would have been the case under the old regulatory framework of compensable value.

In the *Ohio* decision[19], the U.S. Court of Appeals rejected a strict benefit-cost test for restoration actions, ruling that the goal of the NRDA process should be to restore natural resources. However, the Court allowed an exception to this goal when the costs of restoration are grossly disproportionate to the benefits. This exception for grossly disproportionate costs has its foundation in economic efficiency. The NOAA rule should include such an exception to ensure that the lowest cost restoration alternative is not economically inefficient.

The possibility of grossly disproportionate costs is one of the shortcomings of service-to-service scaling using HEA. This approach yields no measure of the magnitude of the benefits generated by the restoration alternatives. It simply determines the number of acres (or other metric) required to compensate for the lost services. Thus, economic efficiency cannot be addressed using HEA.

Relationship between primary and compensatory restoration

To be economically efficient, primary and compensatory restoration actions should not be selected separately because of the interrelationship between those actions. Primary restoration actions are undertaken to shorten the return of services to baseline following an injury, so the extent of primary restoration actions will determine the length of time between the injury and the return to baseline. Compensatory restoration actions are intended to compensate for the loss in services during that time period. Primary restoration actions, therefore, have a direct impact on the magnitude of compensatory restoration required. Thus, it is important to evaluate both types of restoration activities as a combined decision, not in isolation.

---

[19] See *State of Ohio v. U.S. Department of the Interior*, 880 F.2d 432, at 445 fn.9 (D.C. Cir. 1989).

Table 2-2 provides a simplified example with 2 alternative combinations of primary and compensatory restoration alternatives and their respective costs. Suppose that each of these alternatives has been scaled to make the public whole. As shown in this example, primary restoration costs range from a low level of activity costing $100,000 to a high level of activity costing $1,500,000. The gain from the selecting the more intensive primary restoration alternative is to shorten the recovery period from 3 years to 1 year. Therefore, the lower cost primary restoration option would require a greater compensatory restoration effort because the period between the injury and full recovery is longer.

Table 2-2 Selection of restoration alternative based on primary and compensatory costs

Alternative	Description of alternative	Years to recovery	Primary restoration cost	Compensatory restoration cost	Total restoration cost
A	Low level of primary restoration and acquire substantial compensatory acreage	3	$100,000	$500,000	$600,000
B	High level of primary-restoration activity and acquire low compensatory acreage	1	$1,500,000	$100,000	$1,600,000

When evaluated separately, Alternative A has the lowest primary restoration cost, but Alternative B has the lowest compensatory restoration cost. Only by focusing on the total restoration cost can the most economically efficient alternative be selected. Specifically, a comparison of the total restoration cost shows that high level of primary restoration activity in Alternative B does not reduce compensatory restoration costs by enough to justify the selection of that alternative.

Efficiency and trade-offs between public and ecological services

The NOAA regulations provide for resource-to-resource, service-to-service, and valuation scaling to be used in determining the size of the compensatory restoration projects. However, these 3 general approaches provide different kinds of information for use in selection. If we have information on people's willingness to trade off one type of service for another, then it may be possible to reach a more economically efficient restoration decision.

To help illustrate this point, Table 2-3 shows a simplified example with the costs of 3 restoration alternatives, each providing different levels of recreational fishing, brackish marsh habitat, and freshwater marsh habitat. The 3 options presented in Table 2-3 represent restoration alternatives at 3 distinct locations, each with different technical

Table 2-3 Use of trade-off information in evaluating restoration alternatives

		Gains from restoration alternatives		
Types of services	Interim losses	A	B	C
Recreational fishing (angling days)	1,000	1,000	1,000	500
Brackish marsh (acre-years)	100	100	50	125
Freshwater marsh (acre-years)	20	20	200	50
Cost ($)	—	$1,500,000	$1,000,000	$750,000

constraints and cost structures. This table also shows the scale of the interim losses that need to be offset with the restoration alternatives. Assume that all 3 alternatives have been appropriately scaled to provide the same level of utility (i.e., to make the public whole).

In this example, Alternative A would represent the outcome associated with service-to-service scaling because it provides for the same amount of each type of service that is lost.[20] As shown, this alternative is also the most expensive of the 3. The other 2 alternatives represent more cost-effective ways to make the public whole with restoration actions. However, this comparison requires information on preferences across the different services. For example, Alternative B requires information on people's willingness to trade off brackish marsh services for freshwater marsh services. Alternative B provides one-half the amount of brackish marsh that is lost but 10 times the amount of freshwater marsh, implying that the public is willing to trade a decrease of 50 brackish marsh acre-years for an increase in 180 freshwater marsh acre-years. With this information, restoration would be achieved at a cost saving of $500,000 over the service-to-service scaling approach.

Alternative C further broadens the role of the potential use of trade-off information. In this alternative, information is needed on people's willingness to trade among recreational fishing, freshwater marsh, and brackish marsh services. Specifically, this alternative shows that both types of marshes could be increased relative to the interim losses, but with a decrease of 500 fishing days. If such a combination of services provides the same level of utility as Alternatives A or B, then restoration costs would be reduced another $250,000. Of course, the assessment of efficiency would also require that the various transaction costs associated with the different scaling methods be factored into the evaluation. In addition, the costs of these actions must be compared with the value of the benefits generated.

The feasibility of obtaining trade-off information across public and ecological services is uncertain. The psychological literature has shown that people have difficulty making

[20] In this simplified example, we assume the loss time period and the gain time period are the same to avoid the need for discounting. This assumption is a convenience for ease of exposition and does not change the results.

trade-offs between dramatically different goods (Tetlock et al. 1996). This difficulty may mean that a conjoint survey asking for trade-offs across recreation and habitat services, for example, may be too difficult for respondents.

In addition, we have found that biologists, working for either the responsible parties or the trustees, have been unwilling to obtain or use such trade-off information. They are concerned that the general public does not possess the level of understanding about biological processes that is needed to make such trade-offs. This situation has led to the separate evaluation of ecological and public services. As shown in Table 2-3, this separation may lead to less efficient restoration decisions.

An alternative approach that may ease the concerns of biologists would be to have them develop several restoration alternatives that would be biologically equivalent. Then, in a conjoint setting, respondents could evaluate these equivalent alternatives to determine the most preferred combination. Public services would have to be included in order to obtain trade-offs across public and ecological services.

An additional use of trade-off information across various types of services comes in the presentation of the selected restoration alternatives to the public. The NOAA regulations require that public input be obtained on the restoration plan. By collecting information from the public about their preferences, we could show how their input from a conjoint study was used in developing the restoration alternatives included in the plan. Thus, the trade-off information collected from the public could be used both to structure the restoration plan and to justify that plan.

Implications

The NOAA regulations have fundamentally altered the NRDA process by focusing attention on the restoration of resource services. Unfortunately, the regulations also call for restoring resources and services, which is not consistent with economic principles. In addition, the regulations have shifted attention away from the divisive issue of measuring the value of nonuse services and brought more attention to restoring habitats and public use services. They also have suggested the use of methods, such as conjoint analysis and HEA, that offer promise under certain circumstances. Whether these circumstances will prove to be general enough for widespread use in damage assessment is an open issue. The ultimate reliability of these methods for use in damage assessment also remains to be seen. Little will be gained if the divisive CV issue is replaced by new controversies over the reliability of HEA or conjoint analysis. The lack of a guidance document that addresses the reliability of scaling further compounds the uncertainty.

In addition, NOAA has failed to base these new regulations on a firm economic foundation. This paper has developed an economic framework for the new NOAA approach to damage assessment. The key component of this framework is the use of utility as a common metric for evaluating losses and gains. By focusing on the utility lost as the result of an injury and the utility gained from restoration actions (primary and compensatory), the scaling of both public and ecological services can be achieved within a consistent structure. It also provides a basis for assessing the reliability of scaling methods.

Finally, to be consistent with economic efficiency, the compensation of utility losses should be achieved by expending the fewest resources possible. With this concept in mind, the differences between the old DOI approach, the new NOAA approach, and an approach consistent with economic theory are clear. The DOI approach required compensation to take the form of a payment to the trustees equal to the dollar value of the lost services. With NOAA's compensatory restoration requirement, compensation becomes the cost of in-kind replacement. From an economic perspective, compensation should take the form that requires the commitment of the fewest resources. Depending on the situation, efficient compensation could be in-kind replacement of exactly the services lost, in-kind replacement of different services generating the same level of utility, or payment of a sufficient amount of money to offset the utility loss.

References

Adamowicz W, Louviere J, Williams M. 1994. Combining revealed and stated preference methods for valuing environmental amenities. *Journal of Environmental Economics and Management* 26:271–292.

Desvousges WH. 1996. Rebuttal report on potential economic losses associated with groundwater. Expert report prepared for Holland and Hart in the matter of *State of Montana v. Atlantic Richfield Co.* in the U.S. District Court, District of Montana, Helena Division. Case No. CV-83-317-HLN-PGH.

Desvousges WH, Mathews KE, Dunford RW, Russell RR, James HL. 1995. Comments on NOAA's proposed NRDA rule under the Oil Pollution Act. Report submitted to the National Oceanic and Atmospheric Administration, Silver Spring MD. Durham NC: Triangle Economic Research.

Duffield JW. 1995. Revised report and rebuttal: assessment of damages to groundwater and literature review of water use values in the Upper Clark Fork River Drainage. Report prepared for the State of Montana Natural Resource Damage Program. Missoula MT: Bioeconomics, Inc.

Eckstein O. 1961. A survey of the theory of public expenditures criteria. In: National bureau of economic research, public finances: needs, sources, and utilization. Princeton NJ: Princeton Univ.

Hausman JA. 1993. Contingent valuation: a critical assessment. Amsterdam, The Netherlands: Elsevier.

Hensher DA, Bradley M. 1993. Using stated response choice data to enrich revealed preference discrete choice models. *Marketing Letters* 4(2):139–151.

Kopp RJ, Smith VK. 1993. Valuing natural assets: the economics of natural resource damage assessment. Washington DC: Resources for the Future.

McConnell KE. 1986. The damages to recreational activities from PCBs in New Bedford Harbor. Cambridge MA: Industrial Economics, Inc.

Swaite J, Louviere JJ, Williams M. 1994. A sequential approach to exploiting the combined strengths of SP and RP data: application to freight shipper choice. *Transportation* 21:135–152.

Tetlock PE, Peterson RS, Lerner JS. 1996. Revising the value-pluralism model. In: Seligman C, Olson JM, Zanna MP, editors. The Ontario symposium: the psychology of values. Mahwah NJ: Lawrence Erlbaum Associates.

Unsworth RE, Bishop RC. 1994. Assessing natural resource damages using environmental annuities. *Ecological Economics* 11:35–41.

Wisconsin Department of Natural Resources and Wisconsin Division of Health. 1994. Health guide for people who eat sport fish from Wisconsin waters. Publication number IE-019 4/94REV. April.

2a

Discussion Paper I on Scaling and Selecting Compensatory Restoration Projects: An Economic Perspective

*Raymond J. Kopp**

Desvousges, Fries, Hudson, and Dunsford attempt to place the rules for natural resource damages assessments conducted under the Oil Pollution Act of 1990 (OPA) and promulgated by the National Oceanic and Atmospheric Administration (NOAA) (61 *Federal Register* 4, 439–510) within an economic context that is based broadly on microeconomic utility theory. Given the nature of the rules, this is a nontrivial task.

The authors state that the paper makes 2 important contributions. First it provides the conceptual framework with which to view the NOAA rules, and second it provides the context for selecting the most economically efficient projects. They do provide a conceptual basis for viewing the NOAA rules, but they provide a very particular view—the appropriateness of which can be argued. With respect to the choice of economically efficient projects, I think the authors are in error.

Here, I concentrate on those areas of the paper with which I disagree and generally skip over most of the paper with which I do agree. I have ordered my comments using the same headings and subheadings as the paper.

Role of utility in NRDAs

The authors set out the economic context for their arguments and state, "The economic concept of utility provides the necessary organizational construct. Utility is defined as the satisfaction that people receive from using a commodity or engaging in an activity."

This is an extremely restrictive definition of utility, and it leaves the false impression that utility is not dependent upon a vast array of other things as well. One might conjecture that this definition is proposed so that utility losses associated with nonuse value or passive uses of injured resources may be ignored.

If the utility of individuals is negatively impacted by natural resource injuries, then the compensation required is the value of that utility loss, and the cost of providing that compensation is the damages in a natural resource damages suit. There is little to argue with here, but the authors state, "From an economic perspective, therefore, a

*Resources for the Future, Washington, DC

hazardous substance release or oil spill has to result in a loss in utility in order for there to be damages."

This is a dangerous and much too sweeping statement. As an illustration, one of the things my utility depends on is the knowledge that marine wildlife is not being harmed by human activity. Now suppose that a large spill of oil occurs and it causes the deaths of 10,000 sea birds off the California coast. By some strange turn of events the spill is not reported and only the folks who watch the birds notice they are gone. I assume all is right with the world and therefore suffer no loss of utility while in my ignorant state. Are the only damages those associated with the utility losses suffered by the bird watchers?

There is another interesting twist to this same statement by the authors and that has to do with some general guidance provided in the rule regarding restoration actions:

> Trustees must consider a reasonable range of restoration alternatives before selecting their preferred alternative(s). Each restoration alternative is comprised of primary and/or compensatory restoration components that address one or more specific injury(ies) associated with the incident. Each alternative must be designed so that, as a package of one or more actions, the alternative would make *the environment and public whole* (emphasis added). (61 *Federal Register* 4, 507; §990.53 [a]).

This statement, that restoration alternatives should be designed to make the environment and public whole, could be construed as saying that a compensatory restoration should not only compensate the public for interim losses of utility, but should also compensate the environment (other natural resources) for losses in services provided to it. I do not think this is what is meant by the statement, but I do think the statement is quite ambiguous on this point. If it is NOAA's intention to provide a compensatory restoration for interim service losses from one resource to another, than damages can result in the absence of human utility losses.

Utility's relationship to demand

The authors discuss how the notion of a demand curve (a relationship between the price of a good or service and the quantity of that good or service an individual or household would choose to consume) is derived from the concept of utility. They then suggest how the use of demand curves and the estimation of consumer's surplus lie at the heart of economic valuation.

The relationship between utility and demand is not at issue here, rather I simply want to remark on the limitations of traditional demand analysis applied to the services of natural resources as a means of quantifying damages. Specifically, a demand relationship is predicated on the existence of a well-defined quantity measure for the service in question and a well-defined price per unit of that service. In the case of marketed, private goods and services, the price and quantity components are in general readily available (although not always). However, in the case of non-market public goods, the quantity definition can be quite problematic, and without a good quantity measure, it is not possible to have a well-defined price.

Often, when we speak about the degradation in the services provided by a natural resource we describe quite specifically the state of the resource and its services in the injured and baseline state. However, we may not be able to formulate the service reductions in terms of a quantity measure that is meaningful for demand analysis. This is not to say that we should not try to do so, only that it may be more difficult than we would like.

Finally, it is important to repeatedly point out a well-known fact that is increasingly becoming popular to overlook: the traditional demand analyses based solely on observed human behavior cannot capture nonuse value losses due to a natural resource injury.

Scaling methods

Stated-preference models

Contingent valuation and conjoint analysis

The authors' summary of the usefulness of stated-preference valuation approaches to the problem of scaling restoration includes their standard criticism of CV. This criticism states that "CV has many well-documented problems, especially when it is used to measure nonuse values, that stem from its hypothetical nature." Support for this statement is always the same, i.e., the book edited by Jerry Hausman that contains research bought and paid for by the Exxon Corporation as part of its defense in the *Exxon Valdez* oil spill litigation (Hausman 1993). However, there is now a second citation: the report of the panel of experts convened by NOAA to inform the agency as to the reliability of CV for the assessment of nonuse losses in the case of oil spills.

If CV studies followed a set of protocols and procedures suggested by the panel and passed an economic consistency test, now known as a scope test, the report to NOAA states:

> Thus, the Panel concludes that CV studies can produce estimates reliable enough to be the starting point of a judicial process of damage assessment, including lost passive-use values (Arrow et al. 1993, p. 4610).

My judgment on the reliability of CV as a tool for the measurement of economic value parallels that of the NOAA panel and therefore runs counter to the opinions expressed by the authors.

The authors further argue that CV is just not a very useful tool for scaling as envisioned in the OPA rule. They state that the compensatory restoration programs need to be known before the survey is designed and that prohibitively large numbers of respondents are needed since they assume that only one restoration program will be valued at a time.

I do not agree with the authors. If nonuse values are to be considered in setting the level of a compensatory restoration program, then one must first estimate the size of the economic loss (comprised of lost use and nonuse value) so that one has some idea of the "value target" the compensatory restoration program is designed to hit. Contingency valuation is the only valuation tool that has been applied to this task in an actual damage assessment and is a tool whose reliability has been rigorously assessed. The authors argue that conjoint analysis (another stated-preference technique) is better suited to the scaling task than is CV, but to my knowledge, conjoint analysis has never been applied in a damage assessment context where nonuse values are present. Conjoint analysis has not been subject to any level of scrutiny that can be compared meaningfully to the scrutiny of CV.

More problematic for the use of conjoint analysis in damage assessment in the context of litigation is the fairly restrictive assumptions that one must make to map the choices people make in a conjoint experiment to statements about that individual's magnetized utility levels associated with those choices Louviere 1988; Desvousges et al. 1996). These assumptions regarding the form of the utility function, the heterogeneity of preference, the marginal utility of income, the relationship between expressed ranks and cardinal utility, to name just a few, are made on a largely ad hoc basis and are unnecessary when using CV.

Using conjoint techniques to simply rank alternative compensatory restoration programs can prove to be quite useful and can be done without imposing the assumptions noted above. However, in this context one still needs to use a monetary valuation tool like CV to set the scale.

Service-equivalency models: HEA

The apparent attraction of the service-to-service compensation approach is its claim of simplicity—a simplicity that is gained by avoiding all economic valuation of the losses caused by the natural resource injuries or the benefits to be gained through the restoration programs. I am in general agreement with the authors that the set of circumstances that must be obtained for the service-to-service approach be appropriate (that is compensate the public for the losses, while not overcompensating) is so restrictive that the circumstances are likely to be met rarely. Thus in general, one can expect the service-to-service approach to over- or undercompensate the public.

There are 2 other points worth noting. First, service-equivalency models do not adequately capture nonuse values. For example, suppose 10,000 bird deaths occur due to an oil spill and thus reduce a specific colony of these birds by 10,000. Now suppose that we have become very good at breeding and replacing birds and can restock the colony to baseline levels in a few years at low cost. Does that imply that a low-cost bird restocking operation compensates the public for the utility losses suffered by the animal deaths? That is, is the process of breeding and replacing 10,000 birds equivalent in the eye of the public to killing 10,000 birds? In other words, would the public have no preference between 2 programs in which the first would prevent 10,000 birds from being killed by an oil spill and the second would let the birds be killed but would put in place a breeding and replacement program? My guess is that the public would *not* be indifferent and would place a greater significance on the birds' deaths than on the simple replacement cost. If my conjecture were correct, the service-equivalency approach would undercompensate the public for its losses.

The second point has been raised by the authors. The service-equivalency approach never measures the value of the loss, therefore we never know how important the loss was to society. Moreover, it never measures the value of the restoration activities; and therefore, we never know how much value we got for our dollar. By measuring neither the costs of the injuries to society, nor the benefits to be gained by the restoration, it is impossible to assess whether the damages paid by the responsible party are in any sense reasonable.

Implications

The authors state 4 implications of the analysis presented in the paper. First, they argue that the regulations call for the restoration of services in a manner that is not consistent with economic theory. I do not believe this to be entirely true, but the ambiguous nature of the guidance provided by the rules leaves that question open.

Second, the authors claim that the new OPA rules have "shifted attention away from the value of nonuse services." I too believe the rules have shifted attention, but that is not to imply that the rules ignore nonuse value losses. With respect to the compensatory restoration, the rules state that

> To the extent practicable, when evaluating compensatory restoration actions, trustees must consider compensatory restoration actions that provide services of the same type and quality, and of comparable value as those injured. If, in the judgment of the trustees, compensatory actions of the same type and quality and comparable value cannot provide a reasonable range of alternatives, trustees should identify actions that provide natural resources and services of comparable type and quality as those provided by the injured natural resources. Where the injured and replacement natural resources and services are not of comparable value, the scaling process will involve valuation of lost and replacement services (61 *Federal Register* 4, p. 507; §990.53 [c][2][2]).

The term value used in the discussion of compensatory restoration actions is defined as

> Value means the maximum amount of goods, services, or money an individual is willing to give up to obtain a specific good or service, or the minimum amount of goods, services, or money an individual is willing to accept to forgo a specific good or service. The total value of a

> natural resource or service includes the value individuals derive from direct use of the natural resource, for example, swimming, boating, hunting, or bird watching, *as well as the value individuals derive from knowing a natural resource will be available for future generations* (emphasis added). (61 *Federal Register* 4, p. 505; §990.30).

The phrasing "value individuals derive from knowing a natural resource will be available for future generations" suggests to me that lost nonuse values are still on the table.

Third, the authors state that their paper has laid the correct foundation for the interpretation of the new rules and that foundation rests on utility theory. As long as one interprets utility broadly, I do not think there is much to quarrel with here. However, the authors then go on to state that ". . . the scaling of both public and ecological services can be achieved within a consistent structure." This is true if the scaling techniques are the well-known and applied techniques of CV, random utility travel-cost models, and hedonic pricing, but it is not clear whether this statement pertains to conjoint analysis and service-to-service approaches. The service-to-service approach is decidedly problematic. The ability of conjoint analysis to retrieve from choices utility measures that can be defined as willingness-to-pay for compensatory restoration programs has yet to be demonstrated to my satisfaction.

Finally, the authors state that "efficient compensation could be in-kind replacement of exactly the services lost, in-kind replacement of different services generating the same level of utility, *or a payment of a sufficient amount of money to offset the utility loss* (emphasis added)." One must quarrel with the last of these 3 forms of compensation. If one determines that a beach closed due to an oil spill led to a recreational loss of $20 million, but that the most cost-effective compensatory restoration program would cost $30 million, a payment of $20 million by the responsible parties would not compensate the public because the payment cannot be made to the individuals suffering the loss. In this case a "payment of a sufficient amount of money to offset the utility loss," made payable to the trustees and in a form that can only be spent on compensatory restoration programs will not be an efficient form of compensation since it will in fact not be sufficient to compensate the public under the OPA statute.

References

Arrow K, Solow R, Portney PR, Leamer EE, Radner R, Schuman H. 1993. Report of the NOAA panel on contingent valuation. *Federal Register* 58(10):4601–4614.

Desvousges WH, Johnson FR, Hudson SP, Gable AR, Ruby MC. 1996. Using conjoint analysis and health-state classifications to estimate the value of health affects of air pollution. Final Report to Environment Canada, Health Canada, Ontario Hydro, Ontario Ministry of Environment and Energy and the Quebec Ministry of the Environment, Triangle Economic Research, Durham NC.

Hausman JA. 1993. Contingent valuation: a critical assessment. Amsterdam, The Netherlands: Elsevier.

Louviere JJ. 1988. Analyzing decision making: metric conjoint analysis. London, UK: Sage.

2b

Discussion Paper 2 on Scaling and Selecting Compensatory Restoration Projects: An Economic Perspective

*James R. Bieke**

We discussed the paper presented by William H. Desvousges and colleagues from Triangle Economic Research entitled "Scaling and Selecting Compensatory Restoration Projects: An Economic Perspective." They present an overview of the approach embodied in the current natural resource damage (NRD) assessment regulations of the National Oceanic and Atmospheric Administration (NOAA), describe a number of challenges and problems in that approach from an economic standpoint, and present a conceptual framework for a revised approach in an effort to make NRD assessment more consistent with economic theory.

Unlike some of the broader proposals for NRD reform, such as that embodied in Professor Richard Stewart's paper in this volume, the authors assume that the current distinction between primary and compensatory restoration will be maintained. Within that context, the authors offer an economic perspective on NRD assessment, including the determination of what resource injury should be compensable in NRD and the scaling and selection of both primary and compensatory restoration actions, with particular emphasis on the latter.

Here we discuss some of the key points addressed by the authors, including the critical role of services in NRD assessment, the defects in NOAA's approach, and the key components in the authors' revised approach. It then evaluates the authors' approach, identifies a number of issues and challenges in implementing that approach, and makes some suggestions for addressing those issues. Here, we assume that NRD will consist of both primary and compensatory restoration.

Critical role of services in NRD assessment

The authors begin by quoting NOAA's statement that the goal of NRD assessment under the Oil Pollution Act (OPA) is "to make the environment and public whole" for injuries to natural resources (61 *Federal Register* 440). This statement is correct only if "the environment" is included in this goal not as an end in itself but because the environment provides value to society, since ultimately the purpose of our environ-

---

*Shea & Gardner, Washington, DC

mental laws is to protect and benefit human society. It is misleading to speak of making the environment whole as if that were a separate and distinct objective from making the public whole. Rather, the environment is relevant only to the extent it affects the public, and it is to be made whole under OPA only to the extent that doing so contributes to making the public whole. The same is true of NRD assessment under the Comprehensive Environmental Response, Compensation, and Liability Act (CERCLA).

Given this premise, it is clear that NRD must be tied to the loss of something of value to the public and must be designed to compensate the public for that loss. As noted by the authors and recognized by economists generally, the value of natural resources to the public derives not from the physical, chemical, and biological properties per se, but from the services that the natural resources provide. Accordingly, a change in a resource harms society and thus results in a compensable loss, only to the extent that it reduces the services provided by the resource. By the same token, once the services provided by the injured resources are returned to their baseline level, with any additional compensation to the public for services lost in the interim, society is fully compensated for its loss (i.e., made whole), and the goal of OPA and CERCLA is satisfied.

Moreover, given the objective of NRD, this focus on services must relate to services that are provided to the public, either directly or indirectly. As stated by A. Myrick Freeman, ecological functions "do not have economic value unless they help to support service flows to people," and thus "the key to valuing a change in an ecosystem function is establishing the link between that function and some service flow valued by people" (Freeman 1995).

NOAA regulations

The current NOAA regulations do not consistently implement the above principles. Unlike the regulations of the Department of the Interior (DOI) under CERCLA, NOAA's regulations do not require trustees to demonstrate any reduction in resource services in order to claim NRD; indeed, they explicitly allow trustees to quantify injuries without regard to a reduction in services (15 C.F.R. §§990.51, 990.52.[1] Furthermore, again unlike DOI's regulations, NOAA's regulations do not require trustees to formulate and evaluate primary restoration actions in terms of returning the resources' services to a baseline level, and in fact they require such actions to restore both the resources and their services (C.F.R. §990.53[b]).[2]

---

[1]By contrast, DOI's regulations explicitly require trustees to quantify a reduction in the resource services before NRD may be assessed (43 C.F.R. §11.71).

[2]By contrast, DOI's regulations, as interpreted in *Kennecott Utah Copper Corp. v. Dept. of the Interior,* 88 F.3d 1191, 1220 (D.C. Cir. 1996), require trustees to measure restoration of the injured resources by reference to the level of services provided. See 59 *Federal Register* 14262, 14272 (25 March 1994).

As the authors observe, NOAA's new compensatory restoration approach *is* based on replacing service losses with equivalent service gains. While that is appropriate in theory, the authors point out certain respects in which NOAA's approach "lacks the proper economic foundation for evaluating these service losses and gains." First, the authors discuss the various available economic techniques referenced by NOAA as methods for scaling compensatory restoration alternatives and explain that the traditional economic methodologies for quantifying and valuing service losses are not well-suited for measuring service gains. It also describes the significant limitations of newer methods, such as habitat equivalency analysis (HEA), for this scaling exercise. In addition, the authors point out that NOAA's tiered scaling approach involving resource-to-resource scaling, service-to-service scaling, and then valuation scaling is problematic in that these general approaches provide different kinds of information, and thus NOAA's approach does not allow for consideration of peoples' willingness to trade off one type of services for another—especially between direct human-use services and ecological services.

Once a range of primary and compensatory restoration alternatives are identified, NOAA's regulations require that they be evaluated based on a number of listed factors (at a minimum) and that the trustees select the "preferred" alternatives (15 C.F.R. §990.54). As the authors explain, this selection process is not based on sound economic principles, since it does not ensure the selection of the most cost-effective and economically efficient means of achieving the statutory goal of making the public whole.

The authors' approach

The authors' suggested conceptual framework is based on the concept of "utility," which it defines as "the satisfaction that people receive from using a commodity or engaging in an activity". Although this definition refers in terms to direct human uses and activities, it presumably also applies, in theory, to any services provided by a resource that are valued by people and from which people derive satisfaction.[3]

Under the authors' framework, a release must result in a loss in utility in order for there to be NRD. Thus, there must be a chin of linkages from the release to resource injury to a loss in services and then to a loss in utility. If this chain is broken, no NRDs are recoverable. Similarly, under the authors' framework, both primary and compensatory restoration must be based on a gain in utility, through a chain of linkages from the restoration action to resource enhancement to a gain in services and then to a gain in utility.

[3]However, to the extent that this definition applies to non-direct-human-use services, the authors would no doubt agree that such services may be included in NRD assessments only if they are actually impaired by a release and if their utility to the public can be reliably measured. At the present time, as discussed below, there is no available method that can provide a reliable measurement of the utility of nonuse services.

To implement this approach, it is necessary to quantify both losses and gains in services and utility and to estimate their equivalence. As the authors discuss, this first requires an accurate and reliable determination of baseline services (i.e., those that would exist in the absence of the injury), which is often very difficult, particularly in the case of historical releases that occurred decades ago. It is even more difficult to reliably quantify service and utility losses and gains. This is particularly true if, as the authors believe, the methods used should allow for trade-offs among different services that provide the same level of utility. Thus, the authors describe the limitations and deficiencies of traditional economic valuation methods for this task. It also points out the limited usefulness of HEA, since HEA necessarily depends on a number of strict assumptions (e.g., that the lost and replacement services are of the same type and quality, have the same unit value, and are subject to comparable demand and supply conditions) that will seldom hold true, especially in complex ecosystems, and since HEA thus does not allow for trade-offs among different types of services.

Basically, the authors' suggested techniques for making the necessary evaluations under its framework come down to two—random utility models (RUMs) and conjoint analysis. It notes that RUMs are well-suited for valuing different bundles of site characteristics for users and for evaluating users' trade-offs among such characteristics. However, this technique is still limited to evaluating recreational services and cannot assess trade-offs between direct human use and ecological services. For the latter task, which TER views as important, the only technique it identifies is conjoint analysis. Yet TER recognizes that conjoint analysis has not been used for this purpose, and that such use may not be feasible, given people's difficulties in making trade-offs between dramatically different goods.

Finally, in discussing the selection of restoration alternatives, the authors recommend consideration of both primary and compensatory restoration measures in combination due to their interrelationship. Assuming that all such combinations have been scaled to provide the same level of utility (i.e., to make the public whole), the authors generally recommend selection of the most cost-effective feasible combination (i.e., the least costly) to achieve that goal. However, it would add a proviso that if the most cost-effective restoration combination would still involve costs that are substantially greater than its benefits (i.e., the value of the services provided), then selection of that combination would not be economically efficient and should not be the basis of NRD. Rather, in that case, NRD should simply consist of the monetary value of the lost services. The authors thus conclude: "From an economic perspective, compensation should take whatever form requires commitment of the fewest resources. Depending on the situation, efficient compensation could be in-kind replacement of exactly the services lost, in-kind replacement of different services generating the same level of utility, or payment of a sufficient amount of money to offset the utility loss."

Comments on the authors' approach

From a conceptual and economic viewpoint and given the current statutory provisions, the authors' approach based on utility is a generally sound framework for assessing NRDs.[4] However, it raises a number of issues and challenges that must be addressed before such an approach could be implemented.

First, as discussed above and as the authors recognize, it is critical that, before NRDs are assessed, trustees must establish a reduction in the services provided by the injured resources to the public. Otherwise, society has suffered no loss in value that is compensable in NRD. The addition of a requirement to establish linkages between the injury, a service loss, and a utility loss, as suggested by the authors, is a useful way to implement that principle. Alternatively, the relevant regulations could require quantification of a reduction in services (as DOI's regulations currently do) and could define services to incorporate the concept of utility. For example, services could be defined as functions performed by a natural resource for the public, either directly or by performing functions for other natural resources that are used or valued by the public.[5]

Similarly, restoration should be measured by the level of services provided to the public. To achieve this goal, the authors suggest use of required linkages between the restoration actions and a gain in services and utility, and they further suggest that the evaluation of the link between services and utility take account of the public's trade-offs between different kinds of services that provide the same level of utility. On a conceptual basis, this approach seems appropriate. As the authors recognize, however, there are significant difficulties in quantifying the gains in services and utility provided by various restoration/replacement alternatives and comparing those gains to losses in services and utility—especially if trade-offs among services are to be taken into account.

For primary restoration, an exercise involving such trade-offs may be unduly complicated, particularly given the Court's holding in *Ohio v. Dept. of the Interior*, 880 F.2d 432, 449, 459 (D.C. Cir. 1989), that such restoration is to be the primary measure of NRD. Hence, primary restoration should be defined simply as actions that return the resource services (as defined above) to the baseline level, through active on-site restoration, natural recovery, replacement, and/or acquisition of alternative resources or services, as appropriate.

---

[4]Looking at the issue from a broader perspective, attention should be paid to the more expansive proposals for NRD reform, such as that suggested by Professor Stewart.

[5]Under such a definition, a change in ecological functions that affect only individual or certain lower-level biotic organisms but would have no adverse impact on the wildlife population or community or the overall functioning of the ecosystem would not serve as a proper basis for NRD because it would not affect what is valued by society—i.e., the continued maintenance of a wildlife population or community or a sustainable ecosystem (see, e.g., Suter and Barnthouse 1993; McFadden 1995).

For compensatory restoration, it makes sense and is consistent with the statutory basis for such restoration (interim diminution in value) to try to implement the authors' approach, including the concept of trade-offs among services that provide the same level of utility. The difficulty here lies in determining what compensatory restoration actions provide the same level of utility as the interim loss in utility, considering trade-offs. While RUMs allow such an evaluation among similar recreational services, the only method identified by the authors for evaluating trade-offs between different kinds of services (e.g., direct human-use services and ecological services) is conjoint analysis. While this methodology appears to have promise for such an application, it has not been tested for reliability and validity for such use. Indeed, Paul Green, one of the developers of conjoint analysis, has pointed out a number of difficult issues that would be involved in applying conjoint analysis to natural resource services, and he has concluded that the reliability of conjoint analysis for this purpose is unknown (Green 1995). Thus, there is a critical need for research on the reliability of conjoint analysis for evaluating such trade-offs. At the present time, however, this technique has not been shown to be sufficiently reliable for evaluating natural resource services, particularly ecological or other non-direct-human-use services, as to warrant a rebuttable presumption. Given this fact, as well as the lack of demonstrated reliability of contingent valuation for measuring the value of nonuse services[6] and the very limited usefulness of HEA, nonuse services should not be included in the scaling of compensatory restoration alternatives. Rather, compensatory restoration alternatives should focus on direct human-use services, for which more reliable methods are available (e.g., RUMs) to evaluate various levels of the services and trade-offs among them.[7]

Finally, with regard to the selection of restoration measures, the general requirement recommended by the authors is proper. Thus, trustees should be required to select the mix of feasible primary and compensatory restoration actions that achieves the objective of making the public whole (i.e., returns resource services to the baseline level and compensates the public for services lost in the interim) in the most cost-effective manner.

However, the authors' proviso—that if the cost of such combination outweighs the value of the services provided, it should not be selected and instead NRD should consist of the monetary value of the lost services—while economically sound, raises certain problems for use in NRD assessment. To the extent that the authors mean that primary as well as compensatory restoration damages should be based on whatever form requires commitment of the fewest monetary resources—whether on-site

[6]See report of the expert panel appointed by NOAA to evaluate the reliability of CV. 58 *Federal Register* 4601 (15 Jan 1993).

[7]In many cases, in practice, a determination of strict equivalence in utility between such replacement services and the lost services may be unnecessarily complicated. Rather, responsible parties and trustees may agree on compensatory restoration projects that provide roughly similar or equivalent services to those lost without having to resort to economic studies to try to determine the precise value or equivalence of those services.

restoration, off-site replacement, *or monetary damages*—it is very close to the "lesser of" rule invalidated in *Ohio*. Hence, insofar as primary restoration is concerned (and assuming no statutory changes), the selection process should simply be based on the general cost-effectiveness criterion, so long as natural recovery, replacement, and acquisition of the equivalent are given equal consideration with active on-site restoration.

For compensatory restoration, the authors' proviso is proper in theory, but would involve the need to determine the value of the lost services—which would require use of the same expensive and controversial economic valuation methods used in the old compensable value approach, which the compensatory restoration approach is designed to avoid. Perhaps the best solution is simply to make clear that trustees may not select a compensatory restoration action whose cost would exceed the value of the interim lost services *if there is reliable evidence of such value*. Thus, if responsible parties (or the trustees themselves) have some question about whether a compensatory restoration alternative would meet this test, it would be up to them to develop reliable evidence on this issue.

Conclusion

The authors have made a valuable contribution to the consideration of an appropriate framework for scaling and selecting restoration projects in NRD. However, the above-discussed issues still need to be addressed and resolved in order for that framework to be implemented in practice.

References

Freeman III AM. 1995. On valuing the services and functions of ecosystems. Paper submitted to Science Advisory Board, U.S. Environmental Protection Agency.

Green PE. 1995. The role and limitations of conjoint analysis in the preference modeling of constructed markets. The Wharton School, University of Pennsylvania. Submitted to National Oceanic and Atmospheric Administration.

McFadden JT. 1995. Comments on Department of the Interior advance notice of proposed rule-making. Submitted to U.S. Dept. of the Interior.

Suter II GW, Barnthouse LW. 1993. Assessment concepts. In: Suter II GW, editor. Ecological risk assessment. Boca Raton FL: Lewis. p 21–47.

2c

Discussion Paper 3 on Scaling and Selecting Compensatory Restoration Projects: An Economic Perspective

*Wiktor Adamowicz**, *Joffre Swait*†

Desvousges, Fries, Hudson, and Dunford provide a very good basic overview of the economic issues involved in selecting compensatory restoration projects or employing "in-kind" resource compensation rather than monetary measures of compensation. They review the changes to the regulatory structure and provide clear and concise definitions of service gains and losses and the difference between traditional monetary valuation and the new compensatory restoration approach. The authors also provide a simple explanation of the economic theory that supports the compensatory restoration approach. The main body of the paper examines several issues involved in selecting compensatory restoration projects, but my focus is on the following: 1) determining baseline services, 2) economic methods for determining compensatory projects ("scaling approaches"[1]) 3) ecological methods for determining compensatory projects ("service equivalency models: HEA"), and 4) selection of restoration alternatives. I also comment on a few more technical aspects associated with determining compensatory projects particularly relating to the use of stated choice methods (SCMs) (choice experiments, conjoint tasks, etc.).

Compensatory restoration projects

The ability to compensate for damages via compensatory restoration projects is appealing for a number of reasons. As the authors mention, it may be possible to use resources more efficiently by finding a specific project or package of projects that compensates for the damages and costs less (in social cost terms) than any other project that also compensates for the damages. Thus, economically efficient compen-

*Department of Rural Economy, University of Alberta, Edmonton, Alberta, Canada

†Intelligent Marketing Systems Inc., Gainesville, FL

[1]The term "scaling" is used in different contexts. Scaling in the body of the text refers to the determination of the amount of a selected restoration project that compensates for the damages. For example, the restoration project may be construction of a boardwalk on a beach but scaling is required to determine the length of the boardwalk required. In contrast to this use of the work scaling, researchers in stated choice methods refer to the adjustment of models based on different data sources as scaling of data types.

sation may occur. Also, resource compensation (using resources/ecological services as "in-kind" compensation) may be more appealing to the public than the more traditional approach to compensation which employs public trust funds. It has been established in various studies that members of the public prefer in-kind compensation over monetary compensation—even though an economic argument would suggest that monetary compensation has the most flexibility and, all else being equal, should be the preferable option. Furthermore, it may be easier in some contexts to derive nonmonetary compensation as members of the general public often find it difficult to monetize environmental benefits.

However, a move to resource compensation brings with it a number of challenges. First and foremost among the difficulties with resource compensation is the fact that there are now a myriad of potential compensatory mechanisms. The problem becomes one of selecting the resource or ecological service (or combination of resource and ecological services) as well as the level of these resources. This dramatically complicates the problem. Compensating for damage at a particular site by improving a different site will have distributional (equity) implications.[2] Even if compensation is based on resources at the same site (in spatial terms), it is possible that the beneficiaries will differ from those who suffer the loss because the preferences of individuals benefitting from that site may differ. Furthermore, there is some question about how far removed from the original damaged ecological service the resource compensation can be. For example, compensation by enhancing public library facilities may be deemed by the trustees as inappropriate compensation for environmental damage (e.g., beach-use loss) even though it may be supported by the public as valid and efficient compensation. Thus, determination of the appropriate resource compensation will depend on the blending of the assessment of public preferences, the determination of "acceptable" projects by the trustees, and some judgment on the distribution of benefits of these resource compensation projects versus the original distribution of benefits. Note that the latter issue is particularly challenging because economic analysis typically describes only the distributional outcomes but does not offer comment on selection among projects with different distributional impacts.

A further complication in the determination of resource compensation is the fact that the losses and the proposed compensation schemes may have different temporal dimensions. For example, in order to compensate for 10 weeks of losses in recreational fishing, one may propose to construct a new boat launch site. However, the life of the boat launch will far exceed 10 weeks. Some form of standardization (e.g., boat-launch service days) will be required as will careful consideration of the discounting of future benefits and costs of these services. Calculation of a temporal stream of losses due to environmental damage in monetary terms is challenging, but this problem is made

---

[2]The fact that equity may become a significant issue in the determination of resource compensation suggests that consideration of "demand heterogeneity" (being able to assess different preferences across members of society) should be an integral component of the analysis.

even more complex by considering the possible range of future "in-kind" projects that make the public as well off as they were before the loss. Different temporal dimensions of losses (injury) versus gains may also affect the types of projects considered and limit them to small or limited time frame endeavors.

In general, the projects proposed as compensation will be "lumpy" either physically or temporally, and thus the optimum level of compensation will be difficult to determine. Slight overcompensation in these cases may be advisable if the compensatory project still costs less than the equivalent monetary compensation. The preference for in-kind compensation and the potential for goodwill benefits (to all parties) suggests that in cases of lumpy projects the upper bound may be preferred.

Determining baseline services

The authors discuss the importance of determining the baseline services and the importance of the use of the "with/without" framework. These points are fundamental to the construction of compensation measures. However, a significant challenge is the temporal dimensions of the injury and its impacts. In assessing the situation with the injury and without the injury over time, one must examine impacts on levels of use as well as participation. For example, in a recreational fishing context one must consider how levels of recreational use may have been affected plus whether individuals have stopped participating in recreational fishing as a result of the injury. This implies a time-series dimension to the problem that is seldom analyzed because of the lack of data and the cost of collection of such data. This temporal aspect also becomes a significant challenge when determining the appropriate compensation scheme, as described above. A potential approach to prepare for this challenge is to begin to collect panel data (time-series data for a set of households) on the use of natural resources. Parallel efforts exist in labor-force surveys and household-expenditure surveys.

Economic methods for determining compensatory projects ("scaling methods")

The authors discuss several economic methods for "scaling" restoration gains, specifically in cases in which activities or uses of resource have been affected (use values). They suggest that these methods are useful in determining the size or scale of a restoration project that will offset lost services. An additional important use of these techniques is the determination of the type of restoration project.

The authors list several economic approaches that have been used in determining the monetary value of environmental changes. Some of these methods will not be particularly useful in a direct resource compensation exercise. Averting-behavior models, for example, provide the monetary value associated with consumer purchases of goods that defend against environmental harm. However, since this method computes monetary values directly and does not compare services lost and gained, its use in resource compensation will be limited. Hedonic pricing methods may have applicability to the problem, however, as the authors mention these methods are limited to cases in which property values are affected and suffer from the fact that the environmental influences must be separated statistically from other influences on property values. Given market data on property transactions these influences are often difficult to separate. Also, these methods will require that the resource compensation scheme be one that has an impact on property values, and evaluation will be limited to those items that currently exist in the environment. For example, the construction of a new boardwalk cannot be considered if boardwalks do not currently exist at the site and/or if they do not appear to affect property values. Resource compensation schemes that are outside the set of goods/services currently available or whose impact on property values cannot be statistically evaluated cannot be included in the determination of resource compensation.

Traditional travel-cost models are somewhat limited in application because they do not employ varying characteristics. However, travel-cost models that determine the frequency of recreational activity (number of trips) are important elements of a compensation-determination exercise when combined with random utility models (RUMs). Random utility models seem to be the most appropriate method for the determination of resource compensation as they operate on attributes and thus can be used to construct resource-compensation schemes that provide utility to offset losses due to injury. However, RUMs using observed behavior often suffer from the fact that the existing market does not provide enough information to be able to uncover the underlying preferences for the important attributes. Furthermore, RUMs based on existing environmental attributes cannot be used to determine if new attributes (items that do not currently exist at the sites) constitute appropriate compensation. For these reasons several researchers are employing stated preference techniques based on hypothetical choices to augment or substitute for models based on actual choice behavior. Included among stated preference techniques are contingent valuation methods, conjoint methods, and SCMs.

Traditional contingent-valuation methods, since they rely on determining monetary compensation, are not directly applicable to resource-compensation assessment. These methods can be modified to assess the value of attributes of environmental amenities but these approaches are likely not the most efficient methods for the exploration of attribute values. Conjoint analysis in its traditional form uses individual ratings of choice alternatives. While this method is very popular in marketing applications, it requires specific assumptions and statistical analysis to translate the ratings-based outcomes into economic utility theoretic measures. Thus, the value of ratings-based conjoint in resource compensation is limited, especially when one considers that SCMs are available and do not have the limitations that traditional conjoint methods do.

Stated choice methods either alone or in combination with RUMs based on observed behavior may be the most useful methods for understanding individual preferences and determining resource compensation projects. These methods are designed to mimic the actual choice situation and yet provide information on preferences that may not be observable using actual market or behavioral data. Stated choice methods are based on random utility theory but they employ choices in constructed markets rather than actual markets. Stated choice methods are increasing in their application to environmental situations (Adamowicz et al. 1994; Boxall et al. 1996; Louviere 1996; Adamowicz et al. 1997) and are recognized for their flexibility and statistical efficiency. Furthermore, while SCMs have not been used a great deal in damage assessment cases, they are tools that have been used extensively in the market analysis branches of industry and thus should be very familiar to potentially responsible parties. Stated choice methods can be used in situations where new goods/services are being proposed, where the proposal is to offer levels of existing goods and services beyond what currently exists, and where current environmental/market structures are such that individual preferences over specific attributes cannot be identified. These methods rely on careful survey construction and statistical design to closely approximate actual choice environments while also examining situations that do not necessarily exist in today's environment.

The ideal situation for resource compensation involving use value injuries will likely include RUMs based on actual behavior combined with SCMs designed to examine compensation alternatives. Linked to this model of preferences over environmental attributes will be a set of ecological models outlining the changes in ecological services resulting from injury and restoration choices. While such an approach appears to be promising for examining cases in which use values are affected, there may also be promise for SCMs in cases where the restoration alternatives involve passive-use values (or values for restoration of habitats, etc. that do not involve activities or property values). I return to this topic in the section "Selection of restoration alternatives" below.

Ecological methods for determining compensatory projects ("service equivalency models: HEA")

The authors outline the use of habitat equivalency analysis (HEA) as an ecological method for resource compensation. This method has been discussed in several contexts ranging from ecological restoration discussions to analysis of "no-net-loss" policies. The authors clearly outline the assumptions involved in employing HEA as a compensation mechanism. As an elaboration of their discussion, consider the analysis by Watson et al. (1994) in which mitigation using HEA rules was examined for its economic efficiency properties. Watson et al. (1994) assessed the recreational fishing benefits in a case in which fish habitat was replaced on an HEA basis. The results showed that the recreational fishing benefits were significantly lower after the habitat replacement occurred (primarily because the habitat was replaced at sites that were difficult to access and had other detrimental attributes). Also, the cost of the habitat restoration was substantial given the benefits provided.

An additional caution regarding HEA methods is the complexity that the temporal dimension introduces. Given that the method is biological in nature, it is difficult to determine how service flows over time should be treated. For example, if the injury is 3 months of loss of a particular habitat's service flow, how should one compensate with ecological restoration that may exist for very long periods of time? Habitat equivalency analysis provides a useful starting point for restoration-compensation analysis but in order to completely assess the situation the addition of public preference information is crucial.

Selection of restoration alternatives

The authors conclude their paper with a discussion of the selection of restoration alternatives. They raise the issue of trade-offs between habitat restoration options including cases where use values and passive-use values are relevant to the analysis. For example, restoration may involve enhancing recreational fishing opportunities as well as improving ecological conditions at a separate habitat that provides no direct human use. In these situations, there may be several combinations of restoration alternatives that yield utility sufficient to repair the injury. The selection of the economically efficient alternative will involve an understanding of the trade-offs between these services as well as the costs of the restoration alternatives. Several points arise in this context.

First, the authors suggest that primary restoration not be separate in consideration from compensatory restoration. This is a useful recommendation as appropriate combinations of primary and compensatory restoration may provide adequate compensation at lower cost. Economies of scale in restoration activities or thresholds of costs for certain projects may lead to such efficiencies. Second, the authors suggest that compensatory activities be judged in light of the benefits that they yield relative to the cost of damage. The analysis of Watson et al. (1994) provides a useful example. The mitigation effort being examined in Watson et al. (1994) arose primarily because of a loss of $2M in recreational fishing benefits. The mitigation effort was expected to cost nearly $5M to replace the habitat. If there were no other benefits, this would not be an economically efficient restoration. *However, one must be confident that all benefits have been calculated to reach such a conclusion.* If other benefits, including passive-use benefits, are relevant, then these must be included in the economic efficiency calculation. Furthermore, the assessment of the economic efficiency of restoration alternatives in this context requires the determination of the monetary value of the injury, not just the restoration required to compensate "in-kind" for the injury. Thus, economic valuation methods that measure the monetary value of losses as well as the required restoration or resource compensation must be used when determining economically efficient, resource-compensation schemes.

The latter point suggests that an appropriate method for examination of restoration alternatives should be able to assess trade-offs between restoration options (or combinations of options) as well as the monetary value of damages. Since the range of restoration options includes passive-use values and since these types of choices are not made in market settings, some form of stated preference approach is required. Such a multi-attribute based evaluation is not possible in traditional contingent valuation experiments. Traditional conjoint analyses suffer from the difficulties discussed above regarding consistency with utility theory. Thus, SCMs appear to be the most appropriate tool for such evaluation.

The authors provide some interesting suggestions on how the public could evaluate ranges of restoration options, perhaps based on biological science assessments of potential options.[3] They also suggest that individuals often have difficulty in making trade-offs across widely different types of goods. However, SCMs seem to provide the best alternative for structuring choices, perhaps within a referendum context, in order to compare restoration options.[4] The challenges include incentive compatibility, assessment of preference heterogeneity, experimental design considerations (including task design, degree of complexity, and other considerations) as well as the typical sampling and surveying issues. Nevertheless, this seems to be the most promising avenue for practical application of resource compensation methods.

Conclusions

The movement toward in-kind compensation in cases of environmental injury opens up the possibility for more economically efficient and socially desirable compensation schemes. However, there are several significant challenges associated with this change in regulation including the increase in complexity of the compensation determination problem, the definition of the acceptable set of types of in-kind compensation, the examination of compensation on the distribution of benefits, and the development of mechanisms for measuring economically efficient compensation schemes. A further, significant, challenge will be to link rapidly developing economic methods with ecological service flow models. While the determination of resource compensation is a formidable task, the potential payoffs are high, and the recent developments of economic methods provide the tools necessary to take up the challenge.

References

Adamowicz W, Boxall P, Williams M, Louviere J. 1995. Stated preference approaches for measuring passive use values: choice experiments versus contingent valuation. Staff Paper, Department of Rural Economy, University of Alberta, Edmonton, Canada.

Adamowicz WL, Louviere J, Williams M. 1994. Combining stated and revealed preference methods for valuing environmental amenities. *J Environ Econ Manage* 26:271-292

[3] From a social science perspective, the challenge to social scientists and biological scientists is to inform and educate the public about the implications of various restoration options. Such an approach will lead to a better integrated system of compensation determination.

[4] Some researchers have begun to explore the use of SCMs in such contexts. See, for example, Adamowicz et al. 1995.

Adamowicz W, Swait J, Boxall P, Louviere J, Williams M. 1997. Perceptions versus objective measures of environmental quality in combined revealed and stated preference models of environmental valuation. *J Environ Econ Manage* 32:65–84.

Boxall P, Adamowicz W, Williams M, Swait J, Louviere J. 1996. A comparison of stated preference approaches to the measurement of environmental values. *Ecolog Econ* 18:243–253.

Louviere JJ. 1996. Relating stated preference measures and models to choices in real markets: calibration of CV responses. In: Bjornstad DJ, Kahn JR, editors. The contingent valuation of environmental resources. Brookfield MA: Edward Elgar. p 167–188.

Watson D, Adamowicz W, Boxall P. 1994. An economic analysis of recreational fishing and environmental quality changes in the Upper Oldman River Basin. *Canadian Water Resources Journal* 19:213–225.

2d

Discussion Paper 4 on Scaling and Selecting Compensatory Restoration Projects: An Economic Perspective

*Kevin A. Gaynor, Steven R. Johnson**

Alice in Wonderland is an exploration of the unreality of experience. For a potentially responsible party (PRP) facing substantial liability for natural resource damages (NRD), a natural resources damage assessment (NRDA) may seem very much like a trip through the looking glass. While Desvousges, Fries, Hudson, and Dunsford provide a new prism through which the evaluation of damages may be viewed, the paper suffers from the same inherent problem that plagues NRDAs under the National Oceanic and Atmospheric Administration (NOAA) and the U.S. Department of the Interior (DOI) regulations. It does not achieve a consensus on what the "truth" or "reality" is concerning the measure of damages. Like all models, the authors' economic model relies upon assumptions that are, to varying degrees, open to criticism. This susceptibility to criticism is the foundation of litigation.

The critique that follows comes from the perspective of an attorney representing a party alleged to have some or all responsibility for NRDs associated with an oil spill. Before turning to the specifics of the paper, however, it is important to understand the perspective of the PRP. The willingness of a PRP to pay for compensatory restoration projects is directly proportional to the obviousness of the nexus between the PRP's actions or inactions and the alleged damages and the cost of any primary or compensatory restoration projects. In the world of NRDs, the nexus is frequently in question.

Determining baseline conditions—the foundation of the damage calculus

A critical component of establishing the nexus between damages and the PRP is establishment of a baseline. The baseline provides the measure by which service gains and losses are measured and thus the measure of damages. As the authors demonstrate on page 12 of his paper, establishing the baseline is an extremely difficult exercise. Typically, there are no decent data to establish the environmental conditions that existed at a particular point in time that can be used to demonstrate clearly how the environment existed prior to the alleged activity of the PRP that supposedly was

*Kevin A. Gaynor is a partner at the law firm of Vinson & Elkins, L.L.P. Steven R. Johnson is an associate at the same firm. The authors would like to express their gratitude to Mary Jo Kealy at ENTRIX, Inc. for her insights.

the cause of the injury. In dealing with an oil spill that happened in a pristine ecosystem yesterday, it may be possible to have this kind of data, but with the passage of time and with multiple other sources that also could have contributed to injury, it becomes extraordinarily difficult to carry out this exercise. The more imprecise the baseline, the more room there is for the PRP and the trustees to disagree over the degree of the injury and the existence of damages. This makes NRD claims by trustees inherently controversial and likely to result in grave doubts by the PRP that an identifiable injury and damages occurred and, to the extent that they did occur, that the PRP has a significant connection to them.

Moreover, as the authors note, "[t]he first step in correctly establishing baseline is to recognize that baseline services must be examined in terms of 'with and without' the injury, rather than 'before and after' the injury." In the example they give of a release occurring in a pristine environment in 1940, the baseline assumes that one could establish that the environment was in fact pristine in 1940. But this is not possible because other factors unrelated to the release also contribute to the degradation of the environment. The factor they point to in their example is the construction of a highway and manufacturing facilities in the area which caused the previously pristine environment to become heavily industrialized over time. They state, "[a]s a result, the baseline levels of ecological and public services in the area decline over time, completely independent of the release." They continue and state, "[t]herefore, even though the resource was pristine before the release, we cannot assume that the relevant baseline condition is pristine. Because the baseline often is dynamic, its correct establishment must incorporate these types of intertemporal changes." They conclude that "there may be no time period in the past for which the highway existed without the injury, making the determination of baseline services difficult."

These authors continue, noting that an important step in establishing baseline services is to examine the link to the injury. They state

> Whatever the parameter that provides the link to the injury (e.g., fish-consumption advisories), it is important that the baseline level of that parameter be specified correctly. Correctly specifying the baseline level of other site characteristics also is essential. For example, suppose that a mercury release occurs at a lake. Though the lake had no advisories without the release, access to the lake was poor, and, therefore, the site had little recreation demand, even at baseline. Thus, the injury may not have caused a change in the services provided by the lake, breaking the chain to damages.

Their point is critical. There is frequently an assumption among regulators that where a release occurs there must be an injury, and where an injury occurs there must be damages. Depending on the quantity and value of services at baseline, this is not always the case. They correctly point out regarding damages that "[t]he linkages that result in damages should not be assumed. Even in the presence of injury, it is possible that no losses in utility, and thus no damages, have occurred."

Trustees, in examining whether to commence NRD actions, need to carefully examine each step of the chain from release to injury to damages from the perspective of the "appropriate" baseline. Only where this chain clearly exists should the trustees then look to whether a PRP could be liable.

Valuations of service and utility losses—are there damages?

The next step in the NRD calculation is the valuation of service losses and, for purposes of compensating those losses, the value of service gains. The authors' contribution to the NRD calculation is to value service losses and gains from the perspective of utility. However, they fail to provide a consistent and well-supported basis for measuring utility. The authors provide no model or measuring stick for achieving consensus on how to measure utility or to compare utility losses and gains by different people across the range of possible services. As a result, PRPs who face significant damage claims will have plenty of ammunition to challenge damage assessments on the basis of how service losses and gains are calculated. Moreover, the focus on utility as a unit of measure could conceivably result in the kinds of compensatory restoration projects that would be likely to antagonize PRPs and make reaching consensus extremely difficult. For example, because from a utility perspective it makes no difference which members of the public receive compensation, it could constitute efficient compensation for a natural resources injury in South Dakota for trustees to require a restoration project in New York. The further removed the restoration project is from the injury, however, the less obvious the nexus to the PRP and the more likely litigation will ensue.

At heart, the NRDA is an ethereal search for "truth" about service losses, where probably no truth exists. Will the calculation of utility losses aid in the search for this truth? This may not be so. There is no consensus on how to measure utility losses and gains and which losses and gains are relevant. As an example, take the authors' example involving an injury to a lake that results in a reduction in demand for fishing services because the quality of the fishing experience is reduced. According to the authors, this reduction in demand is a way to evaluate utility changes. However, the example highlights the problems inherent in the utility calculation. For example, the reduced demand at the lake may result in increased utility for the surrounding community which will experience less traffic to the lake, less congestion, less air pollution, and less of the kind of development (i.e., fast food restaurants) attracted to the flow of traffic. Similarly, those who continue to use the lake may experience significantly higher utility, albeit in less "pristine" conditions, because of the reduction in people using the lake.

The authors do not provide any guidelines for what utility losses and gains are to be measured and which are compensable. For example, are utility losses that derive from injuries to private properties considered in the damage calculus? Such utility losses may result directly from a release or they may result from behavioral changes by affected people. As in the example discussed above, if additional access to a lake is provided to compensate for service losses resulting from an injury to the lake, this access may result in injury to private property as more people travel to the site and place a strain on the surrounding community. How are these utility losses and gains to be measured? The broader the utility inquiry, the greater the scrutiny by PRPs and their experts. Models used to quantify utility losses and scale potential restoration gains are also ripe for attack by PRPs armed with alternative models and economic experts.

Is the PRP liable for these damages? A litigation perspective

An additional link in the chain concerns whether the potentially responsible party is liable. Even if a trustee can show a release, an injury, and damages, the PRP has the following defenses which a trustee must evaluate before involving the PRP in a NRD case. PRPs may claim that they are not liable because the release was caused by 1) an act of God; 2) an act of war; or 3) an act or omission of a third party. See 33 U.S.C. §2703(a) (OPA); 42 U.S.C, §9607 (b)(CERCLA). In addition, a PRP may dispute liability on the basis of a lack of causation, that a NRD claim is presented after the applicable statute of limitations, and that the trustees' claim exceeds the $50 million dollar limit of a PRP's liability for NRDs. See 33 U.S.C. §2717(1)(B); 42 U.S.C. §9607(c)(1)(D), 9612cx (d)(2). Finally, where there is injury to private property and the Trustee claims damages, the Trustee must demonstrate that the private property is managed by, controlled by, or appertaining to the United States, a state, political subdivision, or an Indian tribe. See 33 U.S.C. §2706 (a). Potentially responsible parties will often contest liability arguing that for damages to private property to be compensable such damages must be related to the government's management and control over the property. For example, where the government regulates private wetlands for dredging and filling purposes, any damages to the services provided by the wetland must be related to the government's regulation of it for purposes of dredging and filling. This is often a contentious issue that is highly dependent on facts.

Even if the Trustee can overcome these defenses, disputes concerning the determination of baseline, allegations of injury, nexus to the PRP, and alleged damages raise substantial issues of fact, as discussed above. The extent to which there are questions about the facts associated with the injury, the linkage of the injury to the PRP, and damages flowing from the injury, the Trustee can anticipate that a PRP will vigorously litigate any NRD claim.

These issues of fact will be dealt with in a complex litigation context whereby trustees will have to prove their case through a battery of experts that are susceptible to attack by the PRP. Each link in the chain leading to a PRP ultimately being adjudged liable for a certain amount of damages in a NRD case has to be defended by the Trustee to obtain damages. In many cases, the trustees' experts will have to rely on modeling to support their conclusions. Invariably, models are predicated upon assumptions that may or may not be valid and are always susceptible to attack and discredit in litigation.

In selecting compensatory restoration projects, it is imperative that trustees keep in mind the real potential for litigation in this area. To the extent the trustees approach compensatory restoration projects in a rational sense such that the PRP can readily understand the rationale behind a compensatory restoration project and the project is cost-effective, the PRP will be far more willing to reach an agreement with the trustees to either implement or pay for the project rather than litigate over the trustees' NRD claim.

With this in mind, we endorse the conclusions reached by the authors. They conclude:

> The NOAA regulations have fundamentally altered the NRDA process by focusing attention on the restoration of resource services. The regulations also have shifted away from the divisive issue of measuring the value of nonuse services and brought more attention to restoring habitats and public-use services. They have also suggested the use of methods, such as conjoint analysis and HEA, that offer promise under certain circumstances. However, NOAA has failed to base these regulations on a firm economic foundation.

In explaining to a client a trustee's NRD claim, it is far preferable to base the explanation on restoration of habitats and public-use services than it is on the more theoretical value of nonuse services, which the average decision-maker in corporate America cannot readily grasp from a common sense perspective. Nevertheless, as the authors point out, while the NOAA regulations are a step forward, they need to have a firm economic foundation.

How much compensation is reasonable?

To be consistent with the tenets of economic efficiency, the authors conclude that the compensation of utility losses should be achieved by spending the fewest resources possible. With this concept in mind, the differences between the old DOI approach, the new NOAA approach, and an approach consistent with economic theory are clear. The DOI approach required compensation to take the form of a payment to the trustees equal to the dollar value of the lost services. With NOAA's compensatory restoration requirement, compensation becomes the cost of in-kind replacement. From an economic perspective, compensation should take whatever form that requires the commitment of fewest resources. Depending upon the situation, efficient compensation could be in-kind replacement of exactly the services lost, in-kind replacement of different services generating the same level of utility, or payment of a sufficient amount of money to offset the utility lost.

It makes little sense from an economic or common sense perspective to not compensate for utility losses by spending the fewest resources possible. Consequently, there needs to be some flexibility on behalf of trustees in applying, for example, the HEA model. As the authors point out, the public may be better compensated by replacing a lost service with a somewhat different service. However, the HEA approach forces a concentration by the trustees on identifying what services are in fact lost. From a PRP's perspective, this exercise is important as it grounds the NRD process into some biological framework from which rational discussions can flow. In terms of replacing the services, the trustees and the PRPs should be working cooperatively to evaluate the least-cost way these services can be replicated or how enhancements on aspects of these services can be identified that will benefit the public more and cost the PRP less. This process results in the most rational expenditure from an economic standpoint of society's resources. Table 2-3 of their paper shows these trade-offs.

The authors imply that making these trade-offs is something that biologists are not willing to do because they are concerned that the general public does not possess the level of understanding about biological processes that is needed to make such trade-offs. While that may be true, through the application of common sense, decision-makers within the trustees and PRPs should be able to make common-sense choices, which may not be "pure" in a biological sense but reflect public preferences. Where there are doubts on public preferences, conjoint analysis can be performed. It is also possible, as the authors point out, to have biologists develop "equivalent" biological alternatives and have decision-makers choose from among these alternatives. While this approach could have a stronger biological basis, it might also unduly restrict decision-makers and result in enhancements that the public would prefer not being considered and for which PRPs would be unwilling to pay.

Conclusion

For the system to work, trustees and PRPs need to recognize that there is no "truth" and that an NRDA is an exercise to value lost services that are difficult to discern and more difficult to value. Valuing such services in terms of utility while adding a consistent unit of measurement does not change the inherent amorphousness of the calculation. Ultimately, the more "unreal" damages seem and the higher the damage claim, the more vigorously PRPs will contest a trustee's claim.

3

Net Environmental Benefits Assessment for Restoration Projects After Oil Spills

*Jenifer M. Baker**

Net environmental benefits assessment process

Most documented shore ecological recovery times are over time scales of 1 to 5 years, regardless of whether the sites were cleaned or not. Prolonged recovery times of up to 20 years or longer may result from extremes of either aggressive cleanup or heavy oiling that has not been cleaned up. If moderate shore cleanup is necessary for overriding human-use considerations, this can be done in most cases without prolonging the shore ecological recovery. However, in some cases there is the possibility that oil can be removed only by aggressive methods that damage the shore structure and organisms. The net environmental benefits assessment (NEBA) process accepts that some cleanup responses may cause damage but may be justifiable because of overriding human-use benefits. Beyond a certain point, expenditure of money on cleanup and restoration will not have a beneficial effect because inherent time scales for some ecological processes cannot be accelerated.

Restoration following oil spills can be viewed as a 2-stage process comprising cleanup (during which oil is removed to minimize the loss of human use and damage to the environment); and rehabilitation (during which attempts are made to facilitate the natural recovery processes after cleanup, back to the baseline condition). However, restoration methods may in some cases damage flora, fauna, or human use; benefit one environmental component at the expense of another; or in the long term be insignificant compared with natural recovery. The advantages and disadvantages of different restoration options therefore need to be weighed and compared with each other and with the advantages and disadvantages of allowing natural restoration to take its course. A NEBA is recommended for screening projects.

The NEBA process typically involves the following actions:

1) Collect information on human use and natural characteristics of the area of concern and details of the proposed restoration methods.
2) Review previous spill case histories and experimental results that are relevant to the area and restoration methods being assessed.

---

*Shrewsbury, United Kingdom

3) Predict the likely outcomes and time scales if the proposed restoration methods are used and if the area is left for natural restoration.
4) Review the advantages and disadvantages of the proposed restoration methods by comparing one with another and also by comparing with those of natural restoration.
5) Weigh advantages and disadvantages with reference to the highest priority resources in the area of concern, to arrive at the optimum restoration response. All parties must accept that the optimum response often cannot avoid all disadvantages.

The NEBA process takes time, which may be available after a spill in the case of some oiled-shoreline scenarios, but which will not be available for typical near-shore scenarios (e.g., a slick moving over shallow water toward a mangrove swamp). It is therefore important to use NEBA as early as possible during the contingency planning process.

It is now possible to look back over 30 years of experience since the Torrey Canyon accident (the first supertanker accident) and find information helpful for NEBA. This information comes from post-spill case studies of cleanup and rehabilitation (in some cases involving long-term monitoring), field experiments, and laboratory experiments including toxicity tests.

Human uses sensitive to oil spills

Possible types of damage include fouling of shorelines, boats, and fishing gear (and resulting loss of economic and recreational activity); tainting of fish and other food organisms; death of sensitive species and alterations to life stages; and ecosystem disruption. It is best if they are shown on sensitivity maps (IMO/IPIECA 1996) as part of the oil spill contingency planning process and as aides to pre-spill NEBA. The following are examples of human-use features liable to damage:

- near-shore, shallow-water fishing areas for finfish, crabs, lobsters, shrimps, or other species;
- seaweed gathering areas;
- shellfish beds in the intertidal zone or near-shore shallow water;
- fish and crustacean nursery areas;
- beaches with fishing activities, e.g., hauling in nets;
- permanent or semipermanent fish traps and fishing platforms;
- aquaculture facilities for fish, molluscs, crustaceans, or seaweed, e.g., floating cages, floating long-lines, fish, and crustacean ponds;
- seaward entrances of rivers important for migratory fish, e.g., salmon.
- ecosystems important for supporting fisheries, e.g., salt marshes, mangrove swamps, seagrass beds, kelp beds, coral reefs;
- educational sites, e.g., rocky shores used for shore zonation studies;

- recreational resources such as amenity beaches, bathing enclosures, water sport and game-fishing areas;
- sites of cultural or historical significance, on or close to the shore;
- boat facilities, e.g., harbors, marinas, moorings, slipways and boat ramps;
- industrial facilities, e.g., water intakes for power stations and desalination plants, coastal mining, and salt evaporation lagoons; and
- attractions for eco-tourists, e.g., coral reefs, seabird and marine mammal colonies, estuaries important for migrating shorebirds, and turtle nesting beaches. It is likely that some areas important for wildlife will have protected status (e.g., nature reserve or national park)

Physical characteristics of an area related to natural restoration

The natural physical characteristics of an area are important considerations for NEBA because they influence natural restoration times. Factors that have a bearing on the course of events include the type of water body and a variety of shoreline features.

In the open sea there is scope for oil slicks to disperse, and some large spills (e.g., the *Argo Merchant* and the *Ekofisk* blowouts) have caused minimal damage. Close to shore, damage is likely to be more pronounced in sheltered shallow water bays and inlets, where oil in the water may reach higher concentrations than in the open sea. This is also likely to be true of inland lakes and some rivers. Such areas are likely to have both greater biological productivity and greater human use than the open sea.

On the shore, the following features may influence the course of events:

- Localized exposure/shelter—even on an exposed shore, cracks, crevices, and spaces under boulders can provide sheltered conditions where oil may persist.
- Steepness/shore profile—extensive, gently sloping shores dissipate wave energy.
- Substratum—oil does not easily penetrate fine sediments, especially if they are waterlogged, but can penetrate shingle, gravel, and some sand beaches (e.g., see Hayes et al. 1979; Long et al. 1981).
- Exposure of the shore to wave energy—from very exposed rocky headlands to sheltered tidal flats, salt marshes, and mangroves. This in turn depends on a number of variables that include fetch; speed, direction, duration, and frequency of winds; and open angle of the shore (Ballantine 1961).
- Clay particles in sediments that can result in clay-oil flocculation—this process reduces adherence of oil to shore substrata and facilitates natural cleaning, as has been described for Prince William Sound after the *Exxon Valdez* spill (Jahns et al. 1991).

Many sensitivity maps classify shorelines using a vulnerability or environmental sensitivity index (ESI), which is typically based on the original index of Gundlach and

Hayes (1978). These maps arrange shoreline types on a 10-point scale, following the basic principles that sensitivity to oil increases with any of the following:

- increasing shelter of the shore from wave action,
- penetration of oil into the substratum,
- natural oil retention times on the shore, and
- biological productivity of shore organisms.

The least sensitive shorelines are rated ESI 1 and are typically exposed rocky headlands; the most sensitive (ESI 10) include sheltered marshes and mangroves.

There is sufficient case history evidence to give a reasonable indication of natural cleaning time scales in different types of habitat. For open water sites, the International Tanker Owners Pollution Federation (ITOPF) (1987) provides graphs illustrating the rate of removal from the water surface (by processes including evaporation, physical dispersal and biodegradation) of different oil types ranging from the lightest oils (Group I) such as kerosene to the heaviest (Group IV) such as Bunker C oil. The ITOPF model can be expressed in half-lives (the time taken for natural removal of 50% of the oil from the water surface), and these half-lives typically range from about half a day for Group I oils to > 7 days for Group IV oils. However, for large spills near coastlines, some oil typically is stranded on the shore within a few days; once oil is stranded, the natural cleaning time scale may be greatly prolonged.

Selected case histories covering a range of shore conditions are summarized in Baker et al. (1990) and Baker (1997). In summary, observed time scales for natural cleaning range from a few days (some case histories for very exposed rocky shores) to more than 20 years (some case histories for very sheltered marshes). Given that in extreme cases (e.g., Baker et al. 1993) thick deposits of oil may remain after about 20 years, it is reasonable to extrapolate that natural cleaning may take several decades in some sheltered environments.

Similarly, there is wide variation of time scales for natural ecological recovery. With open sea plankton communities, recovery may be within days, and there are many reports of good recovery within 1 or 2 years for the more exposed rocky shores. With sheltered shores within 1 or 2 years of oiling, there are more reports of "recovery started" than "recovered." In extreme cases, the recovery times may be much longer (< 20 years) for sheltered shores than for exposed shores.

Oil-spray cleanup methods

This section describes the more widely used oil-spill cleanup methods together with their advantages and disadvantages. No method is foolproof, and the limitations of water-surface methods mean that shore oiling almost is inevitable in any large coastal spill. This shore oiling, in turn, may lead to highly visible and often labor-intensive shore cleanup and the possibility that some oil can be removed only by aggressive methods that can damage the shore structure and shore organisms.

Booms and skimmers

Booms and skimmers can be successful if the spill is promptly reported and the diversion or containment of the oil starts before the oil has had too much time to spread over the water surface. Booms tend to work well under calm sea conditions, but they are ineffective in rough seas. When current speeds are greater than 0.7 to 1.0 knots (with the boom at right angles to the current), the oil is entrained into the water, passing under the boom, and lost (though in some cases it may be possible to angle the boom to prevent this).

Booms also can be used for shoreline protection, e.g., to stop oil from entering sheltered inlets with marshes or mangroves. The time available for protective boom deployment depends on the position and movement of the slick and can vary from hours to many days.

The efficiency of skimmers depends on the oil thickness and viscosity, the sea state, and the storage capacity of the skimmer. Skimmers normally work best in sheltered waters. Some can be used in open seas, but generally their efficiency is low when waves are higher than 2 m. Some newer skimmers follow the wave profiles and therefore can be used with larger waves. The overall effectiveness of skimmers is also dependent on the efficiency of pumping the collected oil to appropriate water separation/storage/disposal facilities. Because of their limitations, recovering 10% of the oil at a large spill in open seas is considered good for these mechanisms.

Dispersants

Dispersants, which contain surfactants (surface active agents), reduce interfacial tension between oil and water. They promote the formation of numerous tiny oil droplets and retard the coalescence of droplets into slicks. They do not clean oil out of the water but can improve biodegradation by increasing the oil surface area, thereby increasing exposure to bacteria and oxygen. The U.S. National Research Council (NRC 1989) concluded, "In a few carefully planned, monitored and documented field tests, as well as in laboratory tests, several dispersants have been shown to be effective—that is, they have removed a major part of the oil from the water surface when properly applied to oils that were dispersible."

In at least some situations dispersants appear to remove a greater proportion of oil from the water surface than mechanical methods. Moreover, they can be used relatively quickly and under sea conditions where mechanical collection is impossible. Dispersants, however, do not work well in all circumstances. For example dispersant spraying was ineffective on heavy fuel oil from the *Eleni V* off the east coast of England in 1978 and the *Vista Bella* in the Caribbean in 1991 (IPIECA 1993). Moreover, even for initially dispersible oils, there is only a short window of opportunity, typically 1 to 2 days, after which the oil becomes too weathered for dispersants to be effective. Other factors affecting dispersant effectiveness include oil viscosity, pour point, degree of oil weathering, dispersant formulation, dispersant:oil ratio, temperature, turbulent energy, and droplet size.

In situ burning

Burning (either contained or uncontained) can continue only as long as the oil is thick enough to support sustained combustion—usually a minimum of 2 to 3 mm. If a relatively thick layer of oil (approximately 5 cm or more) can be ignited, it is quite common that burning will remove over 95% of the oil. If oil continues to maintain its thickness during the combustion process (e.g., from continued spillage or herding within a boom configuration) burn efficiencies likely will exceed 98%. The small percentage of burn residue remaining after extinction of the fire almost always is buoyant and recoverable with hand tools, nets, or viscous oil recovery devices.

Burning has some shortcomings as a response technique, such as:

- it requires the use of special containment booms,
- it needs relatively fresh oil with low water content (preferably less than 20% water-in-oil);
- it requires that the sea be fairly calm with short-period wind-waves of 1 m or less; and
- it generates smoke.

As with dispersants, the window of opportunity is short, typically a few hours to a day or two, depending on the oil type and the environmental conditions at the time of the spill. When it is safe and logistically feasible, in situ burning is highly efficient in removing oil from the water surface.

Non-aggressive shore cleaning

Non-aggressive methods of shore cleaning, methods with minimal impact on shore structure and shore organisms, include the following:

- physical removal of surface oil from sandy beaches using machinery such as front-end loaders (avoiding removal of underlying sediment);
- manual removal of oil, asphalt patches, tar balls etc., by small, trained crews using equipment such as spades and buckets;
- collection of oil using sorbent materials (followed by safe disposal);
- low-pressure flushing with ambient temperature seawater; and
- bioremediation using fertilizers to stimulate indigenous hydrocarbon-degrading bacteria.

In appropriate circumstances these methods can be effective. However, they also may be labor-intensive, and cleanup crews must be careful to minimize trampling damage.

Many cases demonstrate how non-aggressive shore cleaning can remove most or all visible oil from sandy beaches, e.g., in Mozambique and Malaysia following the *Katina P* and *Nagasaki Spirit* incidents (respectively) in 1992 (ITOPF 1993a, 1993b). In a field experiment involving low-pressure flushing of fuel-oil mousse from sheltered sand in a Welsh inlet, about 85% of the applied mousse was cleared and collected (Howard and Little 1987). During the cleanup of the Kolva Basin oil spills in the Komi Republic, as much as 90% of the oil that could be easily dislodged came off in the first 4 to 5 passes with a low pressure hose. Further cleanup eroded soil and vegetation (Owens and Sergy 1996).

Fusey and Oudot (1984), who tested bioremediation of crude oil in a sheltered sandy site in France, found that physical loss of oil dominated initially. They concluded that fertilizers should be applied only after oil contamination falls below a threshold value. This rationale was used after the *Exxon Valdez* spill, where fertilizer application was used as a polishing technique after removal of bulk oil. On well aerated, porous, stony shores of Prince William Sound, this treatment was effective (Chianelli et al. 1991; Atlas 1995). In particular, accelerated degradation of subsurface oil was demonstrated. This is encouraging because subsurface oiling in porous shores presents a very difficult cleanup problem (Hoff 1993).

Non-aggressive methods do not work well in all circumstances. Low pressure flushing, for example, is ineffective on weathered, firmly adhering oil on rocks; and bioremediation is ineffective for subsurface oil in poorly aerated sediments.

Aggressive shore cleaning

Aggressive methods of shore cleaning, those that are likely to damage shore structure and/or shore organisms, include the following:

- removal of shore material such as sand, stones, or oily vegetation together with underlying roots and mud (in some cases the material may be washed and returned to the shore);
- water flushing at high pressure and/or high temperature; and
- sand blasting.

In some cases these methods are effective at cleaning oil from the shore. High-pressure hot water was efficient at removing oil from a Baltic rocky shore (Broman et al. 1983). Hot water was more effective than cold water for removing weathered, viscous *Exxon Valdez* oil from rocks (Nauman 1990). Following the *Apollo Sea* incident off the coast of South Africa (Jackson et al. 1996), dry sand blasting was identified as the only rapid, effective technique on supratidal rocks, with the advantage that it did not produce large quantities of oily waste.

However, heavy machinery, trampling, and high-pressure water all can force oil into sediments and make matters worse. Broman et al. (1983) concluded that high-pressure hot water was not effective on a Baltic gravel shore. In Alaska, *Exxon Valdez* oil flushed from the higher intertidal areas sometimes contaminated lower shore areas that previously had little oil and caused more oil to move underneath cobbles and boulders where it became trapped (Foster et al. 1990). Owens and Foget (1982) describe how high-pressure flushing changed a firm marsh substratum into a poorly consolidated waterlogged sediment, still containing oil that was incorporated into previously uncontaminated deeper sediments.

Rehabilitation

Oil-spill cleanup can be viewed as the first stage of environmental restoration. Once this has been accomplished, other restoration actions (rehabilitation) to encourage recovery should be considered. The most obviously successful actions are coastal wetland replanting schemes (mangroves and salt marshes) which can benefit human use of an area in various ways. However, rehabilitation programs are not a complete solution for badly damaged ecosystems because there is no way of accelerating recovery faster than the natural time scales for many ecological processes (e.g., growth, reproduction, dispersal, settlement and establishment of species interactions for perhaps hundreds of different species at different trophic levels). It is probably inevitable that rehabilitation schemes will have to focus on one or a few key species, e.g., mangrove tree; restoration of the full complexity of the ecosystem will depend upon subsequent natural processes.

Human use values of coastal wetlands

Human uses of coastal wetlands that may be lost following oiling may be direct or indirect. The importance of wetlands as nursery grounds for fish (including many of commercial importance) is now recognized, moreover plant material from wetlands contributes to the food webs that sustain near-shore fisheries. In some parts of the world, salt marshes provide valuable grazing areas for sheep, cattle, or horses. Products from mangrove trees include fuel wood, charcoal, stakes for fish traps and fishing platforms, material for roof thatching, bark for tannin, and traditional medicinal products and dyes.

In recent years the significance of wetlands in dissipating wave energy has come to be realized. Experimental work has shown the effectiveness of marshes acting as natural berms in front of sea walls (Allen and Pye 1992). Maintenance of salt marshes thus becomes a strategy for cost-effective coastal protection, especially now that there are concerns about rising sea levels and increased coastal erosion.

Wetlands are also, generally in an unplanned way, used as treatment systems for wastes discharged into estuaries and near-shore waters. In particular, they remove and assimilate sewage nutrients such as phosphorus, which can cause problems if the estuaries become overloaded. Gosselink et al. (1974) attempted to place a value on the various functions of tidal marshes and concluded that the value of marshes for waste assimilation was particularly high—bearing in mind the high cost of artificial treatment.

Wetlands may be valued for conservation reasons, for example because they provide feeding and roosting grounds for wading birds, and this sometimes has a human-use aspect in the form of eco-tourism.

Mangrove replanting

A particularly good example of a mangrove replanting scheme is the Refineria Panama project (Teas et al. 1989). In this case, more than 75 hectares of oil-killed mangrove forest were successfully replanted using more than 86,000 nursery-grown mangrove seedlings and propagules.

The time that must elapse after an oil spill for the soil to become sufficiently nontoxic for natural propagules or replanted mangroves to survive depends on factors such as the kind of oil spilled, the type of soil, local tidal flushing, and rainfall. The ability of mangroves to grow does not require that all oil has been eliminated from the soil. Mangroves can become established and apparently grow normally at oil-spill sites where there is residual weathered oil. In the case of the Refineria Panama spill, soil condition was tested both by chemical analyses and by pilot planting of red mangrove propagules (the term "propagule" in this case refers to seedlings growing out of fruits; they start doing this while the fruits are still attached to the trees and are the normal, tidally dispersed propagating organs of the red mangrove). Those propagules planted 3 months and 6 months post-spill all died; however, some of the propagules planted 9 months post-spill and larger fractions of those planted later survived. Thus the main replanting scheme did not start until 1 year after the spill.

Cylinders of oiled mangrove soil were removed by use of post-hole diggers and nursery-grown seedlings planted in the holes, or the holes were filled with upland soil and propagules were planted. In either case the developing roots of the seedling plants were protected from residual oil in the soil by a buffer of non-oiled soil in which the roots of a seedling could grow while the toxicity of oil in the soil continued to decrease through weathering and tidal and rainfall washing.

As an aid to restoring a mangrove forest as rapidly as possible, it is useful to set up a nursery where mangroves can be grown in order to have plants ready to plant out in the field when the oil toxicity has attenuated. Both planting of nursery-grown mangrove seedlings with their packets of upland soil and planting propagules in upland soil within the oiled mangrove forest proved successful in Panama. Two years after the spill, when the first natural regeneration was beginning to appear in the form of newly rooted propagules, planted nursery stock were already about 1 m tall. Survival of planted mangroves was typically > 90%.

Salt marsh replanting

Restoration schemes have focused on Spartina (a widespread robust grass) or a few other key species. Sediments to be planted must be at an appropriate height relative to tidal datum, and in some cases backfilling with suitable sediment is an option for achieving appropriate sediment height. Aggressive cleaning can lower the marsh surface to the extent that plant growth is not possible, as has been shown by the *Amoco Cadiz* case history (Vandermeulen et al. 1981; IPIECA 1994; Gilfillan et al. 1995a). In contrast, Krebs and Tanner (1981) successfully planted Spartina on marsh from which oily sediments had been stripped to a depth of not more than 10 cm. This removed most of the oil (which in high concentrations killed plants), and the residues remaining did not preclude good plant growth. In cases of doubt, initial small-scale experimental transplants are useful. These indicate if concentrations and degradation of oil residues are such that the sediments are suitable for full-scale planting.

Revegetation may be accomplished using seeds, young "bare-root" nursery seedlings (i.e., not potted), or older potted nursery seedlings that are planted into the sediments in their biodegradable pots, thus avoiding root damage. Use of nursery stocks avoids the damage that would be caused by digging up plants directly from existing local healthy marsh. However, the original propagation material used by the nursery should be as local as possible because there is considerable geographical variability in most salt marsh plant species.

Older potted seedlings are comparatively costly but are more resistant to erosion than seeds and young seedlings, are more vigorous, and have a higher survival rate. Costs will also be influenced by density of planting, e.g., a 1-m planting grid may be suitable for a very sheltered marsh and a denser pattern with plants at 1/3 m intervals may be suitable where the marsh is more exposed to wave action or tidal currents. Monitoring of transplant performance should be included in the program (IPIECA 1994).

Setting priorities for response

Typically following a spill there are a variety of both human-use and ecological resources to be considered, and if each one is considered separately it is found that the optimum spill response is not the same for all of them. In some cases there are conflicts of interest, and it is necessary to set priorities for response. In other words, the optimum overall response may nevertheless entail some disadvantages to particular resources. The following relationships may exist:

- The area contains mainly human-use interests (e.g., harbor facilities), so there is no potential conflict with purely ecological interests. However, there may be conflict between different human-use interests (e.g., near-shore dispersant spraying may be of benefit to protect amenity beaches, but it may lead to tainting in near-shore fisheries).
- The area contains both ecological and human-use interests, but the optimum response for one is not the optimum response for the other. For example, the area contains both birds and fish culture facilities. Dispersant spraying might be the best way of reducing the threat to birds, but it would increase the risk of fish tainting.
- The area contains both ecological and human use interests, but the optimum response for one is the same as the optimum response for the other. For example, a mangrove swamp may be of importance both ecologically and for shellfish collection. In both cases, the highest priority would be given to preventing or reducing the amount of oil entering the mangroves.
- The area of concern contains resources which are mainly of ecological interest (e.g., bird colonies), so there is no potential conflict with other human-use interests. However, there may be conflict between different ecological resources

(e.g., aggressive shore cleanup may benefit seals about to breed there, but it may prolong the recovery of shore organisms such as seaweed and mussels).

The contingency planning process should identify areas of potential conflict and attempt to resolve them before any spill and include consultation among all the interested organizations. A guide to contingency planning that includes the roles of different organizations and response team members and proposals for plan sections and subsections is provided by IPIECA (1991). It is worth considering the rationale of Lindstedt-Siva (1991), who used ecological criteria to define environmental sensitivity. This reasoning was on the grounds that "ecological impacts are both longer lasting, and once they have occurred, harder to repair than most other kinds of impacts (e.g., aesthetic, economic)."

NEBA for oiled shorelines

Consider a stony shore with subsurface oil that gradually is leaching into the near-shore waters. Information collected for the NEBA shows that near the shore are shallow subtidal beds of shellfish that were used for food by local people before the spill. Biological recovery on the shore has started (e.g., there are algal sporelings, and there has been some settlement of new barnacles) but the shellfish are tainted. If the shore is not thoroughly cleaned, some tainting will continue for up to 5 years, making the shellfish inedible for this period of time. Does this justify aggressive removal of the oil?

From a purely ecological point of view, there is no justification; previous case-history evidence (e.g., Rolan and Gallagher 1991) indicates that the recovery of the shore would be set back. Moreover, it is unlikely that there would be any purely ecological benefit to the shellfish populations, which can survive even though they are tainted. However, there would be a benefit for the people who collect shellfish as food if the source of tainting was removed as quickly as possible. The main problem for the NEBA is weighing the disadvantages of aggressive cleanup to the shore organisms against the advantages for use of an environmental resource—the shellfish. There would have to be a compelling human-use benefit of cleanup to override the ecological point of view, but in some cases (depending on the size and importance of the shell-fishery), the human-use consideration might justifiably prevail. This might include cultural factors, e.g., subsistence use of shellfisheries by ethnic minorities.

As illustrated in the above scenario, it is possible to distinguish 2 groups of reasons for possible shore cleanup, 1 group relating to the actual shore and the other to interacting systems. The shore comprises the physical features that form habitats for organisms, and the shore organisms themselves, meaning those species that only live on the shore and are sessile or of limited mobility (e.g., algae, barnacles, mussels, limpets, and periwinkles). The interacting systems impinge on, use, or are related to the shore in some way, but are not generally regarded as a permanent shore feature. They include human activities such as water sports, shellfish collection, or near-shore fisheries and aquaculture that may receive runoff from a polluted shore. Other examples are the following:

- marine mammals, e.g., seals using the shore as a haul-out and breeding area;
- near-shore habitats, e.g., coral reefs, seagrass beds, and kelp beds, which may receive oily runoff from a polluted shore; and
- salmon streams which debouch over the shore, so that salmon entering a stream might have to swim over an oily shore at high tide.

Prince William Sound is rich in examples, which in some cases provided justification for aggressive shore cleanup after the *Exxon Valdez*. For example, seal haul-out sites, with birth of pups in May and June, had high priority for cleanup of bulk surface oil after pollution in March 1989 (Lowry et al. 1994). This is in contrast to a later study on the advisability of excavation and washing of rocks on shores with subsurface oil residues (NOAA 1990). The study concluded that the proposed treatment would indeed remove subsurface oil but for most shores it did not offer a net environmental benefit because it would alter the shore structure and delay biological recovery (which already had begun). In this case, the negative aspects of the proposed cleanup were not judged to be outweighed by either the positive aspects of cleanup treatment or negative aspects of no treatment.

Possible shore scenarios

The following discussion is of possible shore scenarios bearing in mind the above distinctions.

Lightly to moderately oiled shores

Sell et al. (1995) analyzed all adequately documented case histories and showed that 85% of rocky shores and 75% of salt marshes showed good ecological recovery within 3 and 5 years respectively, regardless of whether they had been cleaned or not (these figures exclude a few extreme cases which are discussed in the following section). It is unreasonable to expect cleaning to reduce natural recovery time scales significantly below 3 and 5 years, simply because most recovery processes of immigration, settlement, and growth cannot be accelerated (evidence concerning the time scales of these natural processes in the absence of any oil and cleanup impacts is presented in Sell et al. [1995]). Therefore, if there are no interacting systems that take precedence, there is little justification on the basis of current evidence in carrying out any sort of shore cleanup operation on rocky shores or salt marshes. Evidence for other types of shores has not yet been analyzed.

On the other hand, the evidence also shows that if moderate cleanup is carried out for the sake of interacting systems, this can be done in most cases without prolonging the biological recovery time of the shore in an unacceptable way.

Extremely oiled shores

In a minority of cases, the shore oiling may be so severe that, on the basis of current evidence, the predicted natural recovery times may be unacceptably long. It may therefore be decided to clean the shore even if there are no important interacting systems. In other cases there may be a requirement to quickly achieve a shore as free of oil as possible for the sake of some interacting system. An interesting comparison is provided by marshes heavily oiled by the *Metula* and *Amoco Cadiz* spills, with the latter being aggressively cleaned and the former not cleaned at all.

In the case of the 1974 *Metula* spill in the Strait of Magellan, Chile (Baker et al 1993), one very sheltered marsh received thick deposits of oil and mousse (water-in-oil emulsion). The marsh is in a remote area with very little human population. In 1994 oily deposits were still visible on the marsh surface, with the mousse quite fresh beneath the weathered surface skin. There has been little plant recolonization in the areas with the thicker deposits (mean oil depth 4.1 cm). Thus natural recovery times for such an extreme scenario can be predicted as substantially more than 20 years.

In the case of the 1978 *Amoco Cadiz* spill in Brittany, there was similar heavy oiling of a marshland, but in an area with much greater human use including shellfisheries. The decision was taken to clean the Ile Grande marshes using heavy equipment. As much as 50 cm of sediment was removed, at the same time channels were widened and straightened. Subsequently it was realized that the treatment was harmful because some of the marsh surface was lowered to the extent that it was at the wrong intertidal height for plant growth. In 1990, 3 marshes still had 26, 35, and 39% of their pre-spill surface areas missing (Vandermeulen et al. 1981; IPIECA 1994; Gilfillan et al. 1995).

There are other examples of aggressive cleanup of heavy oiling having apparently prolonged the ecological recovery time, notably the 1978 *Esso Bernicia* spill in Sullom Voe, Shetland. In areas where there was substantial mechanical removal of rocks and gravel, biological communities had not fully recovered after 9 years (Sell et al. 1995).

What would happen if it were necessary to deal with a new case of very thick oil deposits on a shore? On the basis of the above evidence, if the main considerations were ecological, it seems that in some cases neither natural cleanup nor intense treatment would give the best environmental benefit. It seems likely that the greatest benefit would result from a moderate level of cleanup—sufficient to remove most of the bulk oil, but gentle enough to leave the surface of the shore intact and to avoid churning oil into underlying sediments. This could be achieved by using small crews and avoiding the use of heavy machinery. The appearance of the shore after such treatment is likely to be somewhat oily and therefore not optimal from an aesthetic viewpoint, but there are numerous examples of biological recovery taking place in the presence of weathered oil remnants (Baker et al. 1990). If marsh plants were smothered to death before removal of the bulk oil, a replanting scheme should be carried out.

If there is an overriding requirement to achieve a clean shore as quickly as possible because of human-use considerations, it needs to be borne in mind that this may delay ecological recovery. Even if a replanting scheme is carried out, this typically relies on one or a few species, and it cannot quickly recreate the complexity of the original ecosystem.

NEBA for near-shore waters

Consider a slick moving over shallow near-shore water in which there are coral reefs of particular conservation interest and eco-tourism importance. The slick is moving toward sandy beaches important for tourism. Assume that the only logistically feasible response in the limited time available is aerial dispersant spraying. This should minimize pollution of the beaches, but it is predicted that some coral species will be damaged by dispersed oil. From an ecological point of view, it is best not to use dispersants but to allow the oil to strand on the beaches, from where it may be quickly and easily cleaned using front-end loaders and crews with hand tools. If dispersants are used, damaged corals could take many years to recover. Widespread degradation of fringing reefs could in turn alter the dynamics of nearby sandy beaches, with possible adverse consequences.

A closer look at the subject of dispersant use in shallow tropical waters provides some interesting examples of the potential complexity of NEBA considerations. The TROPICS experiment (Ballou et al. 1989) compared the effects of untreated and chemically dispersed oil in an area with mangroves, seagrass beds, and corals. The average water depth was less than 1 m, and concentrations of dispersed oil reached as high as 222 parts per million (ppm). With the dispersed oil treatment, there were declines in the abundance of corals and other reef organisms, reduced coral growth rate in 1 species, and minor effects on seagrasses and mangroves. Fresh, untreated oil had severe effects on survival of mangroves and associated fauna, and minor effects on seagrasses, corals, and associated organisms. However, it would be premature to jump to the conclusion that not using dispersants would be the best action if corals were considered to be the highest priority. The Refineria *Panama* oil spill (IPIECA 1992; Cubit and Connor 1993; Garrity et al. 1993) provides further essential information. In this case, untreated oil caused damage to both mangroves and corals, including corals at a greater depth (3 to 6 m) than those affected in the TROPICS experiment. Branching corals appear more susceptible than massive corals, and recovery has been slow. The impacts on corals have been attributed to the slow release of oil from nearby mangrove sediments and subsequent depression of coral viability because of the chronic low-level contamination of near-shore waters (IPIECA 1992).

Further information on field experiments that provide useful input to NEBA for dispersant use (Gilfillan et al. 1983, 1984; Page et al. 1983 Lai and Feng 1985; Sergy and Blackall 1987; LeGore et al. 1989) is summarized in Baker (1995), and the *Braer* spill adds unique case history information on "worst case" concentrations of dispersed oil in near-shore waters.

Braer spill

The *Braer* grounded on the southern tip of Shetland on 5 January 1993, and the cargo of 84,700 tonnes of Norwegian Gullfaks crude oil was nearly all dispersed into the water because of the turbulent sea conditions. Though 120 tonnes of dispersant were sprayed on the oil, most of the dispersal was through natural physical processes. Published data (ESGOSS 1994) show that initial concentrations of oil in the water near the tanker were measured at some hundreds of ppm, and the sea was described as having a brown "coffee-like" coloring typical of dispersed oil. The droplet size of this oil was similar to that of chemically dispersed oil (Rycroft personal communication). In the following days, values as high as 50 ppm were reported near the wreck, but oil concentrations decreased with time and returned to background concentrations 60 to 70 days after the grounding. These data show that oil exposure (concentration x time) (NRC 1989) for water column organisms greatly exceeded anything previously reported (NRC 1989; IPIECA 1993) for field trials or case histories involving application of chemical dispersants. Moreover, according to Rycroft et al. (1994), it would never be possible to disperse the sort of quantity of oil spilt from the *Braer* with chemicals (for logistical reasons). Thus the *Braer* represents an extreme scenario for considering the advantages and disadvantages of dispersing oil in near-shore waters.

The fate and effects of the oil have been described by ESGOSS (1994). Some summarized findings that are of relevance for dispersant use and NEBA are given below. The overall conclusion was that the impact of the spill on the ecology and environment of South Shetland has been minimal, and that damage would have been greater if the oil had not dispersed but had formed slicks and coated shorelines and structures such as aquaculture facilities.

- Salmon in farms 20 to 25 km from the wreck site were tainted but did not suffer unusual mortalities. However, many of the farms had to be destroyed because they could not be sold. By the end of July 1993, samples from all the affected sites had no taint, and virtually normal values for polycyclic aromatic hydrocarbons (PAHs).
- Many dead wild fish, mainly wrasse and sand eels, were washed up on the beaches near the wreck during the first few days after the spill (SNH 1993 as quoted by Moore (1994). For sand eels (a species of critical importance to several food chains), there was no change in distribution around South Shetland, and no evidence of effect on populations. For all species of wild fish, contamination in samples fell rapidly, and by April 1993 the ban on fishing was lifted.
- For shellfish, there was still evidence in May 1994 of low levels of contamination in some species, and the fishing ban had not been lifted by summer 1994.
- For near-shore and intertidal areas, there is little evidence of lasting hydrocarbon contamination, and residual sediment toxicity is negligible. Questions remain about the degradation rate of oil in fine sediments in relatively deep water and in some of the southwestern voes.

- The oil does not appear to have affected coastal macrobenthos significantly. For benthic communities in areas of fine sediment affected by oil, there were some increases in opportunistic and oil-tolerant species; abundance of some indicator meiofauna species declined.
- For seals, otters, and cetaceans, the short-term effects of the spill have been negligible.
- For all species of birds, mortality was low by comparison with other spills, and there were no signs of sublethal toxic effects apart from some minor effects on kittiwakes.

Conclusions

- The human and ecological advantages and disadvantages of different cleanup and rehabilitation responses (including restoration by entirely natural processes) should be weighed for any area of concern using the NEBA approach. As this process takes time, it is best done before a spill as part of the contingency planning process. Decisions need to be reached through consensus.
- Many years of international experience have demonstrated the limitations of cleanup methods (human intervention). No method is a panacea, and in the case of any large coastal spill, shore oiling is almost inevitable. In some cases, dispersant spraying in near-shore waters offers the best hope for reducing shore oiling, but it increases the risk to subtidal organisms.
- Most documented shore recovery times are over time scales of 1 to 5 years, regardless of whether they were cleaned or not. Prolonged ecological recovery times of up to 20 years or more may result from extremes—either of aggressive cleanup or of heavy oiling that has not been cleaned up. If moderate shore cleanup is necessary for overriding human-use considerations, this can be done in most cases without prolonging the shore recovery. However, in some cases there is the possibility that oil can be removed only by aggressive methods that damage the shore structure and/or organisms. Net environmental benefit assessment accepts that some cleanup responses may cause damage but may be justifiable because of overriding human-use benefits.
- Human-use considerations include the potential need to clean up amenity beaches and boats, and minimize the tainting of fish and shellfish. In some cases, the optimum response for human use is not the optimum response for ecological resources. Net environmental benefit assessment should identify areas of potential conflict and attempt to resolve them as completely as possible before any spill occurs.
- Beyond a certain point, expenditure of funds, time and effort on cleanup, and rehabilitation will not have beneficial effects on ecological recovery because inherent time scales for some ecological processes cannot be accelerated.

Acknowledgments—Alan Allen, Spiltec, Woodinville, USA and Ed Owens, OCC, Bainbridge Island, USA, are gratefully acknowledged for providing information on in situ burning and low-pressure flushing, respectively.

References

Allen JRL, Pye K, editors. 1992. Saltmarshes: morphodynamics, conservation and engineering significance. Cambridge UK: Cambridge Univ.

Atlas RM. 1995. Petroleum biodegradation and oil spill bioremediation. *Mar Pollut Bull* 31:178–182.

Baker JM. 1995. Net environmental benefit analysis for oil spill response. Proceedings, 1995 International Oil Spill Conference. Washington DC. American Petroleum Institute,. p 611–614.

Baker JM. 1997. How clean is clean? Issue paper presented at the 1997 International Oil Spill Conference. American Petroleum Institute, Washington DC.

Baker JM, Clark RB, Kingston PF, Jenkins RH. 1990. Natural recovery of cold water marine environments after an oil spill. Paper presented at the 13th AMOP Technical Seminar. Environmental Protection Service, Environment Canada, Ottawa.

Baker JM, Guzman LM, Bartlett PD, Little DI, Wilson CM. 1993. Long-term fate and effects of untreated thick oil deposits on saltmarshes. Proceedings of the 1993 Oil Spill Conference. Washington DC. American Petroleum Institute. p 395–399.

Ballantine WJ. 1961. A biologically defined exposure scale for the comparative description of rocky shores. *Field Studies* 1:1–19.

Ballou TG, Hess SC, Dodge RE, Knap AH, Sleeter TD. 1989. Effects of untreated and chemically dispersed oil on tropical marine communities: a long-term field experiment. Proceedings of the 1989 Oil Spill Conference. Washington DC. American Petroleum Institute. p 447–454.

Broman D, Ganning B, Lindblad C. 1983. Effects of high pressure, hot water shore cleaning after oil spills on shore ecosystems in the northern Baltic proper. *Mar Environ Res* 10:173–187.

Chianelli RR, Aczel T, Bare RE, George GN, Genowitz MW, Grossman MJ, Haith CE, Kaiser FJ, Lessard RR, Liotta R, Mastracchio RL, Minak-Bernero V, Prince RC, Robbins WK, Stiefel EI, Wilkinson JB, Hinton SM, Bragg JR, McMillen SJ, Atlas RM. 1991. Bioremediation technology development and application to the Alaskan spill. Proceedings of the 1991 Oil Spill Conference. Washington DC. American Petroleum Institute. p 549–558.

Cubit JD, Connor JL. 1993. Effects of the 1986 *Bahia Las Minas* oil spill on reef flat communities. Proceedings, 1993 Oil Spill Conference. Washington D: American Petroleum Institute. p 329–334.

[ESGOSS] Ecological Steering Group on the Oil Spill in Shetland. 1994. The environmental impact of the wreck of the *Braer*. Scottish Office, Edinburgh, Scotland: Ecological Steering Group on the Oil Spill in Shetland. 207 p.

Foster MS, Tarpley JA, Dean SL. 1990. To clean or not to clean: the rationale, methods, and consequences of removing oil from temperate shores. *Northwest Environ J* 6:105–120.

Fusey P, Oudot J. 1984. Relative influence of physical removal and biodegradation in the depuration of petroleum-contaminated seashore sediments. *Mar Pollut Bull* 15:136–141.

Garrity SD, Levings SC, Burns KA. 1993. Chronic oiling and long-term effects of the 1986 Galeta spill on fringing mangroves. Proceedings, 1993 Oil Spill Conference. Washington DC: American Petroleum Institute. p 319–324.

Gilfillan ES, Page DS, Hanson SA, Foster JC, Hotham JR, Vallas D, Gerber R, Pratt SD. 1983. Effect of spills of dispersed and non-dispersed oil on intertidal infaunal community structure. Proceedings, 1983 Oil Spill Conference. Washington DC: American Petroleum Institute. p 457–463.

Gilfillan ES, Maher NP, Krejsa CM, Lanphear ME, Balls CD, Meltzer JB, Page DS. 1995. Use of remote sensing to document changes in marsh vegetation following the *Amoco Cadiz* oil spill (Brittany, France, 1978). *Mar Pollut Bull* 30:780–787.

Gosselink JG, Odum EP, Pope RM. 1974. The value of the tidal marsh. Baton Rouge LA: Center for Wetland Resources, Louisiana State University.

Gundlach ER, Hayes MO. 1978. Vulnerability of coastal environments to oil spill impacts. *Mar Technol Soc J* 12:18–27.

Hayes MO, Gundlach ER, D'Ozouville L. 1979. Role of dynamic coastal processes in the impact and dispersal of the *Amoco Cadiz* oil spill (March 1978), Brittany, France. Proceedings, 1979 Oil Spill Conference. Washington DC: American Petroleum Institute. p 193–198.

Hoff RZ. 1993. Bioremediation: an overview of its development and use for oil spill cleanup. *Mar Pollut Bull* 26:476–481.

[IMO/IPIECA] International Petroleum Industry Environmental Conservation Association. 1996. Sensitivity mapping for oil spill response. London, UK: International Petroleum Industry Environmental Conservation Association.

[IPIECA] International Petroleum Industry Environmental Conservation Association. 1991. A guide to contingency planning for oil spills on water. London, UK: International Petroleum Industry Environmental Conservation Association.

[IPIECA] International Petroleum Industry Environmental Conservation Association. 1992. Biological impacts of oil pollution: coral reefs. London, UK: International Petroleum Industry Environmental Conservation Association.

[IPIECA] International Petroleum Industry Environmental Conservation Association. 1993. Dispersants and their role in oil spill response. London, UK: International Petroleum Industry Environmental Conservation Association.

[IPIECA] International Petroleum Industry Environmental Conservation Association. 1994. Biological impacts of oil pollution: saltmarshes. London, UK: International Petroleum Industry Environmental Conservation Association.

[ITOPF] International Tanker Owners Pollution Federation. 1987. Response to marine oil spills. London: International Tanker Owners Pollution Federation Ltd., Witherby and Co. Ltd.

[ITOPF] International Tanker Owners Pollution Federation. 1993a. *Katina P. Ocean Orbit*. April 1993. p 2.

[ITOPF] International Tanker Owners Pollution Federation. 1993b. *Nagasaki Spirit. Ocean Orbit*. April 1993. p 2.

Jackson L, Dernier W, Woodend J, Needham G, Cooper S, Moldan A. 1996. South African experience of building a response capability. IMO/Industry Oil Spill Planning Meeting, Cape Town, South Africa, 12–15 March 1996.

Krebs CT, Tanner CE. 1981. Restoration of oiled saltmarshes through sediment stripping and Spartina propagation. Proceedings, 1981 Oil Spill Conference. Washington DC: American Petroleum Institute. p 375–385.

Lai HC, Feng MC. 1985. Field and laboratory studies on the toxicity of oils to mangroves. Proceedings, 1985 Oil Spill Conference. Washington DC: American Petroleum Institute. p 539–546.

LeGore S, Marszalek DS, Danek LJ, Tomlinson MS, Hofmann JE, Cuddeback JE. 1989. Effect of chemically dispersed oil on Arabian gulf corals: a field experiment. Proceedings, 1985 Oil Spill Conference. Washington DC: American Petroleum Institute. p 375–380.

Long BFN, Vandermeulen JH, Ahern TP. 1981. The evolution of stranded oil within sandy beaches. Proceedings, 1987 Oil Spill Conference. Washington DC: American Petroleum Institute. p 519–524.

Lowry LF, Frost KJ, Pitcher KW. 1994. Observations of oiling of harbor seals in Prince William Sound. In: Loughlin TR, editor. Marine mammals and the *Exxon Valdez*. San Diego CA: Academic. p 209–225.

[NRC] National Research Council. 1989. Using oil spill dispersants on the sea. Washington DC: National Academy.

Nauman SA. 1990. Shoreline cleanup techniques - *Exxon Valdez* operations. Proceedings, 13th AMOP Technical Seminar. Environmental Protection Service, Environment Canada, Ottawa. p 431–438.

[NOAA] National Oceanic and Atmospheric Administration. 1990. Excavation and rock washing treatment technology: net environmental benefit analysis. Seattle: WA: National Oceanic and Atmospheric Administration. 199 p.

Owens EH, Foget CR. 1982. A small river oil spill: a large step back for cleanup technology. Spill Technology Newsletter. Jan/Feb 1982, p 7–10.

Owens EH, Sergy G. 1996. Oil on shorelines and shoreline treatment: a state-of-knowledge review. Proceedings, 19th AMOP Technical Seminar. Environmental Protection Service, Environment Canada, Ottawa. p 1105–1116.

Page DS, Foster JC, Hotham JR, Pendergast E, Hebert S, Gonzalez L, Gilfillan ES, Hanson SA, Gerber RP, Vallas D. 1983. Long-term fate of dispersed and undispersed crude oil in two nearshore test spills. Proceedings, 1983 Oil Spill Conference. Washington DC: American Petroleum Institute. p 465–471.

Rolan RG, Gallagher R. 1991. Recovery of intertidal biotic communities at Sullom Voe following the *Esso Bernicia* oil spill of 1978. Proceedings, 1991 Oil Spill Conference. Washington DC: American Petroleum Institute. p 461–465.

Rycroft RJ, Matthiesson P, Portmann JE. 1994. MAFF Review of the UK Oil Dispersant Testing and Approval Scheme. Ministry of Agriculture, Fisheries and Food: Directorate of Fisheries Research, Lowestoft. 89 p.

Sell D, Conway L, Clark T, Picken GB, Baker JM, Dunnet GM, McIntyre AD, Clark RB. 1995. Scientific criteria to optimize oil spill cleanup. Proceedings, 1995 Oil Spill Conference. Washington DC: American Petroleum Institute. p 595–610.

Sergy GA, Blackall PJ. 1987. Design and conclusions of the Baffin Island oil spill project. *Arctic* 40(Supplement 1):1–9.

Teas HJ, Lasday AH, Luque E, Morales RA, De Diego ME, Baker JM. 1989. Mangrove restoration after the 1986 Refineria *Panama* oil spill. Proceedings, 1989 Oil Spill Conference. Washington DC: American Petroleum Institute. p 433–437.

Vandermeulen JH, Long BFN, D'Ozouville L. 1981. Geomorphological alteration of a heavily oiled saltmarsh (Ile Grande, France) as a result of a massive cleanup. Proceedings, 1981 Oil Spill Conference. Washington DC: American Petroleum Institute. p 347–351.

3a

Discussion Paper I on Net Environmental Benefits Assessment for Restoration Projects After Oil Spills, or Science, Environmental Damage Assessment, and Restoration: Putting First Things First

*John A. Wiens**

The focus of this conference is on restoration of lost human uses of the environment following environmental contamination. To develop and implement the most effective restoration actions, we must first determine the nature and magnitude of environmental impacts and whether these impacts affect natural ecosystem processes or alter direct human uses of the environment (see contributions from Stewart, McHugh, and Hyatt in this volume). We must also assess the likelihood that natural processes will foster recovery of the system without active restoration efforts. Accurate determination of impacts and recovery is therefore a necessary precursor to restoration efforts. Although there will always be some uncertainty in the assessment of environmental impacts and recovery (Schmitt and Osenberg 1996; Lemons 1996) (see King, this volume), our goals should be to reduce this uncertainty as much as possible and then to deal with the remaining uncertainty as objectively as possible. In this way, restoration efforts may be directed where they will do the most good. This is the foundation of the net environmental benefit assessment (NEBA) approach discussed by Baker (this volume).

How do we do this? Reducing uncertainty requires rigorous scientific design and analysis, while objectivity requires that we recognize preconceptions and advocacy and minimize their influences on the assessment process. Here, I'll discuss each of these topics. Although my points apply to any sort of environmental contamination, I will cast my comments in the context of oil spills, using examples from studies of the *Exxon Valdez* oil spill, with which I have direct experience (Wiens 1996a). I will focus my comments on the scientific determination of environmental impacts of spills and will not address the economic valuation of lost human uses of resources or the aesthetic dimensions of changes in human perceptions of the environment. These are

*Department of Biology and Graduate Degree Program in Ecology, Colorado State University, Fort Collins, CO

also important components of restoration efforts, but they ultimately relate closely to the natural resources and ecosystem functions that are my focus here.

Assessing damages and recovery

When an oil spill occurs in a coastal or marine environment, some damages, such as oiled beaches or dying seabirds, are immediate and obvious. The ecological system has been altered. To determine whether restoration efforts may be justified, however, 2 questions must be addressed.

- What is the likelihood that natural processes will lead to a recovery of the damaged resources, and how long will such recovery take?
- Are some damages to resources less obvious, or are some of the obvious damages more apparent than real?

Answering these questions requires, first, that "injury" and "recovery" be defined objectively and operationally. The NOAA Natural Resource Damages Assessment (NRDA) regulations consider injury and recovery (or restoration) in terms of departure from and return to a "baseline," respectively. Conditions of the resources are related to those that would have existed if the release or discharge had not occurred.

Environments and the organisms that occupy them vary over time. It is therefore likely that the condition of resources will change whether or not a spill has occurred. The challenge becomes one of identifying a change associated with a spill against the background of natural variation, which makes baseline conditions a moving target. Elsewhere (Wiens 1995, 1996b) I have argued that injury should be defined in statistical terms, as a statistically significant difference between samples exposed to the contaminant and reference samples that encompass the normal range of variation in the system. Recovery is then the disappearance through time of this statistically significant difference. Definitions of recovery based upon a return of the system to pre-spill baseline conditions (e.g., *Exxon Valdez* Trustee Council 1993) may therefore be unrealistic (Paine et al. 1996).

A statistical approach to defining injury and recovery has the advantages of being objective and operational, and it also permits the detection of spill effects that may not be so obvious as oiled beaches or dead seabirds. But drawing valid statistical comparisons rests on using a sound study design. Environmental contamination events are unplanned and unreplicated. Therefore, we cannot predict when (or often where) they will occur. Because they are associated with specific activities (e.g., the extraction, transport, or processing of oil releases) that also do not occur randomly in time or space, these attributes of spills pose formidable challenges in developing a study design that will permit valid statistical comparisons to evaluate injury or recovery.

The most obvious design, to compare the condition of the resources following the spill with that before the spill, is also probably the least useful (Wiens and Parker 1995; Wiens 1996b). Spills have a way of occurring where good baseline data do not exist, so it is generally unlikely that suitable "before" information will be available for comparison. When such information does exist, it usually has been gathered some years (or decades) before the spill event, and therefore forms a suitable baseline for comparison *only* if one assumes that the environment has not varied during the interim. Given what we now know about environmental variations, assumption of equilibrium is clearly untenable.

An example of the problems with simple before/after comparisons is provided by attempts to assess the effects of the *Exxon Valdez* oil spill (which occurred in March 1989) on murre (*Uria* spp.) populations breeding on the Barren Islands, Alaska. This area was directly in the pathway of the spreading oil, and concerns were expressed shortly after the spill that the breeding colonies might have been devastated (Piatt et al. 1990; Fry 1993). As part of a larger study to assess spill effects on murres, Boersma et al. (1995) compared counts of birds at breeding sites made after the spill, in 1990 through 1992, with counts made at the same sites before the spill, in the mid- to late 1970s. The early estimates (obtained by different investigators using different procedures) ranged from 61,000 birds in 1975 to 19,000 birds in 1978. Boersma et al. (1995) estimated that there were 31,000 birds in this location in 1990, which could represent a 51% decrease or a 39% increase, depending on which "before" estimate is used. Moreover, during the more than 10 years between the early surveys and the oil spill there were 2 El Niño events, one the strongest in this century. Boersma et al. (1995) concluded that "the pre-spill information available is not good enough to detect either the amount or the direction of change in the murre population."

Other study designs follow the lead of experimental sciences and regard the spill area as a "treatment" and areas outside of the spill zone as "controls." Here the underlying assumption is different, but equally tenuous. Because spills do not occur in random locations, it is likely that the affected area will differ systematically from other nearby areas that might be used as controls. Thus, even though sampling stations may be randomly distributed within the two areas, the differences between the areas make the control area an inappropriate baseline for comparison. For example, studies of harlequin ducks (*Histrionicus histrionicus*) conducted following the *Exxon Valdez* spill compared the western part of Prince William Sound, where the spill occurred, with the eastern Sound, which was unoiled (Patten 1993). Because breeding activity was greater in the eastern control than in the western treatment, it was concluded that the spill had adversely affected harlequin reproduction. The environments of eastern and western Prince William Sound differ in many respects, however; coastal currents are different, mainland topography and stream lengths differ, more stream headwaters are glaciated in the western Sound, and the western Sound contains many more small islands and fewer shallow lagoons and tidal mudflats than the eastern Sound. Thus, the conclusion that reproductive differences between the areas reflect spill impacts is compromised by the other differences between the areas. In general, then, one cannot deduce the effects of a contamination event (or gauge recovery) by comparing 2 areas that would differ whether or not the spill occurred.

All study designs make assumptions of one sort or another (Wiens and Parker 1995; Schmitt and Osenberg 1996). However, designs that incorporate a quantitative measure of contamination intensity (i.e., a "dose-response" approach) instead of casting the analysis in a contaminated/uncontaminated framework are likely to be more effective in revealing spill-related injuries, especially if the effects are subtle. For example, when Day et al. (1995, 1997) used a quantitative measure of oiling intensity to assess the effects of the *Exxon Valdez* spill on habitat use by birds, they recorded initial effects of the spill on substantially more species than did studies that simply compared oiled and unoiled areas.

Designs that include measures of environmental features other than oiling as covariates in the analyses can also reduce the confounding effects of systematic spatial differences among areas and permit more robust statistical determinations of variations associated with the contamination. By conducting repeated sampling over time following a spill, one can assess the effects of natural variability of the system more accurately, and such a design also enables one to detect recovery over time or delayed impacts of the spill. Thus, although Day et al. (1995, 1997) documented initial impacts of the *Exxon Valdez* spill on nearly one-half of the bird species they considered, their approach also showed that the statistical evidence of spill effects disappeared within 1 or 2 years for most of the affected species.

The choice of a study design to assess the extent of injuries to resources from environmental contamination inevitably will involve trade-offs between feasibility, cost, speed of implementation, effectiveness, statistical power, and the degree of resolution or level of certainty required in the conclusions. Because everything that is done in the restoration phase depends on the documentation of initial injuries and damages, however, it is imperative that the assessment of contamination effects be as rigorous and sensitive as possible. Unfortunately, the quickest and easiest approaches may not always be the best.

Coping with preconceptions and advocacy

The release of hazardous materials or pollutants into the environment gives rise to immediate concerns about damage to resources or the integrity of ecological systems. We expect that the spill will have negative effects on at least some components of the environment, and there is abundant evidence to support this preconception. We fear the worst. If the spill is large, these preconceptions of spill damages may be reinforced by strong emotional responses to the apparent spill damages. It is impossible to remain emotionally detached when confronted with oiled beaches and blackened, struggling seabirds. Indeed, these are the images used by the media to portray the effects of spills to the public at large. They are real, and they are powerful. But it is not always certain that such images are an accurate reflection of the extent of overall damages of a spill. Documenting spill damages requires that one set aside preconceptions and emotions and assess what has really happened as rigorously as possible. Careful selection of an effective study design is so important. The pull of our preconceptions is both powerful and subtle, and it can easily lead to studies that seem superficially sound but contain strong underlying biases. In a treatment-control study, for example, the selection of an inappropriate area as the control for comparison can virtually assure that the contaminated treatment area will be different, playing nicely into our preconceptions about what should be. Such biases may be quite unintentional, but they are biases nonetheless, and they may severely compromise the accurate assessment of spill damages and the likelihood that we will ever document recovery.

One often hears arguments that such biases are permissible because it is better to err on the side of documenting damages that did not really happen than to miss detecting some damages that actually did occur. It is better to be safe than sorry. This is the basis for the ongoing debate about whether one should be concerned about Type I or Type II errors in statistical analyses of contamination effects (Shrader-Frechette and McCoy 1993; Wiens and Parker 1995; Mapstone 1996). However, this argument should not be used to justify inadequate study designs that may be predisposed to provide results that coincide with our preconceptions. Restoration efforts, some of them massive in scope (see McCammon, this volume), may rest upon such findings. It is the responsibility of those assessing injuries to provide an accurate and objective foundation for these efforts. This requires that emotional responses be set aside and preconceptions recognized for what they are, and that the assessment of damages be immune to their influences.

Contamination events may affect the environment and particular resources that are important to humans, but they also occur within a complex biological-sociological-economic-political context. Spills attract media attention and not infrequently lead to litigation, and they also may provide funding opportunities for research. Collectively, these forces can create a situation in which there may be substantial pressures to become an advocate for a particular position, be it environmental, corporate, political, or some other agenda. Advocacy in and of itself is not necessarily wrong, but it can easily become intertwined with the scientific process. When this happens, the integrity and credibility of science are diminished, and the foundation of restoration efforts may be correspondingly eroded (Wiens 1996a).

Advocacy can affect the scientific process in several ways. Some of these influences can be minimized by careful selection of an appropriate and rigorous study design, but others are more subtle and difficult to control. After results are obtained from a study of possible spill damages, they must be interpreted. Because of the difficulties of implementing a pure design for an unplanned environmental accident and the effects of natural environmental variations in space and time, there is usually uncertainty in the results. Unfortunately, the degree of uncertainty often increases with the importance of the issue. Such uncertainty leaves ample room for alternative interpretations, and it is easy for the favored interpretation to be influenced by one's advocacy position, whether one realizes it or not. Suppose, for example, that one documents a marginally significant impact of a spill on a resource of interest. The statistical variance may be high, so there is considerable uncertainty about the result. Whether one then interprets this finding as real evidence of a spill effect or instead discounts it may be strongly influenced by whether one tends to advocate the position of the natural resource trustees or of the responsible party. Scientific objectivity demands neither: the results should be interpreted without regard to the implications for the damage assessment or restoration processes. Only if this is done will those responsible for implementing the NRDA regulations have accurate information on which to base their decisions.

Advocacy also can become incorporated into conclusions through scientific speculations. Most scientists at some point speculate about what their results might mean, or about what chain of events might have produced the results. Because speculations deal with possibilities rather than actualities, they are particularly prone to the intrusion of advocacy positions. I have described elsewhere how speculations made following the *Exxon Valdez* spill became transformed into "facts" (Wiens 1996a). Suffice it to say that this can happen, particularly when the speculations are accepted and reported uncritically by the media; it is the scientist's responsibility to ensure that this does not happen.

Conclusions

If restoration efforts are to be founded on an accurate assessment of damages and recovery, it is essential that this assessment be based on scientific studies that are carefully designed to take into consideration the complicating effects of temporal and spatial variations in the environment. The studies and the interpretations of their results must be free of biases that result either from an inappropriate study design or from advocacy of one or another position. These points bear repeating, for in the rush to "do something" following a spill careful thought may not always prevail. Emotions can overwhelm objectivity, and principles of sound scientific design may be viewed as an extravagance that time and circumstances do not permit. When this happens, there are no winners, and well-intentioned restoration efforts may turn out to be ineffective.

References

Boersma PD, Parrish JK, Kettle AB. 1995. Common murre abundance, phenology, and productivity on the Barren Islands, Alaska: the *Exxon Valdez* oil spill and long-term environmental change. In: Wells PG, Butler JN, Hughes JS, editors. *Exxon Valdez* oil spill: fate and effects in Alaskan waters. Philadelphia PA: American Society for Testing and Materials. ASTM STP 1219. p 820–853

Day RH, Murphy SM, Wiens JA, Hayward GD, Harner EJ, Smith LN. 1995. Use of oil-affected habitats by birds after the *Exxon Valdez* oil spill. In: Wells PG, Butler JN, Hughes JS, editors. *Exxon Valdez* oil spill: fate and effects in Alaskan waters. Philadelphia PA: American Society for Testing and Materials. ASTM STP 1219. p 726–761

Day RH, Murphy SM, Wiens JA, Hayward GD, Harner EJ, Smith LN. 1997. Effects of the *Exxon Valdez* oil spill on habitat use by birds in Prince William Sound, Alaska. *Ecolog Appl* 7:593–613.

Exxon Valdez Trustee Council. 1993. Draft restoration plan. Anchorage AK: *Exxon Valdez* Trustee Council.

Fry DM. 1993. How do you fix the loss of half a million birds? In: *Exxon Valdez* Oil Spill Symposium Abstracts. Anchorage AK: *Exxon Valdez* Oil Spill Trustees Council. p 30–33

Lemons J, editor. 1996. Scientific uncertainty and environmental problem solving. Cambridge MA: Blackwell Science.

Mapstone BD. 1996. Scalable decision criteria for environmental impact assessment: effect size, Type I, and Type II errors. In: Schmitt RJ, Osenberg CW, editors. Detecting ecological impacts. Concepts and applications in coastal habitats. San Diego CA: Academic. p 67–80.

Paine RT, Ruesink JL, Sun A, Soulanille EL, Wonham MJ, Harley CDG, Brumbaugh DR, Secord DL. 1996. Trouble on oiled waters: lessons from the *Exxon Valdez* oil spill. *Annual Rev Ecol Systematics* 27:197–235.

Patten Jr SM. 1993. Acute and sublethal effects of the *Exxon Valdez* oil spill on harlequins and other seaducks. In: *Exxon Valdez* Oil Spill Symposium Abstracts. Anchorage AK: *Exxon Valdez* Oil Spill Trustees Council. p 151–154

Piatt JF, Lensink CJ, Butler W, Kendziorek M, Nysewander DR. 1990. Immediate impact of the *Exxon Valdez* oil spill on marine birds. *Auk* 197:387–397.

Schmitt RJ, Osenberg CW, editors. 1996. Detecting ecological impacts. Concepts and applications in coastal habitats. San Diego CA: Academic.

Shrader-Frechette KS, McCoy ED. 1993. Method in ecology. Strategies for conservation. Cambridge UK: Cambridge Univ.

Wiens JA. 1995. Recovery of seabirds following the *Exxon Valdez* oil spill: an overview. In: Wells PG, Butler JN, Hughes JS, editors. *Exxon Valdez* oil spill: fate and effects in Alaskan waters. Philadelphia PA: American Society for Testing and Materials. ASTM STP 1219. p 854–893

Wiens JA. 1996a. Oil, seabirds, and science. *BioScience* 46:587–597.

Wiens JA. 1996b. Coping with variability in environmental impact assessment. In: Baird DJ, Maltby L, Greig-Smith PW, Douben PET, editors. Ecotoxicology: ecological dimensions. London, UK: Chapman & Hall. p 55–70.

Wiens JA, Parker KR. 1995. Analyzing the effects of accidental environmental impacts: approaches and assumptions. *Ecolog Appl* 5:1069–1083.

3b

Discussion Paper 2 on Net Environmental Benefits Assessment for Restoration Projects After Oil Spills, or Some Reflections on the Decision Process

*Robin Cantor**

Jenifer Baker addresses the use of net environmental benefits assessment (NEBA) for the purposes of planning and evaluating alternative cleanup and rehabilitation options for oil-spill injuries to natural resources. A basic question I have stems from the NEBA terminology; is it being used as a general methodological term, or is there some formal reference for its source? As discussed in the paper, NEBA seems to be the author's recommended process for screening proposed restoration projects. How does it differ, for example, from an environmental impact assessment of alternatives, or a benefit-cost analysis of alternatives, or even a cost-effectiveness analysis, given a more narrow range of benefits? It would help the reader to have this recommended assessment process put into a decision-analytic context. It might also be appropriate to place it in a well studied response context, i.e., natural disaster planning, so that we could have a sense of the empirical basis for planning of this type.

It is encouraging to learn that there is 30 years of experience upon which to base an analysis of restoration alternatives. Methodological issues notwithstanding, that kind of empirical database can be very useful for informing purely theoretical or analytical claims about alternatives (actual demand-side management data has been valuable for engineering and economic estimates of performance). However, Baker does not provide a more formal analysis of this data. Where is the typology or schema to compare different cleanup and rehabilitation options? Presumably there are identifiable interactions with the characteristics of the damaged ecosystem, to which Baker alludes, but her discussion of advantages and disadvantages would benefit from parallel structuring of the factors considered.

I do not, however, want to criticize the natural science and engineering components of the paper. I will leave that to others and simply accept that cleanup and rehabilitation options differ in their rate, scope, and extent of resource restoration following an oil spill. I wish to address the other major conceptual aspect of the paper—the planning and decision implications of NEBA.

---

*Law & Economics Consulting Group

Baker's description of NEBA emphasizes that it is an approach which "weighs advantages and disadvantages of different cleanup and rehabilitation methods" (Baker, this volume). The author also suggests that NEBA is capable of identifying "areas of potential conflict and attempts to resolve them as completely as possible before any spill occurs" (Baker, this volume). Baker does not suggest how benefit categories are selected, how benefits are measured, how weights are determined, or how conflicts over weighting might be resolved.

In these respects, the paper avoids the hardest parts of the problem, which are the normative and methodological bases for measuring net benefits. How do we know when a change results in a benefit or a cost? Against what standard of measurement are we evaluating the change or ecological results of any rehabilitation option? How do we measure the social implications of different ecological changes? In more familiar terms, Baker has avoided the "which benefits?" and "benefits to whom?" questions that have confounded resolution of the environmental valuation debate.

Baker lists a number of human-use features liable to damage that might be considered in net benefits. This first step may mislead the reader, however, by indicating that once listed, it is a straightforward task to examine the comparative implications of different options across these features. Quite the contrary is known from decision analysis; a long and comprehensive list of consequences probably makes the task more difficult since it expands the number of comparative measures required for a complete evaluation of options (Kirkwood 1997).[1] To some extent, NEBA is facilitated by honing the list to the most critical features of comparison. This raises the obvious issue of how to determine the critical set.

"If you don't know where you're going, any road will do."

Kirkwood (1997) offers a succinct description of analytical steps for the strategic approach to decision-making:

1) specify objectives and scales for measuring achievement with respect to these objectives,
2) develop alternatives that potentially might achieve the objectives,
3) determine how well each alternative achieves each objective,
4) consider trade-offs among the objectives, and
5) select the alternative that, on balance, best achieves the objectives, taking into account uncertainties.

This description also oversimplifies the problem, but there is quite a bit of formal analysis that could have helped structure Baker's analysis. Formal structure will only help with the organization task, and it may do very little to assist with the social process of planning (contrary to some of the claims in Baker's paper). The social process necessarily involves a complex interaction among stakeholders, and my

[1] Careful thought should be given to the decision to exclude any objective, value, or area of concern.

remaining my comments will address what social science has to offer practitioners of NEBA.

Why is NEBA first and foremost a normative issue?

As presented by Baker in the paper and in the more general concept of the approach, NEBA involves a fundamental value judgment about good and bad. We all understand that benefits are good and costs are bad. The issue is which benefits and which costs? Many people have argued that nonuse values should not be part of the good–bad equation. What about benefits to other nations? What about global costs? What about future generations? What about highly uncertain benefits and costs? The list goes on, but the point is clear: every decision framework must set its boundaries as in Step 1 of Kirkwood's list, and often it is the selection of objectives that can be the show-stopper in complex environmental decision-making.

Each and every decision analytic framework is normative. We are not attempting to state how decisions *are* or *were* made, but rather prescribe how they *should be* made to maximize one or more objectives.[2] This is a fundamental but poorly understood feature of decision models and planning processes.

The concept of being best, optimal, or even "good enough" has no meaning in the absence of objectives. Just as there are different cleanup and rehabilitation options for responding to an oil spill, there are a number of different technologies for decision-making. Which one makes sense in the context of an actual decision problem is also a matter of comparing advantages and disadvantages. Like technologies, decision models require some commitment on the part of the user. Alternative frameworks impose different judgments about objectives and different underlying assumptions about key features of the decision process itself.

Let me describe a simple model of this particular problem. Years ago, during the height of a number of risk-assessment debates such as the coal versus nuclear choice, Funtowicz and Ravetz (1985) proposed a heuristic tool based on their extensive experience with difficult science policy decisions. They argued that the right assessment model depended on 2 factors present in all social planning and decision-making: *systems uncertainty* and *decision stakes*.

Systems uncertainty refers to the inexactness, uncertainty, and ignorance encountered by analysis of technological or natural systems. Decision stakes refer to the costs and benefits of the various policy alternatives as evaluated by the numerous, interested parties. The heuristic tool combined these factors and predicted the style of scientific analysis appropriate to the policy problem (see Figure 3b-1).

---

[2] I do not mean to suggest, however, that decision analysis is unconcerned with descriptive and predictive knowledge of decision-making. In fact, this is the basis of behavioral decision science. While I might argue that the best decision models are those that are well-grounded in the science of decision-making, this is nonetheless a value judgment.

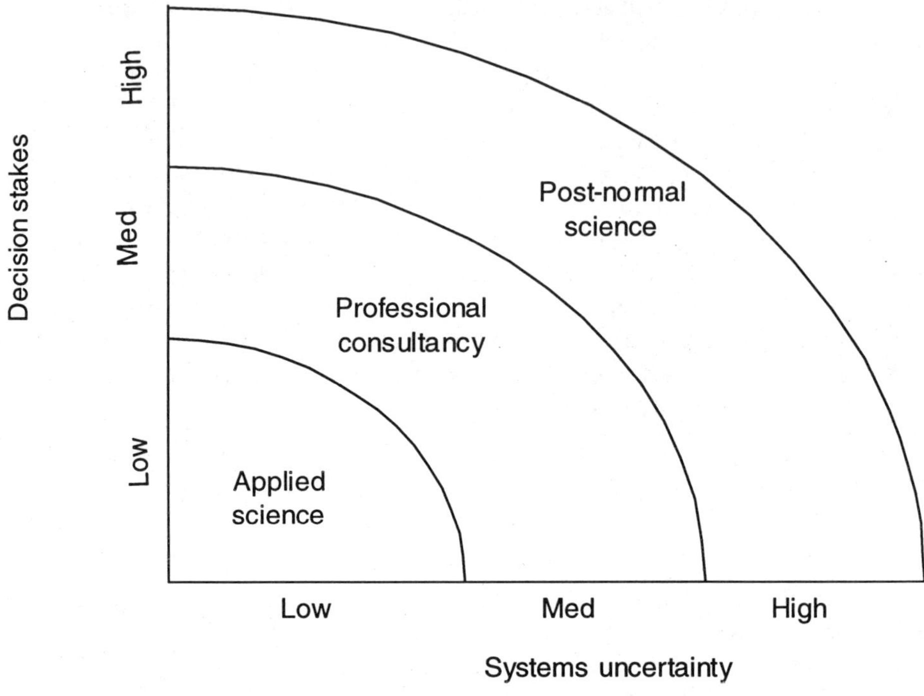

Figure 3b-1 Different types of scientific assessment

The Funtowicz and Ravetz heuristic articulated an awareness that many practitioners in the field of risk analysis had been developing for some time, that "the science involved in risk assessments is somehow radically different from that of classical lab practice" (Funtowicz and Ravetz 1992). Whereas the traditional approach in risk assessment was to "get the science right" for good decision-making, the combination of high systems uncertainty and high decision stakes led to decision processes which appeared to be immune from such appeals to scientific wisdom.

Funtowicz and Ravetz concluded that the real problem was with the formulation of the decision model. Applied science, they argued, viewed every problem as a well-defined puzzle, with a unique solution within its own terms. Professional consulting, as formalized by environmental assessment, environmental impact analysis, NEBA, regulatory impact analysis, and benefit-cost analysis among other techniques, recognized the complex and value-laden character of many problems, but maintained a presupposition of a stable and manageable context. In contrast, post-normal decision models not only recognize, but formally address, the roles of uncertain facts, disputed values, high stakes, and urgency in decision-making. Post-normal science comprises "a dialogue among stakeholders in a problem, regardless of their formal qualifications or affiliations" (Funtowicz and Ravetz 1992).[3]

Practical application of a post-normal science decision model requires

> an *extended peer community*, and they will use *extended facts*, which include even anecdotal evidence and statistics gathered by a community. Thus, the extension of the traditional elements of scientific practice, facts, and participants creates the elements of a new sort of practice. This is the essential novelty of post-normal science. In this way we envisage a democratization of science, not in the sense of turning over the research labs to untrained persons, but rather bringing this relevant part of science into the public debate along with all the other issues affecting our society (Funtowicz and Ravetz 1992).

The point is clear that this kind of dialogue, necessary as it might be, will be a challenge for those of us charged with defining objectives and measuring the net benefits of alternative planning options. Post-normal decision models are no less than a call to balance technocratic and democratic ideals. Net benefits are the result of such a balance, whether the analyst chooses to recognize this or not.

Is it more difficult to apply the net benefits concept to environmental planning?

Putting aside the general observation about decision stakes and systems uncertainty, is there good reason and science to believe that environmental decisions (such as planning for oil-spill response) represent a special class of decision problems? In other words, is there something special about environmental decisions that fundamentally affects the conceptualization and measurement of net benefits?

Baker sees a valuable role for NEBA in contingency planning and suggests it may help identify areas of potential conflict over which interests (e.g., ecological or human) receive more weight in the response plan. Missing from her discussion is a consideration of the extent and intensity of these conflicts, and here we can learn something from similar efforts to reconcile the interests of diverse stakeholders. In particular, we can make use of some empirical generalities about conflicts in environmental decision-making. Controversies about lost-use values, and environmental valuation more broadly, are instructive even though NEBA need not reduce alternatives to monetary outcomes.

Implicit in the author's discussion for setting priorities for response is an understanding that trade-offs are likely to be the rule, not the exception. Although some literature (e.g., Porter and vand der Linde 1995) about "no-regrets global change policies" and environment-competitiveness relationships suggests there may be some free lunches

---

[3]Other labels for this type of decision model exist; for example, the National Research Council (NRC) uses the term analytic deliberative process (NRC 1996).

in life, most environmental choices involve difficult and sometimes severe trade-offs. What seems to be special about environmental decision-making is not the magnitude of the trade-off, but the type of trade-off involved. In this sense, environmental planning shares with risk management the problem of multidimensionality.[4]

We know from 2 decades of research in risk perception that particular dimensions of the risk problem elicit very different and sometimes extreme behavioral responses. An easy dimension to understand is the child or infant receptor, where risks to children elicit higher concerns than risks to adults. A harder dimension to interpret is the manmade versus natural source of the hazard.[5]

What dimensions of the environmental planning problem are likely to cause conflicts among stakeholders? While this area lacks the empirical base supporting our knowledge of risk, the following dimensions have been widely discussed in the context of valuing environmental assets and consequences:

- Unfamiliar goods and unfamiliar institutions: to the extent that people do not come into contact with particular environmental goods and services, or their managing institutions (through the market or otherwise), these aspects of the planning problem may be unfamiliar. People worry more about unfamiliar risks than familiar ones, and this may transfer to risks of unfamiliar environmental resources.
- Time scale: environmental improvements occurring at different and much separated points in time will need to be placed in a common context. Discounting to reflect the trade-off between current and future values is the traditional approach. Discounting affects the selection of public investments and the rate at which society depletes natural resources. The higher the discount rate, the more we will favor investments that yield rewards sooner than later. This discrimination against the future has generated a long history of debate about the right rate of discount for social investments, especially in the context of environmental planning.[6]
- Intergenerational consequences: closely linked to the time scale dimension, a number of ethical and practical concerns stem from how we treat future generations.[7] To what extent do our decisions show that we have been good stewards for future generations? Is it morally wrong to subject future generations to potentially catastrophic risk? Again, we know that people react more

[4] The concept of multidimensionality and attributes of choice are closely related. A central difference, however, is the scope of analysis. Psychologists have tended to focus on the dimensions, while economists have tended to focus on the object, good, or service.

[5] For a summary, see Covello (1985).

[6] See Pearce and Turner (1990) for a nontechnical summary of the issues and Lind et al. 1982 for a more technical treatment.

[7] For a summary of the arguments, see Spash (1993).

intensely to catastrophic and irreversible risks; why should we not anticipate similar reactions in the context of environmental changes?

- Individual and group perspectives: traditional approaches to measuring benefits emphasize the aggregated returns to self-interested individuals. It has been argued that some environmental evaluations derive not from the norm of consumer sovereignty, but they involve an alternative collective norm. Acceptance of community norms may lead to planning rules such as the precautionary principles or safe minimum standards, even where such rules appear to be at odds with private rewards.[8]
- Cultural conflicts and systemic functions: even when implementing a planning exercise within a single, well-contained community, analysts often encounter a number of cultural views on nature. Anthropological research demonstrates a strong link between social organizations and particular views of nature as fragile, robust, resilient, or capricious.[9] Different views are likely to generate conflicts among stakeholders that cannot be easily predicted by attention to the benefit categories alone. (See Table 3b-1 for a summary of viewpoints by different social organizations.)

Table 3b-1 Social organization and preferred environmental principles

Social organization	Image of nature	Moral imperative	Response strategy
Egalitarian	Fragile	Don't mess with nature	Prevention
Market	Robust	Don't curb growth	Adaptation
Bureaucracy	Resilient	Preserve choice	Sustainable development
NIMBY	Capricious	Don't tread on me	Fatalism

Source: Cantor and Rayner 1994

Summary

Baker's paper presents a reasonable recommendation that different cleanup and rehabilitation options for oil-spill response planning can be productively evaluated with NEBA. The paper appears to be sound technically, but it falls short of examining the difficult issues confronting any process of decision-making. I would have preferred to see more consideration of objectives, trade-offs, and potential conflicts. I hope my brief review of insights from the decision and risk sciences helps readers appreciate the complexity and challenge entailed by NEBA and other formal decision models when they are faced with a contentious planning problem.

---

[8] In fact, concern for the system, rather than the individual, is at the core of many arguments in ecological economics (see Daly and Cobb 1989). Similar arguments support rationales for recycling even in the face of poor economics (see Ackerman 1997).

[9] For an extensive empirical study of the issues, see Kempton et al. (1995).

References

Ackerman F. Why do we recycle? Markets, values, and public policy. Washington DC: Island. 210 p.

Cantor RA, Rayner S. 1994. Changing perceptions of vulnerability. In: Socolow R, Andrews C, Berkhout F, Thomas V, editors. Industrial ecology and global change. Cambridge, UK: Cambridge University.

Covello VT. 1985. Socila and behavioral research on risk: uses in risk management decision-making. In: Covello VT, Mumpower JL, Stallen PJM, Uppuluri VRR, editors. Environmental impact assessment, technology assessment, and risk analysis. New York NY: Springer-Verlag.

Daly HE, Cobb JB. 1989. For the common good: redirecting the economy toward community, the environment, and a sustainable future. Boston MA: Beacon.

Funtowicz SO, Ravetz JR. 1985. Three types of risk assessment. In: Whipple C, Covello VT, editors. Risk analysis in the private sector. New York NY: Plenum.

Funtowicz SO, Ravetz JR. 1992. Three types of risk assessment and the emergence of post-normal science. In: Krimsky S, Golding D, editors. Social theories of risk. Westport CT: Praeger.

Keeney RL, Raiffa H. 1993. Decisions with multiple objectives: preferences and value tradeoffs. Cambridge UK: Cambridge Univ. 589 p.

Kempton WM, Boster JS, Hartley JA. 1995. Environmental values in American culture. Cambridge MA: MIT. 336 p.

Kirkwood C. 1997. Strategic decision-making. Belmont CA: Wadsworth. 270 p.

Lind RC, Arrow KJ, Corey GR. Discounting for time and risk in energy policy. Washington DC: Johns Hopkins Univ. 468 p.

[NRC] National Research Council. 1996. Understanding risk: informing decisions in a democratic society. Washington DC: National Academy Pr.

Pearce DW, Turner RK. 1990. Economics of natural resources and the environment. Baltimore MD: Johns Hopkins Univ. 392 p.

Porter ME, van der Linde C. 1995. Toward a new conception of the environment-competitiveness relationship. *J Econ Perspect* 9(4): 97–118.

Spash CL. 1993. Economics, ethics, and long-term environmental damages. *Environ Ethics* 15:117–132.

3c

Discussion Paper 3 on Net Environmental Benefits Assessment for Restoration Projects After Oil Spills, or An Appeal for a More Quantitative NEBA

Thomas A. Campbell, Andrew L. Strong

The *Exxon Valdez* net environmental benefits analysis

If we had it all to do over again, would we steam clean the cobble beaches of the Prince William Sound?

We would hope the answer now would be "no." In the early days of the *Exxon Valdez* response, a group of scientists approached upper management of the National Oceanic and Atmospheric Administration and asked for funding to conduct a net environmental benefits analysis (NEBA). Their hypothesis was that the steam cleaning of the cobble beaches was actually doing more harm than good. Their testable hypothesis was that the diversity and density of species at the control site would, over time, exceed the diversity and density at steam-cleaned beaches. Seven control sites were cold-water cleaned only; the remaining beaches were steam cleaned.

To no one's great surprise, the steam-cleaned beaches through the years have had consistently fewer species present than in the control areas. The densities of any given species have also been depressed. The conclusion is apparent. From a biological perspective, one would have to conclude that the steam cleaning of the majority of the beaches in the Prince William Sound did not provide a net environmental benefit. From a public policy perspective, it may be fair to say that Exxon was forced to pursue a cleanup strategy, at the cost of more than $1 billion dollars, that may have produced a significant environmental detriment.

The need for NEBA supported by testable hypothesis

The environment is like a patient and the cleanup team is like a physician. The Hippocratic Oath of medicine dictates that the physician's first concern should be to "do no harm." Those charged with cleanup should abide by the same rule. The burden should be upon those who would seek a cleanup or remedial action to show that it would produce a net environmental benefit. If the action would not, then the action should not be pursued.

The leading edge of a steam rake can do every bit as much harm to a cobble beach as oil. The good intentions that placed the steam into motion will not protect the beach from injury.

If it was all to be done over again, would we have the tools to allow a public policy-maker to make a different choice? Net environmental benefit analysis, as described by Baker, would be of marginal use. As described, it is purely qualitative. It weighs unrelated factors without description of how they might be compared. The paper presents a truly insightful collection of examples of cleanups that have gone too far and of other instances where cleanups have not gone far enough. The upside and downside of a number of cleanup methodologies are skillfully discussed. The author points out some of the factors that might be considered, but provides precious little guidance as to how they might be weighed. In essence, we are told that they should be weighed, but not how.

Net environmental benefit assessment can be more quantitative and can provide results that are supported by testable hypotheses. These results could in turn be used by policy-makers to "do the right thing" in controversial situations.

NEBA can compare biological and human-use service losses by incorporating concepts developed from the use of habitat equivalency analysis

Baker states that "NEBA weighs advantages and disadvantages of different cleanup and rehabilitation methods (including restoration by entirely natural processes)." While weighing advantages and disadvantages is a useful endeavor, Baker acknowledges that the NEBA process, as she envisions it, is a purely qualitative endeavor. A slight change in this proposed definition would add a very important quantitative dimension that would be helpful in both making and defending NEBA decisions.

The following is an alternative definition:

NEBA weighs the risk of ecological and human-use service losses that may result from different cleanup and rehabilitation methods (including restoration by entirely natural processes).

The problem often presented when making quantitative NEBA comparisons has been the lack of a common metric. Habitat equivalency analysis (HEA), an economic model developed by NOAA and the Department of the Interior (DOI) for scaling restoration options, was founded on the basic concept that ecological service losses could be compared against ecological service gains. Why couldn't the service losses that would result from one cleanup approach be compared to the service losses from another approach in order to determine the superior approach? Moreover, wouldn't it also make sense to compare the service losses of a cleanup approach to the service losses associated with a natural recovery approach? To demonstrate how this is done, it is necessary to introduce some basic concepts.

Ecological services

Habitat equivalency analysis expresses anthropogenic influences (or the risk of influences) in terms of ecological services. Ecological services are those services provided by natural resources, e.g., the capture of sunlight for food, shelter, nutrient recycling, recreational uses, commercial uses, etc., that are valued directly or indirectly by humans. Ecological services derive from habitats.

How habitat equivalency analysis works

Habitat equivalency analysis models the economic value of losses and gains in ecological services and has been used as a metric to quantify environmental obligations for restoration compensation. It has been applied to many different types of habitats (riverine, wetlands, forest, fields, marshes, bogs, etc.). Habitat equivalency analysis relies on a unit of measurement that takes into account temporal and spatial gains and losses in ecological services. The unit of measurement is a service acre year (SAY).

In the example below, the environmental debit associated with a cleanup alternative is evaluated using the SAY metric. In this example, there is the risk of reduction of service of approximately 25%. It is projected that this reduction in services will persist for 5 years, but that within 2 years, the impacted system will begin to recover. Based upon past experience, the rate of recovery is projected which defines the shape of the recovery curve. In order to account for the fact that some of the services will be lost at some time in the future, a discount rate of 3% is applied so that the service losses can be evaluated in their present value. Figure 3c-1 takes into account only a single acre and represents the services lost in an impacted acre over the years.

The model projects the service losses over the total number of acres impacted over time. The model result is expressed in units that are discounted to represent their present value—a discounted SAY. In this example, the result was a deficit of 4400 SAYs.

A number of factors must be considered to project the percentage reduction in ecological services that would occur as a result of a particular activity. Figure 3c-2 describes the suite of ecological services that come from a warm-water stream habitat. The team conducting the NEBA would have to evaluate the relative importance of the services provided by that habitat. Then an assessment of the potential risk to those services is made.

This is followed by a projection of the likely reduction to each of those services. This in turn is translated into a weighted average that allows the team to project the percentage of ecological service reduction that would result from a given alternative.

The weighted service reduction figure is then used in the HEA model. When comparing cleanup options, the same approach is used for each alternative to ensure consistency and a fair comparison.

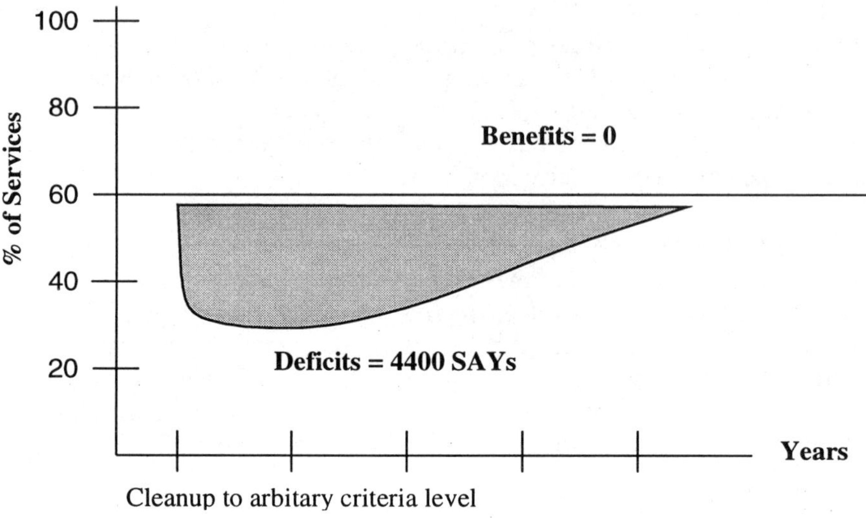

Figure 3c-1 HEA calculates lost ecological opportunity cost of performing cleanup activity

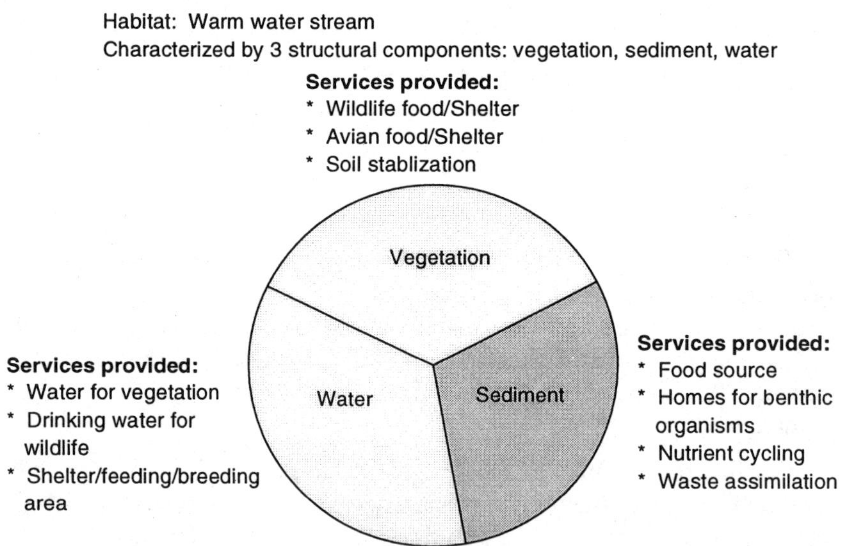

Figure 3c-2 Weighted averages of multiple services

Comparing cleanup alternatives

Habitat evaluation analysis was created to scale restoration efforts to injuries to habitats. However, there is no reason that SAYs cannot be used to compare the risks associated with alternative cleanup options. In Figure 3c-3, a natural recovery alternative is compared against a more aggressive cleanup approach. The natural recovery alternative projects an 800 SAY loss in ecological services, while the more aggressive cleanup alternative projects a 3300 SAY loss. The result of pursuing the more aggressive alternative would be a loss of 2500 SAYs greater than the loss that would be created by allowing natural recovery to occur.

Looking at this for a moment from a natural resource damage (NRD) perspective, the NEBA would also project that the cleanup alternative would significantly increase a potentially responsible party's (PRP) exposure for resource damages. The irony of this type of situation is that if the PRP were compelled to pursue the more aggressive

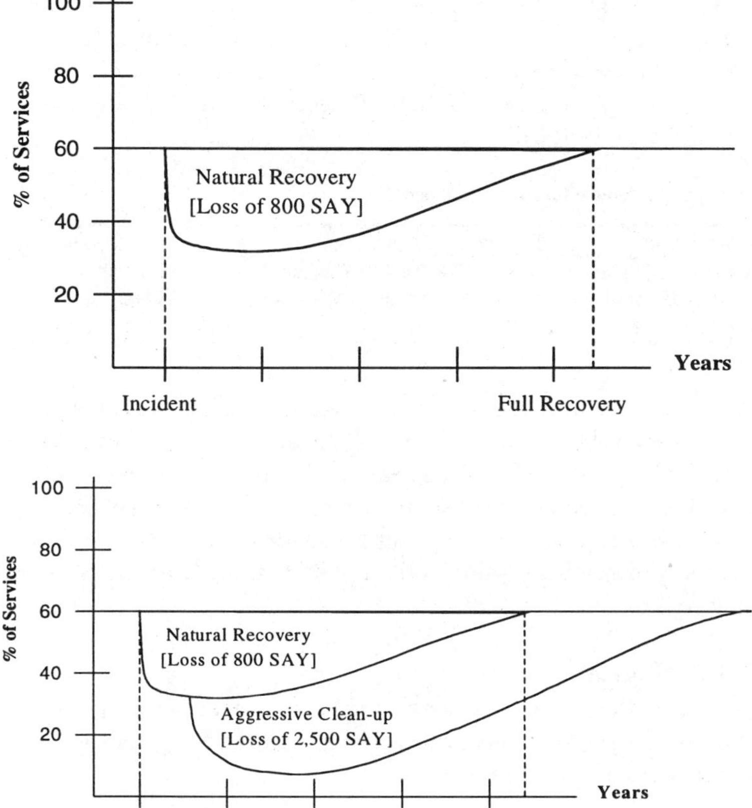

Figure 3c-3 Case study: natural recovery versus aggressive cleanup approach

cleanup approach, it would essentially be paying cleanup contractors to increase its NRD liability. From a public policy perspective, a NEBA would project that the more aggressive cleanup alternative would do more harm to the environment than good and, therefore, should not be pursued.

More quantitative NEBA provides opportunity for interim corrective restoration measures

In some instances, the use of the SAY metric in the NEBA process will fail to provide a clear choice. The aggressive cleanup alternative may only produce a marginal benefit over natural recovery alternative (or some other alternative). In such an instance, it may be good public policy to allow the PRP to proffer an interim corrective restoration measures (ICRM) alternative. Continuing with the previous example, if the NEBA did not rule the "aggressive alternative," but rather it was recognized that there was the risk of significant continuing loss of ecological services for which some action was necessary, and if there was significant expense associated with that alternative, the PRP could be given the option of proffering an ICRM. That ICRM, in many cases, would be a restoration alternative that provides the same service benefits that the continuing presence of residual oil contamination would create. The ICRM, in many cases, would provide far more real benefit than the aggressive cleanup alternatives at a much reduced cost (see Table 3c-1).

Table 3c-1 Cleanup options and associated costs/benefits

Cleanup/restoration option	Ecological benefits/costs	Transactional costs
Natural recovery + restoration	(800 SAY) + 5000 SAY = 4200 SAY	$1,000,000
Cleanup (small scale) + restoration	(1500 SAY) + 4000 SAY = 2500 SAY	$3,000,000
Aggressive cleanup (large scale)	(3300 SAY)	$10,000,000

The public would benefit because the "aggregate performance" of the ecosystem can be restored or improved. When dealing with human health issues, the health and well-being of the individual is paramount. When dealing with an ecosystem, our central concern should be for the health of the system as a whole. The removal of anthropogenic influences (e.g., agricultural runoff, loss of detritus) on one part of an ecosystem can aid in the recovery of another portion of the system that has been damaged or impaired by an oil spill.

Restoration of ecological services

When functions and services in an ecosystem component are impaired, those injuries can be compensated for elsewhere in the ecosystem so that the ecosystem aggregate performance is either restored or improved.

Conclusion

A more quantitative NEBA can be performed using concepts borrowed from HEA. Policy-makers need to focus public concern on the direct and indirect services that the affected area provides the public. The risk of service losses from alternative cleanup methodologies should be compared using the SAY metric (or other service-based metric). The alternative that produces the smallest SAY debit should be given the greatest weight in the ultimate decision process. Natural recovery should always be considered as an alternative.

If a relatively costly alternative produces a relatively marginal additional benefit, then the PRP should be given the option to proffer interim corrective restoration measures that would offset the service losses created from leaving residual contamination in place. The goal of providing this alternative would be to ensure that the aggregate performance of the affected ecosystem be continued to the extent possible at pre-spill levels.

A quantitative NEBA using a service loss metric will assist in making and defending controversial cleanup decisions. It will also allow us to understand the risk of ecological and human-use service losses early in the cleanup process, and it will provide the opportunity to consider interim corrective restoration measures, thereby reducing cleanup costs and ensuring the continued undiminished aggregate performance of the affected ecosystems.

4

Enhancing Damaged Public Assets: Perspectives from Landscape Architects and Planners

Diana Balmori, Michael T. Huguenin†, Robert E. Unsworth†, Anton P. Giedt§[1]*

This conference focuses on restoration of human uses of the environment lost because of the release of a hazardous substance or the discharge of oil (hereinafter termed "incident"). Natural resource trustees seek to compensate the public for loss of use and enjoyment through projects that will enhance future public uses of the injured environment. Such projects are termed "compensatory restoration" in the National Oceanic and Atmospheric Administration's (NOAA) natural resource damage assessment regulations for oil spills and are recognized as addressing "compensable value" under the Department of the Interior's (DOI) natural resource damage assessment (NRDA) regulations.[2]

Here, we address questions of how compensatory restoration projects for lost human uses can best be identified and evaluated. We consider

- What kinds of projects are appropriate to restore human uses that are commonly lost?
- What features of projects are most important to people?
- How can projects be connected to the specific human uses lost and the environmental setting that was injured?
- What kind of public involvement is useful?

To these questions we bring the perspective and knowledge of landscape architects and planners—disciplines with a core concern to enhance human use and enjoyment of outdoor environments in an ecologically sound manner. In so doing, we hope to

*Balmori Associates, Inc. & Yale University

†Industrial Economics, Incorporated

§National Oceanic and Atmospheric Administration

[1]The views and opinions expressed in this paper are solely those of the authors and do not necessarily represent the position of the United States Department of Commerce, National Oceanic and Atmospheric Administration, or the United States Government. The authors thank Emly McDiarmid of Yale University for helpful comments on earlier drafts of this paper.

[2]15 C.F.R. §§990.10 — 990.66 (NOAA Natural Resource Damage Assessment Regulations for OPA: §990.30 & §990.53(c) Compensatory restoration); 43 C.F.R. §§11.10 — 11.93, as amended (DOI Natural Resource Damage Assessment Regulations for CERCLA and the CWA: §11.83(c)(1) Compensable value).

add to the thinking of the natural scientists, economists, public resource managers, and attorneys already working on these issues in many settings.

The question of *how much* restoration is necessary to fairly compensate the public for lost use and enjoyment is important but is not our focus here. Ways in which restoration projects might be "scaled" to achieve a fair balance between the public's loss from the environmental injury and gain from compensatory restoration are active areas of research and debate. We offer some insights about scaling compensatory restoration projects at several points in this paper.

We have organized this paper into 5 sections. First, we summarize the statutory basis for compensatory restoration claims and suggest how landscape architecture and planning may provide useful tools for meeting the requirements of the law. Second, we reflect briefly on the nature of the human use and enjoyment typically impaired by the release of oil or hazardous substances to the environment. Third, we propose a general principle of design useful when creating or evaluating projects to enhance human uses of the environment. Fourth, we suggest ways to improve public involvement in the process of developing compensatory restoration projects. Finally, we present 2 illustrations showing how our general principle might be used to create compensatory projects for typical incidents.

Legal basis for compensatory restoration

Claims for natural resource damages under federal statutes such as the Comprehensive Environmental Response, Compensation, and Liability Act (CERCLA or Superfund) (42 U.S.C. §9601 *et seq.*, as amended; §9607(a)(4)(C) and (f) [liability for natural resource damages]), the Clean Water Act (CWA) (33 U.S.C. §1251 *et seq.*, as amended; §1321(f)(4) and (5) ([liability for natural resource damages]), and the Oil Pollution Act of 1990 (OPA) (33 U.S.C. §2701 *et seq.*, as amended; §2702(b)(2)(A) and §2706 ([liability for natural resource damages]) have their genesis in the common law theory of tort in that they provide a mechanism to compensate the public for injury to natural resources resulting from hazardous substance releases or oil spill incidents. Unlike common law, however, natural resource damage (NRD) claims are not necessarily constrained by the common law precedent that recovery be limited to the "diminution in value" of the thing that was lost. Indeed, a key motivating force behind the NRD provisions of CERCLA was Congress' dissatisfaction with the common law and the desire to "make whole" the environment and the public through remedial actions and the restoration of natural resources adversely affected by the release of hazardous substances.[3]

Accordingly CERCLA, CWA, and OPA all provide for the recovery of damages (monetary compensation) by federal, state, or tribal natural resource trustees for injury to, destruction of, loss of, or loss of use of natural resources resulting from an incident. These statutes include the mandate that the primary method for measuring damages

[3] *See State of Ohio v. U.S. Department of the Interior,* 880 F.2d 432, at 445 fn.9 (D.C. Cir. 1989).

is the cost of restoration, rehabilitation, replacement, or acquisition of the equivalent of the injured natural resources and natural resource services to the condition that would have existed had the incident not occurred. The NOAA regulations under OPA have defined this component of the NRD claim as "primary restoration," and this term has begun to find meaningful application in the CERCLA context as well. In addition to the cost of primary restoration, these statutes authorize the recovery of damages for the "interim lost use" or "services" of the injured natural resources pending the completion of primary restoration or natural recovery.[4] The statutes explicitly require that all damages recovered by natural resource trustees, including restoration costs and interim lost use damages, must be used only for the restoration, rehabilitation, replacement, or acquisition of the equivalent of the injured natural resources.

The DOI and NOAA regulations provide standards and procedures for assessing NRDs under CERCLA, CWA, and OPA, respectively (43 C.F.R. §§11.10–11.93, as amended [DOI Natural Resource Damage Assessment Regulations for CERCLA and the CWA]; 15 C.F.R. §§990.10–990.66 [NOAA Natural Resource Damage Assessment Regulations for OPA]). With respect to interim lost human uses, a fundamental principle under these regulations is that trustees must develop alternatives that address the injured natural resources from which human uses flow. The restoration objectives must be specific to the injuries and cannot replace the human uses that were lost in isolation without attention to the underlying environmental injury (see Unsworth et al., this volume). Both agencies have incorporated into their regulations requirements for public and potentially responsible party participation.[5]

Neither the regulations nor the experience of NRD practitioners provide guidance about how best to synthesize the ecological and human-use objectives of the restoration process. We suggest that the general design principle set forth in this paper may serve as one tool to address interim lost human use in a practical and effective way because the principle helps synthesize the ecological and human-use objectives of the restoration process in a manner that also is consistent with the requirements of CERCLA, CWA, and OPA.

The nature of human uses lost

The public derives enjoyment from natural resources in many ways, all of which can be adversely affected by injuries to natural resources. Common lost uses involve beach

---

[4]While this paper focuses on the restoration of lost human uses, note that interim lost ecological services also are included in this damages category, i.e., the services the environment provides to itself.

[5]*See* 43 C.F.R. §§11.82(c) — (d), as amended (DOI Natural Resource Damage Assessment Regulations for CERCLA and the CWA directing trustees to develop a range of restoration alternatives that take into consideration the services provided by the alternatives and 10 factors for trustees to consider in selecting among the alternatives); 15 C.F.R. §§990.53 — 990.55 (NOAA Natural Resource Damage Assessment Regulations for OPA providing detailed guidance on the nature of compensatory restoration, a hierarchy describing how to evaluate and select acceptable projects and evaluation standards for selecting preferred restoration alternatives).

visits; fishing from shores, piers, and boats; boating and canoeing trips; swimming, snorkeling, and SCUBA diving; hiking, camping, visiting national parks and monuments; and wildlife viewing. The impairment or interruption of public uses can range from a complete elimination of the activity in cases where, for example, an oil spill and associated clean up effort force officials to close beaches to any public use, to reductions in the quality of the activity in cases where, for example, fish can be caught but not eaten due to contamination, or visitors to a national park must endure the smell of oil fumes during their visit. Obviously, the range of possible quality reductions is broad.

The time period over which human uses are lost also can vary. Lost uses from oil spills and related clean up activities can continue for weeks or months, with beach and waterway closures ending earlier but fishing restrictions and perceptions of environmental degradation continuing for longer periods. Chronic releases of hazardous substances to the environment, for example the release of polychlorinated biphenyls from contaminated sediments, can impair human uses of natural resources for decades. In these settings, compensatory restoration projects may be needed to enhance the public's use and enjoyment of a resource that remains contaminated while protecting the public from the contamination.

Proximity of the incident to human populations, as well as the specific resource and human uses affected, influence the magnitude of the insult. Oil spills near urban beaches can result in hundreds of thousands of lost or diminished beach visits over a few weeks. Injury to natural resources further from human populations may affect fewer people but diminish human activities of particularly high value if people travel great distances to enjoy the resource or spend considerable time once there.

These factors suggest that a broad variety of restoration projects are required to compensate for lost human uses. Restoration planners must consider

- the specific environmental injury suffered and the types of human activities impaired;
- whether quantity or quality of uses, or both, are affected;
- the duration of the impact, particularly if the environmental injury is continuing; and
- the proximity of human populations, how they travel to the resource, and the duration of their use once there.

A general principle for design of compensatory restoration projects

Two recent developments in the field of landscape architecture—a greater reliance on ecology and the emergence of the linear park—can help us think about compensatory restoration projects. We discuss each of these developments below.

Insights from ecology

Ecology is defined here as the study of the relationships between living organisms and their environment. Ecology has highlighted the importance of scale and shown the greater fragility of small fragmented and isolated pieces of landscape. Ecology also has given us a unit of landscape—the watershed—whose health can be measured. The watershed has become one basic unit by which landscapes are measured and monitored. The work of Herbert Bormann and others at Hubbard Brook has given great specificity to work in the landscape (see Bormann and Likens 1979). Alternatives to the watershed are being examined for this purpose but though we know of the fragility of fragments we do not yet know what size a forest or a prairie, for example, must be to survive. In the face of uncertainty about necessary sizes, the general response has been to create continuity, connecting small fragments.

The work of John Cairns in restoration ecology directly supports the need for continuity of landscapes (Cairns and Heckman 1996). Cairns in addressing restoration of landscapes has listed 5 points that touch on the need for continuity: 1) large systems are more likely to be self-maintaining than fragments of systems; 2) economies of scale are as present in ecological restoration as they are in many other activities; 3) large ecological activities are likely to generate more publicity than restoration of small fragments or patches and thus may be better protected from future damage because of increased public awareness; 4) patch dynamics (e.g., shift of a patch from a source or a sink of a particular species) function well at the landscape level but not as well at the fragment level (which might not even be large enough for a single effective patch); and 5) distribution of seeds and other propagules is more likely to be effective if an array of diverse habitats is available or if heterogeneous habitats at least have the potential to develop in the same area being restored.

The need to create continuity has brought the corridor to the attention of ecologists and landscape planners and has resulted in laws protecting continuous hedges in England and creating passages for wildlife under major highways in the U.S. The main argument for the effectiveness of corridors for wildlife populations centers around metapopulation theory. The argument states that increased immigration among fragmented habitat patches will increase species richness and diversity, increase population sizes of particular species, permit reestablishment of extinct local populations, and prevent inbreeding depression. Corridors also provide increased foraging area for wide-ranging species and provide routes for movement between habitat areas if environmental injuries make current habitats unsuitable.[6]

[6] We note that the utility of corridors for wildlife is currently under debate. The potential disadvantages of corridors are that they may facilitate the spread of epidemic diseases, insect pests, exotic species, weeds, and other undesirable species into reserves and across the landscape. Corridors may also facilitate the spread of fire and other abiotic disturbances or increase exposure of wildlife populations to predators. Further research will partly answer these questions. We refer readers to *Science* 270:1428–1429 for a complete discussion of these issues.

While there is debate about the ecological advantages and disadvantages of corridors, there is consensus that corridors are effective in connecting fragmented landscapes. Linking landscape fragments is particularly advantageous at the edges of streams. When human uses extend to the edge of a stream, these uses can cause fragmentation of the riparian corridor and can thus diminish its function as a connecting element within the landscape. Aquatic ecosystems are degraded along and downstream from bare stretches. Water quality at a given location may be only as good as the most degraded reaches upstream. Restoring the connectivity of riparian corridors can be a strategy for maintaining or improving water quality.

Excessive alteration of upland and riparian vegetation can reduce the movement of fish and other aquatic organisms upstream and downstream. Extreme changes in water quality caused by urban and agricultural development have been shown to isolate populations in stream networks. Intact riparian corridors maintain connectivity and movement pathways for aquatic organisms. Similarly, linking forest fragments is advantageous to plant communities, and the continuity of forest cover aids the overall health of the forest.

The recent San Diego "Model" Nature-Habitat Plan illustrates the importance of continuous landscapes. Under the plan, specific undeveloped sections of land will be acquired and permanently set aside for protected natural habitat while other open land will be set aside for development. As much as possible the land set aside for protection will be continuous in order to create continuous rather than fragmented landscapes. The plan is backed by Secretary Bruce Babbitt of the United States Department of the Interior and has drawn favorable comment from Senators John H. Chafee (Rhode Island) and Dirk Kempthorne (Iowa) who are considering national legislation along the lines of the San Diego plan.[7]

The linear park

The second development in landscape architecture which can be of use in compensatory restoration projects is the linear park, a narrow continuous corridor of land used for walking and biking. Linear parks are being promoted as a new kind of open space by citizens' associations across the country. The popularity of linear parks among millions of Americans seeking places to walk or bike, and the ecological vision of unfragmented landscapes and the value of corridors, join these 2 developments. The linear park socially and the corridor environmentally both can serve the design of compensatory restoration.

People are much less interested today in parks as isolated destination points. They seek paths that make for a pleasant journey, valuing the journey above the destination. The creation of a corridor gives the opportunity to make the damaged area only one of several alternatives and makes the corridor the uniting and predominant experience. At the same time, corridors can serve to unite discontinuous fragmented pieces of

---

[7] The San Diego Plan is described in an article in the *New York Times*, March 20, 1997, page A16.

open space, parks, cemeteries, ball fields, river edges and compose them into a larger healthier continuous green space. Piecemeal treatments of a landscape have not been the best use of resources: erosion of one part of a stream cannot be solved just by treating the place where erosion started. Rather, erosion at one location requires an evaluation of the whole of the stream's watershed. The linear park, in conjunction with the immediate watershed of the area damaged, is a restoration option that has the appropriate scale and specificity.

We argue that a promising approach to compensating for lost human use is the enhancement of the damaged public asset by connecting the area damaged to other facilities or amenities via a corridor of the dominant landscape in which it is contained; to attract users, to diffuse and redirect users to alternate destinations: another beach, forest, marshland, scenic view of similar characteristics or to more than one destination, bestowing in this way a variety of landscapes within walking or biking reach from the damaged area. The damaged area thus becomes part of a system rather than the sole attribute of a place.

A linear corridor that joins the damaged area to alternative and additional locations by means of a beautiful green ribbon such as a walking and biking trail offers compensation for the sense of loss of quality in the environment. It increases environmental health by adding trees and other vegetation with their cooling, noise-abating, and water-absorbent surfaces in a macadamized suburban and urban world. It provides a link from one isolated fragment of landscape to another.

Literature on continuous corridors and linear parks provides support for these ideas. "Corridors perform several other critical functions [than to serve as routes or conduits for movement]—they act as species filters, as habitats for certain species, and as a source of environmental and biological effects on their surroundings" (Forman and Godron 1986). "Since the presence or absence of breaks in a corridor is considered the most important factor in determining the effectiveness of both the conduit and barrier functions, connectivity is the primary measure of corridor structure" (Baudry 1984; Forman and Godron 1984; Merriam 1984). It is connectivity that gives corridors their ecological value. In an interesting parallel it also is connectivity that gives value to human users of linear parks.

Forman and Godron's work on the importance of corridors also has shown how the different origins of a corridor will affect its physical characteristics and the mechanisms by which it is maintained. The origins of a corridor have a direct effect on its physical characteristics and on the species dynamics of its flora and fauna. Environmental resources corridors, which follow faults and streams in the landscape; planted corridors, which are purposefully manufactured; and regenerated corridors, which result from regrowth in areas disturbed by human activity, are all relatively permanent elements of a landscape. Human involvement, whether direct or indirect, may bring an element of constancy to the corridor and become an integral part of its ecosystem (Forman and Godron 1986).

Walking has become the top recreational activity of Americans. Over 100 million Americans walk 2 to 3 times per week. Ninety-three percent of Americans walked outside in the past year. Those walkers averaged 15 walks in the last mild weather month; 75% walk specifically for exercise. The majority of Americans (56%) support increased funding for safe and secure pedestrian and bike pathways. Sixty-one percent of all adults say they would start walking or walk more often if they had access to safe secure pathways. Among cyclists who do not currently commute, 40% or 25 million would start commuting if they had access to safe bike paths.

The Northern Central Rail Trail in Maryland is a good illustration of the popularity of these new kind of corridors. From 10,000 visitors per annum in 1984 it has grown to over 450,000 in 1993, a compound annual attendance growth rate of 53% per year. A survey of users indicated that 94% of the survey respondents feel that the Northern Central Rail Trail is a good use of State funds; two-thirds of respondents like greenways better than traditional, more confined parks; over 95% of respondents view the Trail as an asset to their community; less than 2% of respondents feel unsafe on the Trail; and nearly two-thirds of respondents feel that the trail enhances nearby property values (PKF 1994).

Data on trails being built across the country confirm the experience of the Northern Central Rail Trail and show the popularity of trails and the expenditures associated with them. The quotes below are from one recent study (RTC 1997).

> Just how much can a rail-trail impact a community? One study found that the average user of the Heritage Trail in rural Iowa spends $9.21 per day. The figure for Florida's Tallahassee-St. Marks Trail was $11.02, and for urban California's Layayette-Moraga Trail, $3.97. With use in the tens and hundreds of thousands, the total annual economic benefit for each of the 3 trails ranged from $1.2 million to $1.8 million per year.
>
> The downtown area of Dunedin, Florida was suffering a 35% storefront vacancy rate in the early 1900s until an abandoned CSX railroad track became the phenomenally successful Pinellas Trail. Now, storefront occupancy is 100%, old establishments are remodeling, and business is booming.
>
> Peak-season hotel rooms along Wisconsin's 32-mile Elroy-Sparta State Park Trail are booked up to a full year in advance. A state study of the trail revealed that the destination is so desirable that the average visitor travels 228 miles to experience it. Half of all the trail's users are out-of-state visitors who bring "new" money into Wisconsin.

Another measure of the importance of these new linear parks is the added value to property near them. The Burke-Gilman Trail is one of the oldest of these new linear parks and has yielded the first information on property value impact (City of Seattle 1987).

> Property near but not immediately adjacent to the Burke-Gilman Trail is significantly easier to sell and, according to real estate agents, sells for an average of 6% more as a result of its proximity to the trail. Residents who bought their homes after the trail was opened are most likely to view the trail as a positive factor that increases the value of their home. Real estate advertisements that promote properties as being on or near the trail tend to be from the companies that regularly sell homes near the trail. In other words, people who have recently been involved in the real estate market near the trail are more likely to have experienced the economic assets of the trail.

We turn now to the questions of how large and how close to users must a corridor be to generate human usage. The required scale of the linear corridor and its proximity to users enters into more familiar territory for architects and planners, though there are not yet universal standards (Ryan 1993). A planning standard widely used in the field of landscape architecture and urban design is the half-mile measure. The standard was derived from experiences and observations made on American campuses, and is the maximum distance people will walk to reach their destination; for a longer distance they will get into their car. In linear corridors it is considered the distance that people will veer from the corridor to reach an attraction or destination. In linear parks it defines the area of attraction for the amenities along its length. As to the useful lengths of the corridors, emerging experience indicates 2 to 5 miles for walking and 5 to 10 miles for biking.

The availability of standards from landscape architecture and planning, such as a minimum effective length of a bike path, has direct relevance for scaling projects to compensate for interim losses. The scale of a selected option initially will be determined based on the loss that was incurred. For example, an oil spill that results in a beach closure might have led to the loss of 5,000 beach visits. In this case trustees will look for options that restore 1) the same number of trips (NOAA's "service-to-service" scaling approach); or 2) provide a substitute recreational attribute equal in value to the lost beach visits (the "valuation" scaling approach). However, in scaling options that restore lost services, the trustees should be aware of the standards used by architects and planners. For example, a 2-mile bike path or a half-mile seaside walk may not be large enough to create the value envisioned by the trustees and responsible parties.

Similar concerns have been raised in some cases regarding the minimum scale of proposed wetlands restoration projects and the feasibility of very small scale species protection efforts. The existence of minimum standards for both ecological and human-use restoration projects, combined with the economies of scale achieved in planning for and implementing larger-scale projects, supports the concept of regional restoration plans. For example, a program might be established to create a significant new beach use opportunity in an urban area funded through recoveries from small-scale spills that result in short-term closures or other quality effects at regional beaches.

In our view, fusing these 2 recent developments in landscape architecture and applying them to compensatory restoration yields an important general principle: development and enhancement of continuous unfragmented landscape corridors will increase the quantity and value of human uses of injured areas while promoting ecological health.

Enhancing public involvement

We turn now to the issue of public involvement. Experience with compensatory restoration suggests that trustees generally involve the public in 2 ways. First, trustee representatives often contact local officials to ask for ideas about suitable compensatory restoration projects. This process results in a list of projects of interest to local governments, but the projects often have a limited relationship to the environmental injury and human uses lost. (We are aware of one incident where a new firehouse was proposed as compensation for lost beach visits.) In addition, contacting local officials provides very little information about the preferences and attitudes of the actual users of the resource. Public officials have little time or information to create new restoration project ideas and are hard pressed to predict how the public would respond to such projects.

The second way trustees involve the public is to request public comments on a draft Restoration Plan document. This process, set forth in NOAA's regulations, involves public release of the document, one or more public meetings, and an opportunity for the public to submit written comments to the trustees within a set period of time (usually 30 to 60 days.) The Restoration Plan document describes the nature and duration of environmental injuries, the restoration alternatives considered, and the restoration alternatives preferred by the trustees. Unfortunately, when the Restoration Plan is released for public comment the time for creative thought about compensatory restoration projects may be past. In addition, in our experience there are often very few public comments submitted, suggesting that the public is not particularly engaged in the process.

We believe that users of natural resources have much to offer designers of compensatory restoration projects. The question is how best to involve users in a creative process with planners and resource managers. John Cairns has given us the most compelling reason for public involvement: "no landscape level restoration will endure if undertaken without society's approval and support" (Cairns and Heckman 1996).

Quality of life has emerged as the most important ingredient in the general attraction, success, and viability of an area and a city. Cities and regions that offer quality of life are the ones that surge ahead, attracting population, investment, and new businesses. The conference on cities of North America, held in New York City in 1995, concluded that social and environmental factors are as important as economics to the health of cities (see Anonymous 1995). The elements that make up this quality of life are many, but a beautiful and healthy environment is at the very top followed by opportunities to use it. Here we return to walking and biking trails and their popularity in polls across the nation.

A first step at incorporating public preferences at a very broad level is to look at national trends given by polls as to prevailing public views about use of open space and recreation; then to follow this with regional polls on the use of open space in the area. A local poll in the community affected may be useful in identifying elements that are important to quality of life. It is important to bring in the public early in the process of putting a compensatory plan together and particularly important and useful to bringing in local land trusts or citizens groups involved in clean up, maintenance, or other activities in surrounding public open spaces or trails.

Professionals in the design fields have different methods with which to elicit public response early in projects. First of these is to present options in the form of drawings that make ideas tangible and help the public visualize them. This is an effective form of public education. People in other lines of work do not think of the possible options of design because they have not been trained to do so. But they can respond intelligently and add observations of great value to specific scenarios that they visualize using the drawings.

The second form of public interaction is the public charrette, a more involved process in which options are put up for the public to see. The public is then divided into smaller groups each around a table, and on a map of the area given to each participant, all are invited to mark elements, places, details, and responses which they feel are important. Each map is discussed and the designer and helpers (one at each table) make a composite of the ideas, working them into one design as a written summary at the end of the session. This is followed by another session at which the designer shows visuals of the agreed-upon summary.

There are many variations upon both of these methods. For example, one may start with a brief meeting to provide background information about the region and the environmental problem and examples of design solutions developed for similar problems, followed by a public charrette. Drawings resulting from the public charrette may be made at the session as the discussion is taking place. In all cases, the essential feature of public involvement is the education of the designer by the public and of the public by the designer.

Illustrations

In this section we present 2 very general cases to illustrate how compensatory projects might be designed for typical environmental injuries. The cases involve 1) an oil spill near an urban center that results in several hundred-thousand lost beach visits over a period of 2 weeks, and 2) contaminated sediments in a 20 mile stretch of a river in a populated southern state. The contamination results in a restricted fishery as well as warnings to avoid contact with river and fringing marsh sediments.

The best projects for compensatory restoration in any specific incident would depend on many details specific to the incident. Our purpose here is to illustrate application of our ideas rather than propose specific projects for oils spills or contaminated rivers.

Urban oil spill

An oil spill has resulted in closure of 5 miles of beaches for a period of 2 weeks. The beaches adjoin a major metropolitan area and are heavily used by both residents who walk and drive to the beach and by tourists staying in local hotels. Common beach activities include walking, nature viewing, swimming, sunbathing, and picnicking. There also are paved paths running along parts of the beach for jogging and cycling. The trustees estimate that approximately 200,000 beach visits were lost from the affected beaches during the closure. All signs of the oil were removed from the beaches before they were reopened, and beach usage levels quickly returned to normal.

The most straightforward way to compensate the public for lost beach visits would be to implement projects that result in additional beach visits in the future. In theory at least, such projects could be scaled so that the present value of future incremental beach visits equals the 200,000 visits lost from the spill. We term such projects "quantity-enhancing."

Quantity-enhancing projects are surprisingly difficult to develop. In our experience beaches rarely are capacity or access constrained, so that acquisition of additional beach acreage, improvements to parking areas, better stairways to the beach, and similar projects often will not result in an overall increase in beach visits. Instead, such projects simply draw visitors away from other beaches with no overall gain in usage at all beaches.

The experience of landscape architects suggests a slightly different approach to the design of quantity-enhancing projects. Public corridors such as linear parks may increase use from people who formerly made limited use of fragmented parks or similar destination landscapes. This suggests that well-designed corridors running to or along beaches may increase usage. Some users will stop and enjoy the beach as do present users, engaging in swimming, sunbathing, and similar activities. Other users will enjoy the beach in a different way simply by weaving the sight, sound, and smell of the beach into regular walks or bike journeys. Both types of users will be drawn to the beach by the green corridor that leads there rather than by more traditional access or capacity improvements to the beach itself.

Oil spill restoration often includes projects to protect or improve important habitats such as salt marshes, seagrass beds, and mangrove forests as compensation for ecological injuries. Public access through or adjacent to these areas via linear parks or corridors will generate visits by the public. Although a different experience, such visits may be appropriate compensation for the beach visits lost and will contribute to a sense of improved environmental quality and quality of life in the area injured by the spill. The green corridor connecting restored areas may have ecological benefits as well.

Once restoration planners conclude that quantity-enhancing projects cannot be developed, they often design projects that either 1) increase the value of each beach visit for beach users by improving beach amenities such as vegetation, bathrooms, and so forth; or 2) increase human enjoyment of other environmental resources through acquisition of park lands, nature preserves, and similar resources. Designing and scaling such projects to fairly compensate for lost beach visits is a difficult and controversial undertaking and is not the subject of this paper. We point out, however, that the experience of landscape architects and the design principal of continuity suggest the kinds of projects that are likely to be of most interest and value to the public. At many sites, projects that enhance the continuity of public areas and reduce the fragmentation of the landscape will be favored from both a human-use and ecological point of view.

Contaminated river sediments

Release of a toxic substance from an industrial facility has contaminated the sediments and floodplain along a 20-mile stretch of a river in the southern U.S. The levels of contamination in the sediments and in resident fish are sufficient to prompt public health advisories (i.e., children should avoid contact with the sediments, and all should avoid eating fish from the river). The contaminated portion of the river is located near several towns that are popular weekend destinations.

The trustees estimate that 10,000 additional fishing trips per year would take place but for the contamination and that 1000 recreational boating trips per year have been reduced in value as a result of the contamination. Other forms of recreation also have been affected by the contamination, but have not been quantified by the trustees. In addition, surveys of the public indicate widespread concern regarding the contamination; for example, visitors to a nearby state park frequently express concerns over the perceived health risks to children picnicking near the river, and several local communities have experienced difficulties attracting investors for river front development projects, in part because of the perceived poor quality of the river's environment. While site remediation actions are expected to eliminate future releases to the river, sediment contaminant levels will remain elevated well into the future.

Situations with continuing contamination present special problems for restoration planners. While projects to increase or enhance public uses in other places can be developed, it would be desirable to enhance public use and enjoyment of the injured environment itself. But this must be done carefully in order to protect public health and not interfere with primary restoration efforts or natural recovery.

Compensatory restoration projects might be designed to create access to the river for safe activities such as walking, biking, picnicking, or canoeing but discourage water contact activities such as wading or swimming from shore. Public use areas might be sited along the river but with natural buffer zones such as wetlands to make direct access to the river difficult. This green buffer also will aid the health of the river by providing shoreline vegetation and a floodplain. Constructed overlooks or boardwalks can be developed in some areas to enhance visual proximity to the river. Direct access points to the river for boat or canoe use can be sited in areas where sediments are cleaned and ramps and docks provided to ensure no human contact with contaminated sediments during launching and recovery of watercraft.

Connecting a series of riverside open spaces with trails or bikeways would increase the overall usage and value of these areas to the public. Connectivity to open space amenities as well as public transportation, highways, and urban/suburban attractions would integrate the river as one element of many that attract public usage. A beautiful walk or bike ride with a variety of attractions will enhance overall use of the river.

How best to communicate with public users of these areas through appropriate signs and displays should be an important design consideration. Rather than the usual "Do Not Fish or Swim" signs, displays might be created that tell the story of the river's ongoing recovery, present status, additional actions needed, areas of special concern, and so forth. In addition, public involvement might be fostered by organizing volunteers for river watches, water quality monitoring, and similar activities. The emphasis is not so much education but participation in the process of recovery. Knowing what in fact is happening to the river over time and participating in the recovery process return a sense of confidence to the public.

References

[Anonymous]. 1995. The rise of quality-of-life issues. *Progressive Architecture* October 1995.

Baudry J. 1984. Effects of landscape structure on biological communities: the case of the hedgerow network landscape. In: Brandt J, Agger P, editors. Proceedings of the First International Seminar on Methodology in Landscape Ecological Research and Planning. Volume 1. Roskilde, Denmark: Universitetsforlag GeoDuc. p 55-65.

Bormann FH, Likens GE. 1979. Patterns and processes in a forested ecosystem. New York NY: Springer-Verlag.

Cairns Jr John, Heckman JR. 1996. Restoration ecology: the state of an emerging field. *Annual Review Energy Environment* 21:173.

City of Seattle. 1987. Evaluation of the Burke-Gilman Trail's effect on property values and crime. Seattle WA: City of Seattle Engineering Department, Office for Planning.

Forman RTT, Godron M. 1984. Landscape ecology principles and landscape function. In: Brandt J, Agger P, editors. Proceedings of the First International Seminar on Methodology in Landscape Ecological Research and Planning. Volume 5. Roskilde, Denmark: Universitetsforlag GeoDuc. p 4-15.

Forman RTT, Godron M. 1986. Landscape ecology. New York NY: Wiley.

Merriam G. 1984. Connectivity: a fundamental characteristic of landscape pattern. In: Brandt J, Agger P, editors. Proceedings of the First International Seminar on Methodology in

Landscape Ecological Research and Planning. Volume 1. Roskilde, Denmark: Universitetsforlag GeoDuc. p 5-15.

PKF Consulting. 1994. Analysis of economic impacts of the northern central rail-trail. Annapolis MD: Maryland Greenways Commission.

[RTC] Rails-to-Trails Conservancy. 1997. The economic benefits of rails-to-trails conversions to local economies. Washington DC: Rails-to-Trails Conservancy.

Ryan KL. 1993. Trails for the twenty-first century: planning, design, and management manual for multiuse trails. Washington DC: Rails-to-Trails Conservancy.

4a

Discussion Paper 1 on Enhancing Damaged Public Assets: Perspectives from Landscape Architects and Planners

*Carol E. Dinkins**

When a lawyer critiques a paper that sets forth the perspectives of landscape architects and planners on issues of compensation for damages, the lawyer first must note the legal regime governing liability for such damages. Although litigation has attended claims for natural resources damages (NRDs), considering the magnitude of potential claims and the complexity of legal issues that could be litigated, much remains to be debated concerning these damage provisions of the Comprehensive Environmental Response, Compensation, and Liability Act (CERCLA), the Clean Water Act (CWA) and the Oil Pollution Act (OPA). Construction of these laws and application of the regulations promulgated under them remains to be tested, in large part, in the courts. Although there has been only limited litigation, there has been considerable discussion concerning the concepts and calculations attendant upon assertions of damage claims for natural resources. Balmori, Huguenin, Unsworth, and Giedt have explored an intriguing area—the potential for developing or enhancing environmental corridors and linear parks to compensate for environmental injuries. Rather than explore the underlying legal issues inherent in assertion of NRD claims, this critique instead will examine the suggestions as if the underlying legal issues of whether liability exists, damages are provable, and compensation is calculable are settled issues.

Two sets of regulations govern natural resource damage assessments (NRDAs) and 2 distinct federal cabinet-level departments are responsible for dealing with these situations. The Department of Commerce's National Oceanic and Atmospheric Administration (NOAA) is responsible for events arising under OPA and the Department of the Interior (DOI) is responsible for those arising under CERCLA or the CWA. Their implementing regulations are different, not surprisingly, as NOAA had a decade of DOI's experience to guide development of its regulations. These distinctions make a difference because the NOAA regulations, which on their face are shorter and assign greater discretion to the trustees, govern oil spills, not the presence of hazardous substances that may have been released to the environment decades before the enactment of CERCLA or the CWA.

---

*Vinson & Elkins L.L.P., Houston, Texas

Another circumstance to note is that most damage claims will involve water bodies, water courses, or coastal waters. The Oil Pollution Act establishes liability for the discharge of oil "into or upon the navigable waters or adjoining shorelines." The CWA also includes hazardous substances within its ambit but it too regulates discharges to navigable waters, which is defined as waters of the United States. CERCLA is broadly worded, but many of its NRD claims are associated with waters of the U.S.

The authors make an essential point that always must guide the trustees: "The restoration objectives. . .cannot replace the [lost] human uses. . .without attention to the underlying environmental injury." Thus, although many desirable projects may exist, the trustees always must be mindful of the actual environmental injury in setting restoration objectives.

An essential point the authors omit is that restoration projects can be extremely costly. Their paper was not intended to address calculation of damages, which is an area potentially ripe for debate, but unless the damages that can be proven or agreed upon are quite significant, the types of projects here discussed may be so large that public or other types of funding may be required to supplement a NRD component, unless some number of NRD cases jointly provide the funding.

The authors point out that landscape ecology is an increasingly recognized principle and then set forth a general principle of design in which they describe the importance of continuity of landscapes and how this need for continuity can lead to environmental restoration through the creation of corridors. After noting the importance of continuity, the authors report that consensus exists that "corridors are effective in connecting fragmented landscapes." They reference the San Diego Habitat Plan, which actually is a forward-looking plan to set land aside for conservation purposes prior to development, rather than a restoration plan to reverse impacts and restore habitats.

The authors do not discuss specific corridor environmental restoration projects, but certainly good examples do exist. Although not as part of any NRD case, in the Texas Rio Grande Valley, The Nature Conservancy of Texas has made restoration of South Texas brushland corridors an essential project to restore the big cats—ocelot and jaguarundi—to Texas. The U.S. Fish and Wildlife Service has designated this area as one of its highest priorities. The Conservancy, in cooperation with private landowners, is replanting corridors of native brush such as mesquite and huisache to provide cover for the cats. The Nature Conservancy also owns an excellent example of native brushland, Chihuahuan Woods, and it hopes to connect that preserve to the Rio Grande River to provide the cats with an unbroken conservation corridor to the border. These types of projects can succeed. In the Malpai Borderlands in Arizona and New Mexico, a group of ranchers and The Conservancy are working to restore rangeland through grassbanking, prescribed burning, and managed grazing. Last year a jaguar, long thought to be an extinct species in the U.S., was sighted in the area.[1]

---

[1] *Wall Street Journal*, Sept. 24, 1996, page A1.

But for the matter at hand, the question is whether seeking construction of corridors to restore fragments of such ecological landscapes provides a restoration alternative for damages to natural resources and lost human uses. Conservation or environmental corridors definitely could provide restoration through equivalent resources, but could these be also as effective a compensation for lost human use? Hopefully they could, given their potential importance to natural resources, and thus the authors suggest joining the environmental benefits of corridors with the social benefits of linear parks to design compensatory restoration. They set forth several examples and describe their popularity and economic impact focusing on conversion of abandoned railroad rights-of-way to hike and bike trails as is provided in the Rails-to-Trails Act[2] (Manlange 1989; Ryan; Interstate Commerce Commission 1993).

What the authors did not really discuss, however, is that conversion of these rights-of-way can create substantial controversy. Adjacent landowners are concerned about security, trespassers, and other intrusions. Objections to conversion can quickly dissuade state officials from pursuing such projects.[3]

The authors also did not address a recent development in the Rails-to-Trails program, a development that has the potential to increase the cost of conversion of such corridors. Although the U.S. Supreme Court in *Preseault v. United States*[4] upheld the constitutionality of the Rails-to-Trails Act on its face, it concluded that a remedy might exist for the Preseaults in the Federal Claims Court under the Tucker Act for a Fifth Amendment taking. The plaintiffs subsequently filed such a claim. The trial court found for defendant United States and was initially upheld on appeal to the Court of Appeals for the Federal Circuit.[5] The Federal Circuit thereafter decided to hear the case en banc, and reversed and remanded to the trial court[6], finding that the Preseaults' land had been taken in contravention of the Fifth Amendment, but noting that it was not holding every exercise of government authority under the Act to be a compensable taking.[7] This apparently was a difficult case. The en banc decision came well more than a year after the panel's ruling, and then it was a noticeably split decision, 4 for the majority, 2 concurring, and 3 dissenting. As dissenting Judge Clevenger wrote, "The Preseaults have a victory, but the court's holding has no

[2]The Rails-to-Trails Act was enacted on March 28, 1983, as part of the National Trails System Act Amendments of 1983. Pub.L. No. 98-11, Title II, 97 Stat. 42, 48 (codified at 16 U.S.C. §1247(d) (1994)). The amendments are part of the National Trails System Act, which was first enacted on October 2, 1968. Pub.L. No. 90-543, 82 Stat. 919 (codified as amended at 16 U.S.C. §§1241-51 (1994)). A large amount of material has been published by the Rails-to-Trails Conservancy concerning the conversion of railroad rights-of-way to hike and bike trails.

[3]Telephone interview with Andrew Sansom, Executive Director, Texas Parks and Wildlife Department, April 25, 1997.

[4]494 U.S. 1 (1990).

[5]66 F.3d 1167 Withdrawn (Fed. Cir. 1995).

[6]100 F.3d 1525 (Fed. Cir. 1996).

[7]100 F.3d 1552 (Fed. Cir. 1996).

precedential value."[8] Several cases are pending at the Claims Court under the Rails-to-Trails Act.[9]

Concerning the issue of public involvement, the authors note that the trustees generally have used one of two ways to involve the public and neither appears to work well. They suggest 2 alternatives: to use polls or the public charrette.

I agree with the concept of bringing the public early into the process, and I note parallels with the National Environmental Policy Act alternatives analysis, a generally understood and accepted process. However, in the NRDA context, experience teaches that polls can be expensive, time-consuming and, depending upon the circumstances, of questionable benefit. A reliable, less costly, and altogether simpler course may be to focus this effort with local land trusts, conservation or parks organizations, and similar groups. Their members will include affected users in the community, and they are likely to have a reservoir of knowledge about both historical use and potential project ideas.

The authors suggest that the need for a minimum scale for restoration projects supports the concept of regional restoration plans. This suggestion bears further development, given the necessary scale and cost of various types of restoration projects. One large-scale wetlands restoration project will provide a greater environmental benefit and potentially greater opportunity for human use, such as bird watching, than would several dozen small projects. Better and more extensive public and resource agency input likely could be achieved as well.

One final note is that an aquatic ecosystem can be degraded as a result of many causes, and an oil spill or release of a hazardous substance may not noticeably alter a baseline condition. Significant causes of degradation can include combined sanitary and stormwater sewer outfalls that bypass treatment plants, untreated nonpoint source runoff, atmospheric deposition, and historic massive filling of wetlands adjacent to the watercourses. Any one or all of these examples may make a watercourse or waterbody inhospitable to aquatic organisms and dangerous for public uses such as swimming or fishing. If the area in question has been so impacted, a regional restoration plan in such instances would be costly and necessarily involve a great many more parties and implicate legal regimes beyond those of NRD. In such instances, the restoration plan necessarily must exist in a context greater than that of NRD.

In conclusion, the authors suggest approaches that are practical and that could result in projects beneficial to the environment, the public, and the process. A 5-year retrospective to identify whether any have developed and evaluate whether they actually have come to fruition will be welcome.

---

[8]100 F.3d 1555 (Fed. Cir. 1996).

[9]Telephone interview with James Brookshire, U.S. Department of Justice, April 30, 1997.

References

Manlange CH. 1989. Preserving abandoned railroad rights-of-way for public use: a legal manual.

Ryan KL. Secrets of successful rail-trails: an acquisition and organizing manual for converting rails into trails and trails for the twenty-first century; planning, design and management.

Interstate Commerce Commission. 1993. A guide for public participation in rail abandonment cases under the Interstate Commerce Act. 4th Edition.

4b

Discussion Paper 2 on Enhancing Damaged Public Assets: Perspectives from Landscape Architects and Planners, or Recoverability: Setting the Stages Necessary for Restoration

*Leslie Sauer**

Balmori, Huguenin, Unsworth, and Giedt examine 3 major issues: the legal basis for compensatory restoration, general principles for restoration, and the role of linear parks in restoration. I will address the same topics from the same perspective; as a landscape architect, restorationist, and planner. While the conference in general centers on restoring lost human uses specifically, for the purpose of this paper, I have made no distinction between natural and cultural/social values and uses. I have assumed them to be integrated and interdependent.

Recoverability: the basis for restoration

The primary goal of the U.S. Department of the Interior (DOI) and the U.S. Department of Commerce, National Oceanic and Atmospheric Administration (NOAA) regulations for compensatory restoration is to go beyond defining loss as "diminution in value" to the concept of the need to "make whole" the environments impacted by spills and discharges. The regulatory process is intended to restore, rehabilitate, replace, or acquire the equivalent natural resources and natural resource services after the release of a hazardous substance or the discharge of oil. The objective is to restore the landscape and associated uses to the condition that would have existed had the incident not occurred. The most important assumption underlying these efforts is that full recovery is possible. Therefore the actual recoverability of the landscape is of essential importance to defining and scaling appropriate compensation as well as to developing implementation strategies for restoration projects.

At this time we actually have little evidence that recovery to a prior condition is probable or even possible. Ecosystems demonstrate remarkable resilience, but recovery after major human-induced perturbation is spotty at best. For example, invertebrate and amphibian populations do not return to previous levels even more

*Andropogon Associates, Ltd., Philadelphia, PA

than a century after clear-cut logging. Vernal herbs disseminated by ants also fail to recover, even a century later. Today, many natural ecosystems are degrading rapidly, losing species at accelerated rates, and experiencing pervasive biochemical changes such as high levels of nitrogen deposition from air pollution and eutrophication of soil and water systems. The findings of a survey conducted for the National Biological Service, a research organization within DOI, by Drs. Reed F. Noss, J. Michael Scott, and Edward T. LaRoe finds that scores of ecosystems are imperiled and are dependent on a limited array of fragments that are already too compromised to even sustain existing levels of biodiversity. Each assault further limits recoverability. The reality is that there are many simultaneous disturbances going on everywhere, some chronic, some episodic. In this context it is difficult to talk realistically about recovery to the condition that would have existed had the incident not occurred. Many human uses that are lost are also intimately yoked to the quality of the preexisting landscape and hence to recoverability. Even if the lost number of visitor days is recouped, for example, there is a continued loss of value if the habitat is impoverished. Many quality-related human values are the least likely to be quantified such as the lost educational value of a landscape where students no longer have a chance to observe local examples of once-common native communities, or the loss of that site as a potential source of propagation material for restoring species not easily found elsewhere. We can never truly quantify or scale loss. There is a point at which our energies are better directed toward optimizing for restoration in the broadest possible context.

The goal to make a landscape whole again is, despite the challenges, the most appropriate goal. It is, in fact, the only one that has any chance of working at all; the fragmented approach has already failed. It would be impossible to overemphasize the importance of the context of the landscape to the concepts of restoration and recoverability. You cannot fully restore a fragment of an ecosystem, a small piece of an estuary, or a stretch of a stream. They are still connected to and dependent upon the larger system. Therefore the broadest possible perspective on restoration, not of individual sites or impacted areas, but of ecosystems, will best serve to underpin the intent of the legislation. This approach also has the additional virtue of not being limited by our very narrow understanding of the actual impacts of any incident. Even though we cannot possibly fully quantify impacts or ever compensate for them item by item, we can make a commitment to maximize the opportunity to fulfill this goal of broad-based restoration.

General principles: preconditions for compensatory restoration

The credibility of any effort to determine appropriate compensation is limited by the baseline data available about the site. The concept of compensatory restoration that the agencies subscribe to requires that baseline data be available before, not just after, a mishap. The lack of an adequate national database is a serious flaw that must be addressed if the concept of compensatory restoration is to be fully implemented.

An important corollary to the prerequisite of monitoring is the need to minimize the damage that occurs in the first place. Only when we have identified valuable natural resources, no matter how subtle, are we able to protect those resources. In January 1990 I visited the Arthur Kill, which is the river between New York and New Jersey, 3 days after an oil spill from a ruptured pipeline beneath the river. The air burned my eyes, and the clothes I wore smelled so bad afterward that I threw them away. I could smell the oil on my skin for days.

How much of this damage was not necessary and could have been avoided? The spill was far larger than it might have been because it was undetected for half a day due to failed emergency equipment. The alarm had been ignored because it went off so routinely. Although every wharf and pier was swathed in batting and cordoned off with absorbent booms, the tidal creeks had not yet been boomed off. Even 3 days after the spill, the incoming tide brought in a fresh wave of contaminants, as it had 6 times previously because the creeks were not identified as resources to be protected on the Coast Guard maps. Indeed no natural areas at all were so identified, despite how few and irreplaceable all remaining remnants and derelict lands are in this heavily industrialized waterway. Two-thirds of the colonial shorebirds of the Atlantic Flyway, for example, spend some time on 1 of 3 dredge spoil islands in the Arthur Kill, according to the Trust for Public Lands Harbor Herons Project. Nor was this the last spill in the Arthur Kill; 9 more followed that year alone.

At the same time, the spill brought about important progress toward saving and restoring these remnants through compensatory restoration. Subsequent compensation for this spill has included vital baseline monitoring and has funded innovative restoration efforts. Dr. Marc Matsil of the Natural Resources Group (NRG) of the New York City Department of Parks and Recreation, working closely with NOAA and others, has demonstrated that both clean-up and restoration can be dramatically enhanced by replanting marsh vegetation.

Events such as the ones listed above highlight another aspect of restoration: who actually pays for it? In the end it may be insurers who drive the process of risk reduction. The same factors causing increased losses in property and casualty insurance will also influence costs for hazardous spills and discharges. The increased level of storminess already associated with global warming as well as the associated increase in wave intensity and rising sea level will magnify the impacts of episodic occurrences such as oil spills. The greater magnitude of storms and waves also increases the likelihood of a spill occurring in the first place. Because natural disaster-related claims have created heavy property and casualty losses recently, the need to reduce the damage from hazardous discharges and oil spills, whether it be via double-hulled tankers or effective planning for risk-reduction, must take greater precedence if insurance underwriting for hazardous materials handling is to continue to be available at reasonable cost.

It is important to note at this point that taxpayers are already being asked to take on levels of risk that private insurers are unwilling to accept. In the state of New York for example, taxpayers temporarily carried extra risk (that they were largely unaware of) when private companies failed to meet state deposit requirements for underwriters. The state was forced to suspend its own rules in order to maintain the availability of insurance. As the risk gets greater, more and more of the burden is being transferred to the public. Even as the Red River of the North joins the number of rivers with unprecedented flooding patterns, the federal flood insurance program, which is also inadequately underwritten, was advertising its toll-free number on TV. Simultaneously there are significant political pressures to loosen environmental regulations, undermine wetlands protection, and continue to subsidize sprawl and land speculation by public funding and taxing policies.

In addition to resource monitoring and planning to reduce risk, an effective compensatory restoration program must have a plan for regional-scale ecosystem restoration. At the present time, however ironic, funds from damage awards and settlements represent the most reliable source of funding for restoration. Each incident represents a potential infusion of investment in the form of compensation. Dr. Marc Matsil (NRG) also demonstrates how effectively resource protection can be accomplished by using monies that become available due to damages and settlements that have taken place. The monies are used well when there is both an effective strategy in place to systematically acquire fragments to make a more continuous protected habitat and a program for monitoring and management. A monitoring program would also help distinguish those impacts due to chronic rather than episodic disturbance and better define losses (needed in order to scale compensation appropriately). A strategic plan for regional-scale restoration would require and foster inter-agency cooperation as well as public and private partnerships and community involvement. This strategy greatly enhances the recoverability of the landscape and larger ecosystem as a whole.

Because the local community greatly influences the landscape all the time, any efforts to enhance recoverability and reduce damage must involve the local community as well. Public involvement also is crucial to overcoming problems associated with the intermittent activity and investment derived from damage claims. Consultants brought in to develop a compensatory restoration plan as well as the regulators involved may have very little direct familiarity with the landscape in question, especially if this is a federal-level project in a district spanning several states. Public involvement is an important key to ensuring continuity. In addition, local knowledge of the landscape may avert a costly mistake.

The corridor concept

Linear parks, as proposed by the authors, are an excellent example of the kind of asset enhancement that results from thinking more holistically about compensatory restoration projects and integrating human and natural ecology. The concept of giving emphasis to corridor creation as a vehicle for restoring lost human uses serves to greatly enhance recoverability of the landscape as a whole as well. Connectedness is an absolutely essential quality for restoring and sustaining ecosystems. Corridors managed as natural habitats are not as likely to be lines of invasion as are corridors of disturbed habitat which are unfortunately, now, a far more common condition. The object is to learn how to manage corridors well. They can serve as vital lines of species regeneration after a major perturbation such as an oil spill. The reestablishment of associated species of plants and wildlife in a replanted salt marsh, for example, will be very much impacted by the quality, as well as the presence or absence of, corridors connected to other natural areas.

A common argument against taking on linear projects such as trails, especially where an incident is localized, is the anticipated added complication of a multi-jurisdictional regulatory process. Our experience, in practice, is that compensatory projects of regional significance and value galvanize both public attention and support. A good example is the Cross Jersey Trail that Andropogon developed as compensation for the diversion of public land for a natural gas pipeline crossing most of the state of New Jersey. The right-of-way spanned 2 counties and 17 municipalities, yet the permits were acquired in far less time than expected, largely due to broad support from agencies and institutions as well as the public. The compensation package included coordinated planning for the 75-mile trail as well as complete acquisition and development of a 15-mile stretch of the trail that overlaps with the pipeline and 200 acres of park land in 2 counties. A contractor bankruptcy complicated implementation of the compensation package, but the net effect merely slowed implementation slightly. The trail has been adopted in all the associated municipalities and has been incorporated into the state's official trails plan, largely because the communities all played an important role in its development.

Corridors ultimately are dependent upon the larger natural areas that they connect. A preserve system designed for recoverability must include the richest remaining habitats as well as a large enough total natural area to be of full value. Anyone who depends on the concept of compensatory restoration should invest in assembling large enough bioreserves of critical natural areas, adequate surrounding buffer areas, and connecting corridors in order to fulfill the requirements of the legislation. Those whose activities are to some extent justifiable because of the concept of compensatory restoration should participate to a greater degree in both advocacy and funding for acquisition as well as ecosystem restoration because sustainability goes directly to their bottom line. Indeed, ecosystem restoration, in general, is necessary to support the concept of compensatory restoration.

Conclusions

In conclusion, effective and appropriate implementation of compensatory restoration hinges on fulfilling several vital preconditions. These prerequisites serve as the foundation for assuming we can achieve any reasonable level of recovery at all.

Preconditions for compensatory restoration are as follows:

1) establishment of baseline monitoring,
2) development and implementation of risk and damage reduction strategies,
3) planning and implementation of bioreserves, buffers, and connecting corridor system,
4) advocacy and actions for sustainability in the larger environment, and
5) public involvement and ongoing management by local institutions and community.

We have the opportunity to use the funding and staff time associated with compensatory restoration to pursue a comprehensive program for sustainability, which in some ways is just another word for recoverability. It will take a collaboration of regulatory agencies, as well as the insurers and the handlers of hazardous materials to best achieve an incremental program to enhance the recoverability of ecosystems. Many key individuals who could be instrumental in ensuring landscape recoverability are here at this conference, which is part of the incentive behind this effort. Such an approach, centered on comprehensive restoration, would enhance and restore associated human uses of the broadest kinds, while reducing long-term risk and hence, costs.

4c

Discussion Paper 3 on Enhancing Damaged Public Assets: Perspectives from Landscape Architects and Planners

*Rick Dawson**

The authors offer a unique concept for natural resource trustees to seek compensation for injuries to services. Their ideas have long been debated by ecologists as to how to optimize the benefits of undeveloped habitat in a political and social environment that discourages large, single-block land purchases. The connecting of "habitat fragments" in order to gain an "ecological critical mass" has been advocated by many ecologists as a method to assemble ecologically relevant, sized segments of habitat. The authors' expansion of this concept as a remedy for compensable lost use is novel and deserves careful consideration by trustees in designing solutions for difficult lost-use claims.

The authors targeted what seems to be the most daunting challenge for trustees, i.e., how to compensate for lost use in cases of chronic contamination or long-term interim lost use. The quantification of lost use in both of these circumstances is rather easy, but the fair and equitable scaling is usually difficult. The compensation for thousands of lost or diminished visits always presents the trustees with a problem of how to increase or enhance use without degrading the current user experience. This restoration of use with a fidelity to the area in which the losses occur usually requires creativity. Unfortunately, as the authors point out, these creative impulses of the trustees are expressed most often as an increase in access as a cure for the lost use.

The idea of linking habitats to provide an overall corridor of new uses is an option that few trustees have attempted. The appeal of this concept is that it optimizes the available, undeveloped or underdeveloped lands in an assessment area. These lands then can be connected and perhaps enhanced through rehabilitation to provide a "critical mass" of services over a larger geographic area than was presumably affected by the contamination. This optimization of existing habitats not only will yield ecological benefits, but also will provide a fuller range of uses for the public to enjoy and exploit.

The one problem that the authors do not address is with a site that may be contaminated so extensively that cleanup actions are either very superficial, i.e., made margin-

*Department of the Interior, National Park Service

ally safe for public health, or do not occur at all. In both cases, the problem becomes evaluation of the existing, unlinked habitat segments to determine if it is worthwhile to spend compensation dollars in contaminated habitats. This question of chronic contamination with its continuing loss or diminished use may argue against this habitat-linking approach.

Another issue is the application of a service-to-service scaling for lost fishing use. The linear park concept as presented would not totally compensate anglers for their lost use. In fact, if angler days are lost to fishing closures or angling trips are diminished by fish consumption advisories, then replacing them with bike paths along a contaminated habitat corridor may not seem like a "fix" to the public, especially to the fisherman. The key to this concept will be to demonstrate to the angler the benefits to the fish population of having habitats linked as a way to increase exploited stocks, thereby increasing the "quality" of the fishing experience. Another way to address a service-to service type scaling, including lost angler trips, would be the employment of broad design considerations in the linear park that incorporate fisherman access off paths and from parking areas that is not in interference with biking, walking, etc.

Unfortunately, the authors choose to use the term "linear parks," which implies governmental control and a range of prescribed services. The use of a term such as "habitat corridor" would imply more of an ecological connection, thereby adding to the idea of restoration of full service flows without implying some type of "park-like" development, such as bike paths and parking lots. This concept of habitat corridors also removes the primary impediment that trustees will face in employment of this compensatory technique, i.e., access of the public to all lands within the corridor whether public or private.

In using the authors' example of a watershed, the linking of publicly owned parcels is both sound and economically straightforward. Even the purchase of some property interest of undeveloped parcels is achievable, provided that the funds are available. However, I do not share the authors' optimism that all of the public will embrace a common linear park corridor concept. The task of convincing private property owners to allow expensive waterfront property to return to "natural habitat" will be difficult in and of itself. The hope that many of these same property owners will allow unrestricted access across their holdings will be a much tougher proposition. The highest likelihood of success will be when many publicly owned parcels exist and can be linked.

This idea of reestablishing public lost use on or across private property runs into implementation problems when the trustee is attempting to compensate for lost uses such as fishing. Fishing requires access to the water, which may imply reducing the riparian habitat in some places. Also, fisherman drive cars to their fishing spots, which requires parking. Fisherman generate trash, e.g., food wrappers, bait containers, tangled tackle, beer cans, etc. All of this trash has to have containers that must be emptied. This type of maintenance in someone's backyard is difficult to imagine.

Furthermore, given property values for waterfront land, concerns of liability if a member of the public was injured on their land, and our increasing societal fear of crime by strangers, most private property owners would decline to sign onto a plan to reestablish a natural riparian landscape in their backyard.

If enough experience is available to plan and implement this type of riparian corridor so that the risks of failure are low and the costs of maintaining the corridor over time is minimal, then the future of this type of linear park/habitat corridor concept is limitless. On the other hand, if the techniques for reestablishing riparian corridors are risky and unknown and the costs of future maintenance is high, then the trustees will opt for the sure thing, bathrooms and parking lots.

In conclusion, the application of the concept to allow the "ecological connecting" of habitat fragments is a promising alterative to the safe and sure practice of enhancement of existing public services. This linking of fragmented habitats must not require high or continuous maintenance or any other large, ongoing costs. It must also employ low-risk methods of habitat reestablishment. Finally, the linking of habitats must not require the development of public access across private lands, which seems to be the most formidable obstacle to success.

4d

Discussion Paper 4 on Enhancing Damaged Public Assets: Perspectives from Landscape Architects and Planners

*Gordon A. Robilliard**

In this paper, I provide some observations and comments on the paper of Balmori, Huguenin, Unsworth, and Giedt. My perspective is that of an ecologist with experience in conducting all phases of the natural resources damage assessment (NRDA) process for oil spills and releases of hazardous substances. My emphasis has been and is on the ecological rather than the human-use aspects of the injury and damage assessments and restoration programs.

In general, I support the concept of corridors, as defined by the authors, in urban and suburban areas as a way to connect green and open space by trails, low impact roads, etc. These corridors can certainly enhance peoples' recreational use opportunities as well as improve the overall aesthetic quality of the urban and suburban environment. My personal experience on these corridors in California, with all its roads and millions of people, has been positive. However, I do not go to the corridor for its natural ecological values.

I first provide my comments on the ecological values of corridors as described by the authors. Then I provide comments on specific topics presented in their paper.

The ecological value of corridors in compensatory restoration

One of the authors' main tenets is that corridors have substantial ecological value and that corridors can provide compensatory restoration for both lost human and ecological uses of natural resources injured in the oil spill or release of hazardous substances. In the rest of this section, I discuss the value of corridors as an option for restoring lost ecological services.

First though, a definition of "ecological" as it pertains to NRDA and restoration options, including corridors, is necessary. Ecological as it is usually used by the trustees in an NRDA refers implicitly if not explicitly to the "natural," "native," "undisturbed," or even "pristine" biological community that would be present but for the oil spill or hazardous substance release. Ecological does not usually explicitly include habitats that are created or heavily modified by peoples' activities. In general

*ENTRIX, Inc., Walnut Creek, CA

the trustees have shown less interest in projects in which restoration of lost ecological services would be accomplished with a biological community that is manufactured and expected to be heavily used by people for recreational or commercial purposes. One could argue that restoration of wetlands is an exception, although wetlands are typically not designed for heavy recreational use and disturbance. In the context of the authors' paper, "ecological" seems generally to refer to a landscape in which the habitats are managed so that the corridor is aesthetically pleasing to people and meets project-specific, human-use criteria that focus on recreational use. Maintaining these corridor habitats, especially in urban and suburban areas, as undisturbed and natural ecological communities is not the first priority. Indeed, it seems likely that there is an inherent and possibly irreconcilable conflict between human uses and natural ecological communities in most corridor projects.

Natural ecological communities are often unattractive to people because these communities are usually not open, green, orderly, or predictable. There is dense understory vegetation that precludes viewing of waterways or of long distances. Natural riparian vegetation is typically too dense to see (or hike) through. Animals including many birds are usually not visible because they are wary of human intruders. The public routinely complains about open or green spaces that are overgrown with weeds and occupied by "wild" animals, especially in or near urban and suburban areas. Local public officials typically manage the problem of natural ecological communities by creating a park-like setting.

Some corridors may actually serve the purpose of connecting fragmented and relatively undisturbed habitats and thereby increase the biological diversity and long-term survival of these communities. This is the basic concept behind the Natural Habitat Conservation Plan recently implemented in southern California. However, including trails will certainly attract people and increase the human usage of most corridors. It is exactly this increase in human use that will reduce the value of the habitat for most ecological resources except those that are used to people and to the cultured landscape that these corridors often have.

One obvious solution to the challenge of including both human uses and natural ecological communities is to create corridors that are wide enough to accommodate the habitat requirements of the species of interest and still allow for trails, etc. This solution will require the combined efforts of planners, landscape architects, and ecologists familiar with the local and regional habitats, cooperative trustees and responsible parties, and supportive public officials.

Another solution is to recognize that the real focus is on restoration of human uses, especially where the corridors are relatively narrow and where natural biological communities are not acceptable for whatever reason. This solution requires that all parties accept that restoration of ecological values, as defined previously, will be limited, and to claim otherwise is gratuitous. We should use corridors to restore lost ecological services whenever the corridor can be made large enough to connect fragmented habitats of similar characteristics such that the whole is greater than the sum of the parts and the natural ecological values are sustained or enhanced. Otherwise, we should acknowledge that we are creating linear parks for peoples' enjoyment but that we are not necessarily doing much for the natural ecological values.

Property available for corridors

The corridor option seems to assume and depend upon the availability of property. In most cases, the appropriate property is probably in private ownership, at least in those areas where there is substantial human use that was injured and where corridor restoration is an option. In most oil spills and some hazardous substance releases, the damages are not large enough to buy substantial areas of expensive property let alone put in the improvements and amenities required to develop a corridor. The approach may work for big oil spills or major releases, especially in rural areas near urban or suburban areas.

Scaling injuries and restoration projects

The authors are clear that scaling (i.e., "how much") restoration is not the focus of their paper although it is an active area of research and debate. They could have added "highly charged and often contentious" as well. Scaling is the primary issue in the restoration planning process. Until the appropriate scale of the restoration project is agreed upon be the trustees and responsible party, it is difficult to initiate the restoration planning process. Certainly on the ecological side, there is ample experience to suggest that the trustees and responsible party are likely to be far apart in their initial estimates of injury and thus size of necessary restoration projects. I expect that the same is true for the human-use issues. Therefore, even if we all agree that corridors are a reasonable option to compensate for lost human uses, I submit that scaling the size of the corridor or determining how much corridor is needed will be the major hurdle in most NRDAs for the near future. I strongly encourage planners, landscape architects, economists, and ecologists to focus their research and debate on the scaling issue as well as the selection of appropriate restoration options.

Minimum standards for restoration projects

In discussing the notion of combining damages resulting from numerous small-scale oil spills so that a large-scale project that has been previously identified in a regional restoration plan can be implemented, the authors seem to support the "existence of minimum standards" for restoration projects. The development and promotion of minimum standards may be a double-edged sword. Minimum standards could lead to arbitrary settlements that could be much more (or less) than the damages that might be reasonable given the injuries actually caused by any particular oil spill. With minimum standards could come an ability to make a pre-spill estimate of the damages, and this estimate could then be included as a cost of doing business. The business and nongovernmental organizations are likely to have opposing views on the desirability of that situation. Minimum standards also imply that all small restoration projects in a general category (e.g., wetland habitats or mangrove forests) are of equal value with regard to ecological and/or human uses.

From an ecologist's perspective (and without considering any legal or economic concerns), I generally support the concept of combining damages from small-scale oil spills to accomplish a larger-scale restoration project. My caveat is that the injuries, damages, and restoration proposals for the small spills should be scaled for each spill rather than by applying an arbitrary minimum standard. However, I also believe that, with experience, the NRDA practitioners on all sides will develop a gestalt about the appropriate scale of injuries, damages, and restoration options for small-scale spills. Minimum standards will probably evolve in the NRDA settlement process but I do not advocate codifying them.

Two recent developments in landscape architecture

I agree that "continuous unfragmented landscape corridors will increase the quantity and value of human uses of injured areas." The authors make a strong supporting case in their paper, and I personally enjoy the numerous bike and walking trails near my home in suburban California. However, I am less convinced that the corridors will promote "ecological health" at the same time. The ecological communities along most of the corridors envisioned by this paper are, by definition and for practical purposes, markedly altered and disturbed communities. The health of urban or suburban ecological communities may be promoted but these are not likely to be similar to the ecological communities injured by most oil spills unless the spill occurs in a similar urban or suburban area.

Enhancing public involvement

The last 2 sentences of the first paragraph are not likely to enhance a positive public involvement in a proposed corridor project, and I am surprised that planners would espouse such an elitist attitude that could only be considered insulting to the "local officials." While the local public officials may initially propose inappropriate projects in the context of compensatory restoration, these same officials are very likely to propose entirely appropriate projects once they understand the NRDA framework and goals, and "public outrage" has subsided. The task of the trustees and the planners is to engage all the stakeholders, including the public officials, from the beginning of the restoration planning process so that all stakeholders will propose and support appropriate projects. For example, when trying to estimate the injuries and lost uses from the ecological and natural resource utilization perspectives, we often seek out the local officials as well as the local fishermen, naturalist groups, merchants, guides, and similar local experts to obtain information about the "preferences and attitudes of the actual users of the resource." These local sources have generally proven to be more accurate and reliable than non-local ones, and the local officials are generally more willing to be involved in the restoration process than the public.

Urban oil spill

The authors state, "In our experience beaches rarely are capacity or access constrained, so that [most beach enhancement] projects often will not result in overall increase in beach visits." While this may be generally true, it may not apply to populous urban areas such as southern California, parts of Florida and Hawaii, and similar areas where beach use can be very heavy, especially on holidays and sunny weekends. California has an aggressive Coastal Commission that requires public beach access as a mitigation measure for most projects that impact the coastal zone. In southern California especially, many of these accesses are used to capacity soon after they are opened, based on my personal experience of trying to find uncrowded places to surf fish near urban and suburban areas. At least in these crowded areas, the public may strongly favor quantity-enhancing beach restoration projects over corridors.

Title of paper

To be consistent with the definitions of the NRDA regulations, the title of this paper should refer to *injured* rather than *damaged* public assets. The terms are frequently used incorrectly and/or interchangeably by NRDA practitioners in discussions, reports, and other documents. Usually it is possible from the context to know what the speaker or author means, but not always.

5

Leading Indicators of Ecosystem Services and Values, With Illustrations for Performing Habitat Equivalency Analysis*

Dennis M. King†

An ecosystem can be "any spatially explicit unit of the earth that includes all of the organisms, along with all of the components of their abiotic environment within its boundaries" (Likens 1992). Ecosystems exist and interact at many different geographic scales. The services and products they generate and the benefits they provide depend on these interactions and, as a result, are very site-specific. To compare ecosystems on the basis of their services or values, it is necessary to consider their landscape context as well as their biophysical characteristics.

Unfortunately, conventional ecosystem *assessment* methods are based primarily on ecosystem morphology (studies of their biological form and structure). They are useful for assessing and comparing on-site features of ecosystems and their capacity to provide certain functions. However, they usually do not take account of the interdependencies between ecosystems at higher and lower scales or the effects of landscape context on whether ecosystem functions will take shape or will benefit people.

Ecosystem *valuation* methods are limited in scope at the other extreme. They attempt to assign values to ecosystem services, usually in absolute (dollar) terms, but rarely give consideration to the specific biophysical or landscape features that generate them. Because many of the values of ecosystems are not traded in markets, these methods rely heavily on applications of recently developed "nonmarket valuation techniques." These techniques can be extremely expensive to apply and are reliable only when applied to well-defined products and services in specific contexts. The cost of applying these methods to the full range of services and products provided by even a single ecosystem is usually prohibitive. Moreover, since these services and products and their values are site-specific, estimated values for one site usually cannot be transferred to another site without additional research.

---

*Adapted from King DM. 1997. Comparing ecosystem services and values. NOAA Damage Assessment and Restoration Center. Silver Spring MD: U.S. Dept of Commerce.

†University of Maryland, Center for Environmental and Estuarine Studies, Solomons Island, MD and King and Associates, Inc., Washington, DC

At least for now, the results from ecosystem assessment and valuation methods provide only part of the information needed to compare ecosystems in terms of their services and values. However, research related to wetlands suggests that practical and reliable indicators of relative ecosystem values can be developed based on the fact that the functions, services, and values provided by ecosystems depend in predictable ways on *on-site biophysical characteristics* (e.g., soil, vegetative cover, hydrology) and *landscape context* (e.g., proximity to certain features of natural and human landscapes). On-site characteristics determine the *capacity* of an ecosystem to provide various functions (e.g., support waterfowl). Landscape context determines: 1) if the ecosystem will have the *opportunity* to provide these functions (e.g., attract waterfowl), and strongly influences 2) what *services* will flow from the functions (e.g., hunting and birding opportunities), 3) the *values* that will flow from those services (e.g., how much people are willing to pay), and 4) the *distribution* of benefits to various segments of society (e.g., urban or rural, rich or poor).

I describe how these 2 sets of factors associated with site-specific characteristics and landscape context can provide the basis for indicators of the relative economic value of ecosystems. Such indicators would be useful for 2 reasons. First, they would provide a basis for prioritizing ecosystem protection and restoration efforts and for establishing requirements and trading rules to govern compensatory restoration and mitigation programs. Second, they would provide a basis for applying "benefit transfer methodologies" whereby economic values estimated for one ecosystem might be adjusted to reflect those provided by ecosystems with different characteristics or different landscape contexts.

The paper has 3 sections. Section 1 identifies some typical ecosystem functions and related services and presents some concepts and terms that are useful for comparing ecosystem values. Section 2 identifies 2 sets of criteria for developing indicators of ecosystem value: one based on capacity, opportunity, payoff, and equity considerations under fixed landscape conditions, and another based on factors such as scarcity, vulnerability, sensitivity, and reversibility under changing landscape conditions. Section 3 illustrates why such indicators are important by showing their essential role in performing habitat equivalency analysis (HEA) and in "scaling" primary and compensatory restoration projects as required under the 1996 amendments to the Oil Pollution Act of 1990.

Ecosystem basics

What is an ecosystem?

Strolling the beach you encounter a pile of putrefying organic matter. Whether it is a week-old dung heap or the remainder of a month-old whale carcass, it is an ecosystem. So is the beach you are on (including the pile), the larger estuary of which it is a part, the reef that is breaking the waves you can hear in the distance, and the ocean that you know is just beyond the fog bank. The term *ecosystem* refers to "any spatially explicit unit of the earth that includes all of the organisms, along with all of the components of their abiotic environment within its boundaries" (Likens 1992). Ecosystems exist and can be characterized and analyzed at microscopic or global scales; however, they interact in important ways across many different geographic scales. This fact makes it difficult to assess or compare the services or values of ecosystems without considering their specific landscape contexts.

Sources of ecosystem value

The natural world consists of approximately 250,000 plant species and, excluding insects, about 1.1 million animal species. If insects are included, the number of species ranges from 5 million to 30 million.[1] Each species and its respective habitat exist in hierarchical organizations that combine at various scales to form ecosystems. A few of these individual components of ecosystems contribute in direct and measurable ways to economic welfare (e.g., timber, crops, and edible fish); a few more contribute to the quality of life in other noticeable ways (e.g., dolphins, songbirds, and wildflowers). However, most of the millions of species that exist in nature contribute in obscure and roundabout ways to human welfare (e.g., pollinators and decomposers on land; benthic organisms, plankton, coral, and forage fish at sea). Their lives and functions are so intertwined with each other and with surrounding ecological landscapes that their individual contributions to human welfare, as a practical matter, cannot be isolated. Nevertheless, their contributions can be inferred from the values that people attach to the functions and services provided by the ecosystems of which they are a part. This is why assessing the socioeconomic value of ecosystems, despite all the inherent difficulties, is so important. It is the only way to show how most of the natural world contributes to human welfare. Therefore, it is the only way to use conventional (anthropocentric) concepts of benefits and costs to justify protecting or restoring natural systems.[2]

Limiting the scale of comparison

In scientific literature, ecosystems are often compared on the basis of the "complexity" and "richness" of their internal biological hierarchies and the "interconnectedness" of these hierarchies with each other and with ecosystems at other scales. Here I focus on criteria for comparing the beneficial effects of ecosystems on people. As a result, it will be necessary to gloss over many specific differences in the interconnectedness and richness of ecosystem processes and to maintain a relatively narrow focus on the outcomes of ecosystem processes. However, practical frameworks for comparing ecosystems in terms of their value to humans can be consistent with prevailing

[1]There are disagreements over the exact number of plant and animal species. The numbers used here are from a standard reference on biodiversity by Wilson (1988).

[2]In this paper the terms "benefits" and "values" are used interchangeably and are anthropogenic in the sense that they refer strictly to the beneficial effects of ecosystem functions on people. In strict economic terms this would be measured as the aggregate "willingness to pay" by all individuals for all of the products and services generated by all of the functions of an ecosystem.

ecological theories and models without getting too deeply involved with them. Differences in the complexity of biological hierarchies within ecosystems, for example, are reflected in factors related to their biophysical characteristics, and linkages between ecosystems at different scales are reflected in factors related to their landscape context. Observations about these factors, therefore, reflect some important underlying ecological linkages that are too complex to deal with directly. Fortunately, these same factors also determine the capacities of ecosystems to provide certain functions and the outcomes of those functions, and these capacities strongly influence the services and values that will flow from the ecosystems. Later, the capacities are proposed as the basis of an indicator system that, in the absence of conventional (dollar) measures of value, can be used to compare ecosystems on the basis of their expected values.[3]

Uncertainty of ecosystem functions and values

Ecosystems are constantly changing (e.g., through succession) and adapting to change (e.g., hurricanes, wildfires, oil spills). As they reach certain thresholds, they can also make unexpected shifts from one successional trajectory or evolutionary pattern to another. One important new finding receiving attention in the ecological literature is that ecosystem changes are faster at relatively small scales (e.g., ant pile or pond) than at larger spatial scales (e.g., wetlands or watersheds).[4] Since perturbations affecting populations and communities at different scales ripple through ecosystem hierarchies at different speeds, there are always trends operating on various ecosystems scales that may be difficult to notice at that particular scale. This probably accounts for the high failure rates and wide variability of outcomes from ecosystem restoration projects (NRC 1992; Shabman et al. 1994). It also suggests that comparing expected ecosystem values by considering the mix of functions and services that would be provided by ecosystems in a static landscape context may not be adequate. Changes in landscapes due to changing land-use patterns, weather, and other factors will not influence all ecosystems locations in the same way. As a result, the risks and uncertainties associated with the expected streams of ecosystem services and values from similar ecosystems (even in currently similar landscape settings) may not be the same.[5]

Differences in the susceptibility of ecosystems to landscape changes and in the ability of people to respond to or adapt to those changes affect the risks and uncertainties

---

[3]The difficulties of estimating the use and nonuse values of on-site and off-site services provided directly and indirectly by ecosystem functions are summarized later and described in more detail in Kopp and Smith (1993) and Smith (1996).

[4]"Scale," as it is used here, refers to the spatial or geographic range of an ecosystem. The relationship between ecosystem scale and ecosystem management was addressed in Gunderson et al. (1995) and in Pitelka (1996a).

[5]The important point here is that the risks associated with streams of services and values expected from ecosystems at different sites are different not only because of differences in observable site and landscape conditions, but because of differences in the exposure and vulnerability of different sites to changing landscape conditions.

associated with the expected services and values of different ecosystems. These differences are the reason why the next section outlines 2 distinct sets of criteria for comparing ecosystem services and values. The first addresses expected values under current landscape conditions; the second addresses differences in risk and uncertainty related to the impacts of changes in natural and human landscapes on different ecosystems and on different people. Recent evidence shows the influence of uncontrollable environmental factors such as extreme weather and the spread of noxious weeds is far more powerful in young (recently restored or created) ecosystems than in mature (undisturbed) ecosystems.[6] This has significant implications for the way risk and uncertainty should be factored into comparisons of natural and restored ecosystems.

Focusing on ecosystem comparisons

Scientists who compare ecosystems to learn more about them usually focus their attention on differences in ecosystem processes and ecosystem dynamics. However, because I focus on the contributions of ecosystems to human welfare, factors that reflect differences in the expected outcomes of those processes are relevant. There are 4 attributes of ecosystems that represent building blocks between what is known about ecosystems and the benefits they will provide. They include the following:

Ecosystem features—The site-specific characteristics of an ecosystem (e.g., soil, ground cover, hydrology). These establish its capacity to support various forms of life and perform various biophysical processes.

Ecosystem functions—The biophysical processes that actually take place within an ecosystem. These can be characterized apart from any human context (e.g., fish and waterfowl habitat, cycling carbon, trapping nutrients).

Ecosystem services—The beneficial outcomes that result from ecosystem functions (e.g., better fishing and hunting, cleaner water, better views). These require some interaction with, or at least some appreciation by, humans. However, they can be measured in physical terms (e.g., catch rates, water quality, aesthetics).

Ecosystem values—The aggregate "willingness-to-pay" by all individuals for all of the services associated with all of the functions of an ecosystem. These are usually measured in absolute (dollar) terms associated with specific services. However, they can be expressed in relative terms (e.g., using indicators) for purposes of comparing ecosystems.

These terms describe attributes of ecosystems that are obviously related to one another and are sometimes used to represent one another. (Improvements in fish habitat or in the abundance of fish, for example, are sometimes used to represent improvements in fishery-related values.) However, there are 3 reasons why it is

[6]The evidence that the functions of restored ecosystems are less predictable than those of naturally occurring ecosystems was reported by Kentula and cited in Pitelka (1996a). This national study was based primarily on comparisons of vegetative ground cover at natural and restored wetland sites and yielded results that are consistent with papers presented at symposiums of the Association of State Wetland Managers, Inc. (Kusler et al. 1986).

important to maintain clear distinctions between them. First, the information needed to evaluate each of them and the criteria used to assess ecosystems with respect to each of them are significantly different. The features of an ecosystem that might give it a high capacity to provide a particular function (e.g., suitability as waterfowl habitat) do not guarantee that it will actually provide a high level of function (e.g., attract or support the greatest number of waterfowl). Ecosystems that provide the highest level of function may not provide the highest level of service (e.g., birding, hunting, educational, scientific opportunities). Those that provide the highest levels of service may not provide the greatest value (e.g., aggregate "willingness-to-pay" for birding, hunting, educational opportunities). Lastly, the ecosystem that generates the greatest value may not result in a distribution of benefits considered equitable (e.g., opportunities for rich versus poor or urban versus rural).

Second, there are significant differences in the attributes of ecosystems that allow them to provide different types of ecosystem functions and services. Table 5-1 provides a list of the most often cited functions provided by ecosystems and identifies a few of the associated services. Some of the functions and services listed are provided best by ecosystems that are located away from people and are surrounded by undisturbed natural landscapes (e.g., endangered species habitats); others require that the ecosystem be relatively close to people (e.g., educational and recreational opportunities, flood damage prevention, aesthetics). Similarly, some services, such as those associated with sediment, nutrient, or contaminant trapping, are provided only if the ecosystem is located near disturbed landscapes where runoff is a problem; others, such as breeding habitat for migratory waterfowl, are provided more effectively at sites in undisturbed landscapes. Unless the factors affecting various functions, services, and values of an ecosystem are considered separately, it is impossible to identify important environmental and socioeconomic trade-offs or to compare ecosystems with similar features in terms of the functions, services, and values they can be expected to provide.

The third and most important reason for distinguishing between these terms is that the generally available analytical methods for assessing and comparing ecosystems usually do not strive to make clear distinctions. As a result, many of them tend to mask, rather than clarify, critical linkages between ecosystem features, functions, services, and values, which can differ significantly from site to site. A review of specific methods is beyond the scope of this paper, but a few brief observations can be offered about the 2 most widely used approaches: ecosystem *assessment* methods and ecosystem *valuation* methods.[7]

[7]The brief comments offered here are needed to justify the proposed development of "leading indicators" of ecosystem values in the following section. These indicators are only worthwhile because useful direct measures of ecosystem value are not available and are not forthcoming using other methods. Refer to Freeman (1993), Kopp and Smith (1993), and Smith (1996) for reviews of specific ecosystem valuation methods.

Table 5-1 Ecosystem functions and illustrations of associated services

Ecosystem functions	Associated types of services/values
Fishery habitat	Better commercial and recreational fishing, lower fish prices, improved international trade balance
Waterfowl habitat	Better hunting and bird watching onsite, nearby, and elsewhere
Fur-bearer habitat	Commercial and recreational opportunities
storehouse of biodiversity (onsite species diversity)	Direct, indirect, serendipity value of scientific research, medical discoveries, genetic pools, seed banks, etc
Food chain/Biodiversity support (offsite species support)	Offsite direct, indirect, serendipity value of scientific research, medical discoveries, genetic pools, seed banks, etc
Natural products (e.g., timber, hay, cranberries, peat)	Wholesale and retail market value and associated jobs, incomes
Groundwater recharge/discharge	Drinking water quality, reduced human and environmental health risks
Floodwater storage, conveyance and desynchronization	Reduced soil erosion and property damage
Shoreline anchoring/Erosion control	Protection of beaches, private property, infrastructure, ecosystem
Storm surge/Wave protection	Reduced soil erosion and property damage
Sediment trapping	Protects aquatic ecosystems, reduced dredging, maintains hydropower
Pollution assimilation	Reduced treatment costs, improved public health and environment
Nutrient retention/Filtering	Maintain nitrogen balance, prevent algae blooms and anoxic conditions
Natural area/Open space	Active and passive recreation, research, teaching/learning, general aesthetics, spiritual enrichment, heritage
Micro-climate regulation	General life support; ill-defined but important local/regional linkages
Macro-climate regulation	General life support; ill-defined but important national/global linkages
Carbon cycling	General life support; ill-defined but important national/global linkages

Ecosystem assessment methods were developed primarily by scientists and evolved as extensions of morphological studies-studies of the form and structure of biological systems.[8] These studies focus on ecosystem features and often employ indicators that refer to an ecosystem's biophysical capacity to provide various functions. Although they may refer to "functional values" or "value indices" when describing the "functional capacity" of ecosystems and may use these methods to compare ecosystems, they rarely address ecosystem values as the term is defined above. Ecosystem assessment methods provide only the front-end part of the analysis required to compare ecosystems on the basis of the services and values they provide.

[8]The most modern and fully developed of these methods is the "hydrogeomorphic" or HGM method which was released in late 1995. (See Brinson 1993). HGM, like previously designed morphological methods, provides a basis for comparing wetland features; however it is being used as the basis for guiding wetland mitigation trades under Section 404 of the Clean Water Act and for other purposes that imply that it represents a useful measure of wetland value.

By contrast, ecosystem valuation methods attempt to assign values to ecosystem services, usually in absolute (dollar) terms, but usually without much regard for the specific ecosystem features or functions that generated them. Because many services of ecosystems generate "off-site" and "nonmarket" benefits, these ecosystem valuation methods rely extensively on the application of recently developed non-market valuation techniques to assign values to specific ecosystem services. However, these techniques are far too expensive to be applied to the full range of services listed in Table 5-1.[9] As a result, they have usually been applied to only a subset of them, and therefore serve more to illustrate ecosystem values than to provide a comprehensive accounting of them. The fact that ecosystem values are so site-specific also limits the usefulness of these methods. To be credible, they must be applied to estimate the value of services provided by a specific ecosystem in a particular landscape context. Using the estimates of value developed for the services of one ecosystem at another site requires additional research.[10] Ecosystem valuation methods provide only the back-end part of the analysis that is required to compare ecosystems on the basis of the services and values they provide and are usually too expensive to be used for this purpose.

Landscape context of wetlands

Although exact distances differ from region to region and site to site, Figure 5-1 illustrates 2 important sets of spatial relationships that help establish the effects of location on wetland functions and values. In this figure distance from a wetland site is measured along both the horizontal and the vertical axis. The horizontal axis distance measures the geographic range over which various types of wetland values accrue. Most of the value associated with timber, hay, and cranberry production, for example, require proprietary rights (own or rent); the values associated with on-site hunting and fishing, most scientific and educational uses, and most aesthetic and spiritual benefits require access, or at least near proximity. Other important wetland values, such as spawning, feeding, and nursery habitats for migratory waterfowl and fish extend across much greater regional scales. Still other functions, such as those associated with carbon cycling and biodiversity support, generate values that are national or global in scale.

Similarly, distance measured along the vertical axis in Figure 5-1 reflects the extent to which various wetland functions and values depend on attributes of the surrounding ecological landscape. For example, even though they generate benefits across much

[9]So far, a technique called "contingent valuation" is the only way to explicitly attach "passive-use values" to ecosystem services. A description of the procedures that are required to apply this method to acceptable standards under OPA is provided in NOAA (1992).

[10]Studies aimed at transferring estimates of value developed for one site to another site are generally referred to as "benefit transfer" studies. No generally accepted methodology exists for conducting benefit transfer studies. The approach developed in the following section for comparing ecosystems in terms of their relative values may provide a reasonable basis for conducting benefit transfer studies.

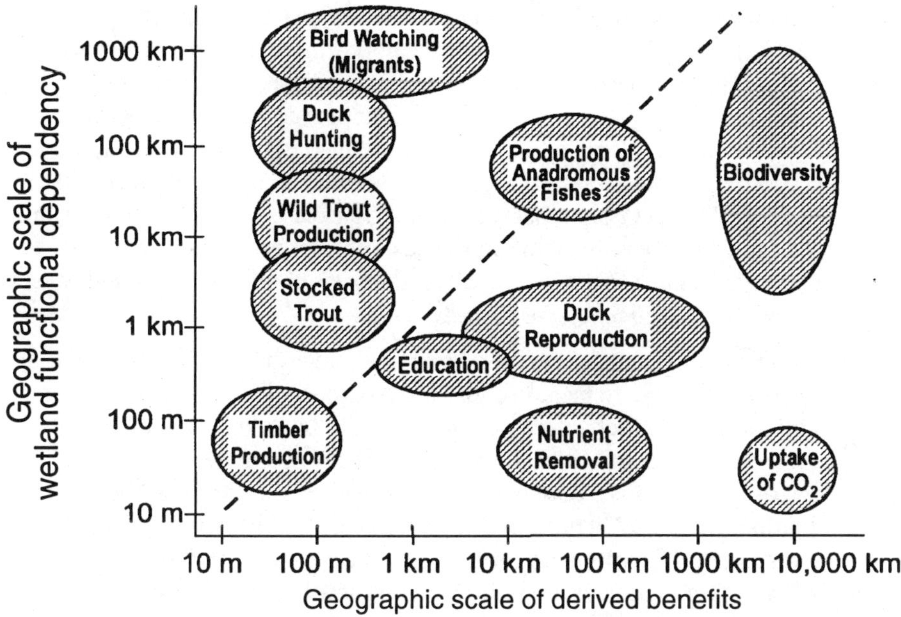

Figure 5-1 Landscape context of wetland functions. These are illustrative ranges only, and they are based on extrapolations of "typical" dependencies and derived benefits. They show how far from the wetland site benefits may accrue (x-axis), and how far from the site features of the natural landscape have influence (y-axis).

different scales, the capacity of a forested wetland to provide timber or sequester carbon are both shown to depend very little on conditions outside the wetland site itself. A wetland's capacity to provide fishery habitat, on the other hand, may depend on water quality in lakes and streams several miles away and on physical connections with them and with the ocean. At the extreme a wetland's capacity to provide waterfowl habitat might depend on conditions along migratory routes and in breeding areas thousands of miles away.

The relationships illustrated in Figure 5-1 with regard to wetlands reveal 2 facts that are important when comparing the services and values of ecosystems. First, the location of an ecosystem can have a significant effect on the mix of functions and values provided by an ecosystem and the levels of services and values associated with them. Second, the location of an ecosystem can have significant effects on the distribution of services and values.

The critical science-policy gap

The analytical problems outlined above are the focus of long-term research. Scientists are giving more attention to landscape context in the development of assessment methods, and economists continue to look for ways to reduce the cost of estimating ecosystem values and improve their reliability. However, these 2 separate areas of research, even if they are successful, may not be of much practical value to policy-makers and jurists making decisions that involve comparing ecosystems in terms of their relative values. These decisions cannot be made on the basis of "value-free" scientific assessments of ecosystems, even if they are improved and expanded to consider landscape linkages. Nor can they be made on the basis of improved estimates of the value of specific ecosystem services, even if they could be provided more reliably and more affordably. The fact is, in most legal and regulatory contexts where decision-makers are asked to compare ecosystems on the basis of their values, they are asked to compare their *expected future services and values* on the basis of information about their *current biophysical features* and *landscape contexts.*

To be useful under these circumstances, there must be some way for the assessment of observable ecosystem features to be linked forward to expected ecosystem functions and services and for the valuation of ecosystem services to be linked backward to observable or measurable ecosystem features. Most of the ongoing research to improve the scientific basis of ecosystem assessment methods and the credibility of ecosystem valuation methods will not fill this gap. Arguably, improving methods for linking current ecosystem features with future flows of ecosystem services is more important for evaluating the socioeconomic trade-offs associated with ecosystems than improving methods of attaching values to services.[11]

Ecosystems as natural capital

Taken together, ecosystems encompass most of what is important to life, so there is no need to justify their overall value. However, all ecosystems are not equal in terms of their environmental or socioeconomic importance and as a result, they do not all deserve the same level of protection or the same level of restoration spending. "Natural capital" is a term used to refer to ecosystems and components of ecosystems as specific assets that contribute in specific ways to economic welfare. Natural capital is comparable to manufactured capital or human capital in the sense that these terms focus on values (measurable or not) stemming from the streams of products and services they are expected to provide over time. This perspective of ecosystems, not as life-support systems but as collections of assets with specific values, is useful for many reasons. It provides a basis for comparing ecosystems in terms of characteristics that affect their capacity and opportunity to provide services and values; it allows investments in ecosystem protection and rehabilitation to be justified on more than purely environmental or emotional grounds; it allows ecosystems to enter social and economic accounting on a par with manufactured capital and human capital; and, most importantly, it permits more realistic assessments of the future costs and risks of

---

[11] There are 2 methods of trying to make this ecological economic link: deterministic models and indicator systems. Deterministic models attempt to describe the link using mathematical equations; these have not advanced to the point that they can be used for this purpose. For a review of these models and their strengths and limitations consult Pitelka (1996a). Criteria for developing indicator systems that might be used to forecast ecosystem values on the basis of ecosystem features are developed later in this paper.

economic development, industrial accidents, and policy decisions that degrade or destroy ecosystems today.

The asset value of ecosystems

There are some important similarities between natural capital and manufactured capital that help illustrate the pathways by which ecosystems generate value. For example, with little or no out-of-pocket costs, ecosystems provide all of the basic services to the economy that are provided separately and at considerable expense by each of the 3 conventional forms of manufactured capital: *inventories, plant and equipment,* and *infrastructure*. Ecosystems have value as *inventories* because they are enormous storehouses of raw materials (e.g., timber, fish, beautiful views). They are valuable as *plant and equipment* because they include all the necessary support systems to replenish these inventories (e.g., wetlands and coral reefs). And ecosystems interact at various scales to provide the basic *infrastructure* that sustains natural and economic systems and supports all other forms of biological and industrial productivity (e.g., biodiversity and water, nutrient, energy, and carbon cycling). The contributions of ecosystems to human welfare can be compared on the basis of how they contribute in each of these basic categories.

When evaluating ecosystems on this basis, it is important to note most decisions involving ecosystems do not involve total losses of ecosystems or the elimination of ecosystem functions without perfect or near-perfect substitutes elsewhere in nature. In some cases, an injured ecosystem may lose only its capacity to provide some functions and services, and it may have the capacity to adapt or recover over time. For purposes of assessing an ecosystem's value as natural capital, therefore, some important and often overlooked questions involve the scarcity of the services it provides, the availability of perfect or near-perfect substitutes for them, the ability of the ecosystem to recover or to be restored or replaced, and the capacity of humans to adjust and adapt to temporary or even permanent ecosystem changes. The answers to such questions provide another basis for what might be referred to as "leading indicators" of ecosystem value.

Critical questions about ecosystem value

The questions about ecosystem features and functions addressed by conventional assessment methods, and the questions about the values of specific services addressed by conventional valuation methods, are only a few of the important questions that need to be addressed when comparing the asset value (natural capital value) of ecosystems. The important questions that need to be addressed for this purpose (including some that are at least partly addressed by assessment and valuation methods) are

1) What functions are provided by this ecosystem?
2) What services, products, and amenities do these ecosystem functions generate?

3) How much value, at least in relative terms, do people place on them?
4) Could they be provided just as well by other nearby or distant ecosystems?
5) Are there man-made substitutes that exist or could be developed?
6) What determines an ecosystem's ability to generate certain services and values?
7) With what reliability, precision, and frequency should ecosystem changes be measured?
8) Do changes in characteristics at one level in an ecological hierarchy reflect changes at other levels (e.g., forage or food fish)?
9) Do changes in an ecosystem at one location (e.g., a single wetland within a watershed) reflect changes at other locations (e.g., all similar wetlands in a watershed)?
10) How can normal fluctuations and cycles in the mix of ecosystem features and resulting services and values be distinguished from significant trends?
11) How reversible are ecosystem changes naturally or through technology?
12) Are biophysical relationships within ecosystems linear or are there important threshold points beyond which there are abrupt shifts in the mix of services and values provided?
13) How can and do people adapt to not having certain ecosystem services?
14) And, most importantly, if waiting to measure actual ecosystems services is impractical or dangerous, what are useful "leading indicators" of them?

Lessons from Wall Street

Providing specific answers to most of these questions would be difficult and in some cases impossible. However, they are still the right questions to be asking. For purposes of this paper the important issue is whether there are practical ways to address them and to organize information about them for purposes of comparing ecosystems. Practical ways of dealing with these kinds of questions, however, are not likely to be found in "scientific" literature aimed at reducing uncertainty about ecosystems and their values. It is more likely to be found in the results of research designed to help people make informed decisions in the face of uncertainty. Clues about how to develop practical methods for comparing ecosystems on the basis of their future services and values comes from what may seem to be an unlikely place: Wall Street.

Ecological systems may be more complex and more difficult to assess than market systems, and the expected values of natural capital may be more difficult to compare than those of manufactured capital. However, the 2 sets of tasks are very similar. Individuals whose livelihoods depend on forecasting the values (earnings streams and future prices) from various mixes of manufactured capital (corporate stocks) consult scientific research; but in the final analysis, the most successful rely on systems of indicators for making comparisons. There is simply too much relevant information about firms, industries, and markets and about financial, legal, and regulatory issues to make sense of investment alternatives in any other way.

The most widely used Wall Street indicator systems employ a variety of composite indicators employing terms such as diversity, resistance, resilience, vulnerability, and volatility. These are terms familiar to anyone exposed to modern literature related to landscape ecology or ecosystem health (see Karr 1992). Wall Street indicator systems also employ concepts of "scale" including links with lower scale labor and input markets and with higher scale intermediate and final product markets. They give attention to "hierarchies" and consider "nested interdependencies" involving firms within industries within industrial sectors within national markets within global trading networks and so on. However, there is one noteworthy difference between the way these terms are used on Wall Street and the way they are used in modern ecological literature. On Wall Street, they are used almost exclusively to provide clues about potential changes in the expected streams of economic returns from manufactured assets. In the ecosystem assessment literature, they are used almost exclusively to describe ecosystem processes or draw inferences about the health or capacities of ecosystems themselves with no specific focus on expected service flows or values.

Some practical differences

The information needs of policy-makers and jurists involved in comparing and trading natural capital are more similar to those of Wall Street investors than to designers of ecosystem assessment or valuation methods. They need practical information to help them deal with unavoidable uncertainty now, more than they need better ways to nibble away at questions that might help them avoid uncertainty some time in the future. As a result there are bound to be differences between the information needs of decision-makers who focus on ecosystem outcomes and those of scientists who are concerned about ecosystem processes. In some cases such differences may merely be a matter of how data are organized and interpreted. Information about vegetative cover at a site, for example, can be used to analyze primary biological productivity and to determine how much the site contributes to fishing opportunities or fishing success in nearby waters. However, some differences are more significant. Information about on-site food web linkages that may be important for scientific studies, for example, may be far less important for purposes of comparing ecosystem values than information about the use of the site by migrating birds or fish or the accessibility of the site to schoolchildren.

There are 2 reasons that differences between the information needs of researchers and decision-makers are far more important in the case of natural capital than in the case of manufactured capital. First, the indicators used by Wall Street decision-makers to develop indicators usually employ the same types of financial and market data that economic researchers use to analyze markets and industries. Second, the financial and market data that they use are collected routinely for other purposes. Unlike the biological components of ecosystems, each individual and corporation that makes up each industrial and market sector of the U.S. economy reports data about their economic and financial health routinely to the IRS and to countless other local, state, and federal agencies. These institutions then sort and aggregate this information in various ways and published it at very little cost.[12] The cost of developing and testing indicators related to manufactured capital, therefore, is very low and usually does not require any dedicated research.

Comparable data about the components of ecosystems, on the other hand, need to be generated from the ground up through directed research and monitoring undertaken at considerable expense. Collecting information about one aspect of an ecosystem usually means that other important information will not be collected. Collecting indicators of how coastal wetlands contribute to fishery values, or what their capacity is to protect property from storms or floods, or what their vulnerability is to future development, or how restorable they are, for example, only marginally improves scientific understanding of wetland ecosystems. There are significant tradeoffs involved in designing research to support scientific studies of ecosystems and to support value-based ecosystem indicators.

The need for careful indicator specification

The fact that there are differences between the types of data needed to support scientific studies of ecosystems and the types of data needed to develop practical indicators of ecosystem services and values is very important. It means that every choice about the focus and scale of an indicator, and the frequency and precision with which the indicator should be measured, has implications beyond just how reliable a predictor it will be. It also determines how much money will need to be spent collecting data about specific ecosystems and, as a practical matter, what data about ecosystems will not be collected. It also means that although general criteria may be developed for designing indicators of ecosystem values, the criteria used to specify indicators-how detailed and site-specific they should be-will not the same under all circumstances.

For purposes of assessing mitigation requirements for wetland permitting, for example, government agencies may make dozens of decisions each month involving small wetland trades within a single watershed. In such cases the stakes involved in each case may be relatively low, the locations and types of ecosystems may be quite similar, and a general-purpose set of indicators based on limited, on-site testing may be adequate. On the other hand, for purposes of settling natural resource damage claims for environmental injuries caused by oil spills, the stakes may be quite high and quite widespread and any basis of ecosystem comparison will need to be capable of

[12]Industry and market indicators rely primarily on data collected and published by the U.S. Department of Commerce, U.S. Bureau of Labor Statistics, and the U.S. Security and Exchange Commission. By contrast, environmental indicators rely primarily on primary data collected specifically for the purpose of developing indicators.

withstanding strong technical and legal challenges. In such cases it may be appropriate to develop detailed sets of indicators to evaluate each type of injury, base them on documented statistical relationships, and apply them carefully using biophysical profiles of specific sites.

The following section develops general criteria for designing leading indicators of ecosystem values. These criteria help identify which attributes of ecosystems will be useful in predicting the services and values it will provide, and they help identify information needs for developing indicators related to them. The criteria should also be useful in selecting indicators that provide an appropriate level of predictive value at an appropriate level of cost. However, they are not used here, and probably cannot be used, to develop a general set of leading indicators of ecosystem values that can be used in all circumstances.

Leading indicators of ecosystem values

Background

An indicator can be defined as "something that provides a clue to a matter of larger significance or makes perceptible a trend or phenomenon that is not immediately detectable" (Hammond et al. 1995). The significance of an indicator extends beyond what is actually measured to larger, more important phenomena. Indicators should serve 2 general purposes: 1) they should *quantify* information so significant changes or differences in the larger phenomena are more readily apparent and can be compared, and 2) they should *simplify* information about complex phenomena to improve understanding and communication.[13]

Indicators can be classified in many different ways on the basis of what they measure and how they are linked to the genuine focus of interest. One important distinction is between *current*, *leading*, and *lagging* indicators (see Anonymous 1992). *Current* indicators refer to measures reflecting phenomena happening now, or more typically, phenomena that happened recently. In the absence of actual estimates of changes in recreational fishing values, for example, it is possible to use changes in the number of anglers, fishing days, catch rates, money spent per trip, distance traveled, or fishing gear purchased as indicators of changes in fishing values.[14] These are current indicators because changes in each of them can be linked with changes in aggregate "willingness to pay" for recreational fishing in the same period. Current indicators, such as

[13]When pondering questions about the future, such as the services and values of natural or manufactured capital, it is not an exaggeration to say the value of measuring anything depends on its usefulness as an indicator.

[14]Because there are so many reliable current indicators of recreational fishing values they are often used as examples of how dependable non-market valuation can be. In the context of this paper it is important to note: 1) recreational fishing provides use value which is much easier to measure than the *nonuse* values associated with most ecosystem functions; and 2) the problem being addressed here is how ecosystem functions can be compared in terms of their ability to provide services such as improved recreational fishing, not the problem of measuring the dollar values of these services once they occur.

these indicators of recreational fishing value, are useful primarily for what might be called "score keeping."

In economics, the term "leading indicators" is used to refer to variables that are measured not because they are good proxies for changes taking place, but because they provide clues as to what important changes are likely to take place in the future. Leading indicators are more useful than current indicators for making investment and management decisions. Typical leading indicators of future conditions in national and regional economies include housing starts, industrial equipment orders, producer price indices, and winter yields of feed corn. The widely used "U.S. composite of leading economic indicators" is a highly reliable indicator of changes in economic income 6 to 9 months in advance. More specialized leading indicators based on trends in demographics, technology, and trade are used routinely on Wall Street to make more long-term forecasts for specific industrial sectors and markets. In ecosystems, leading indicators may be associated with changes in certain "keystone" or indicator species or with changes in political, economic, or land- and water-use patterns known to result in ecosystem change. Declines in forage fish populations, for instance, may be leading indicators of future declines in fish stocks that feed on them. The relaxing of fishery regulations in already overcapitalized fisheries or the backlog of orders for new boats that will enter such fisheries may also be useful leading indicators that a fish population will decline.[15] The range of *potential* leading indicators of changes in the derived value of ecosystem services is limited only by imagination. The range of *practical* leading indicators of ecosystem services and values is limited by cost, reliability, statistical evidence, and other factors discussed later in this section.

Lagging indicators are important primarily as a way to confirm an outcome was the result of the phenomena on which the leading indicators are based. In economics, for example, it may not be clear for many months when increases in gross economic production peaked. However, utilization rates for manufactured capital peak about 1 month after gross economic production, job vacancies peak about 1 month later, growth in net business earnings about 3 months later, and unit labor costs about 5 months later.[16] These same variables lag declines in economic production with a similarly predictable pattern. If an economic upturn or downturn occurred, it could be a critical leading indicator of other important phenomena; the first signs of it may be observed changes in these lagging indicators. In the case of ecosystems, observed changes in invertebrate communities or the size of noncommercial fish populations

[15]The term "leading indicator", as used here, includes factors related to driving forces and pressures that can be expected to result in changes in the state of a resource system. For a review of these factors and their use in other types of indicator systems see OECD (1993a, 1993b) and Bakkes et al. (1994).

[16]The specific lags mentioned here are those used in *The Economist* to report on the status of various national economies and are explained in a book published by the publishers of that magazine; see Anonymous (1992).

may be useful *lagging indicators* that the decline in the previous year's fish abundance index was a result of habitat losses or water quality problems, not overfishing.[17]

Site-specific criteria for developing indicators

Previous sections established that 2 sets of observable characteristics determine whether an ecosystem will generate certain streams of values. *Site-specific features* (e.g., soil type, vegetative cover, topographical features) determine the capacity to provide various functions); and *landscape context* (e.g., proximity to other features of the natural and human landscape) determines if the ecosystem will have the opportunity to provide these functions and strongly influences what services will flow from them, the benefits that will result, and the distribution of benefits.

To focus the development of indicators consider the factors related to capacity, opportunity, payoff, and equity associated with each specific ecosystem function listed in Table 5-1. Each of these factors and general information needs can be summarized as follows:

Capacity: Does the ecosystem have the biophysical conditions necessary to provide this function?

Example: Can it support migratory waterfowl or filter nutrients?

Information needs: site specific biophysical characteristics

Opportunity: Is it located in the ecological landscape where it will serve this function?

Example: Is it situated along a flyway or adjacent to a farming area?

Information needs: location and landscape context

Payoff: How will providing this function at this location result in benefits to people?

Example: How will attracting waterfowl to this site rather than another or improving the quality of adjacent water here rather than elsewhere affect people?

Information needs: location and landscape context

Equity: Who gains and who loses as a result of the ecosystem providing the function at this location, not elsewhere?

---

[17]It may not be possible for many years to establish whether changes in catches or sightings of certain populations in a given year are a result of changes in abundance or changes in availability. Lagging indicators of catches and sightings elsewhere sometimes help establish which it was, and, if it was a result of a decline in abundance, whether fishing-related, habitat-related, or other factors were responsible.

Example: Will attracting waterfowl to this site make them more valuable to some and less valuable to others (intragenerational equity) or more vulnerable to hunting and other pressures (intergenerational equity)?

Information needs: location and landscape context

Building blocks of ecosystem value[18]

Working through an illustration related to one of the many functions provided by wetlands (nutrient trapping) will show how the 4 factors defined above reflect conditions that contribute to services and values of wetlands with specific features at specific sites.

First, consider the *capacity* of a wetland at a given location to filter nutrients and prevent them from having adverse impacts on adjacent water bodies. A wetland's capacity to provide this function depends primarily on its slope and vegetative cover and other site-specific biophysical features; these can be considered independently of its watershed context and are the focus of most ecosystem-assessment methods.

However, the *opportunity* for the wetland to trap nutrients depends on the expected flow of nutrients from adjacent land which is determined almost exclusively by its location within the watershed, in particular its proximity to certain upland land uses (e.g., farms and construction sites versus forests and grasslands). Opportunity determines the "rate of capacity utilization," which is a critical factor in establishing the level of function provided and resulting service flows and values.

Similarly, the *payoff* from the nutrient trapping function depends on the wetland's location, in particular the characteristics of the adjacent (receiving) water body and the resources that exist in it or depend on it. At one location, for example, there may be important water-quality payoffs and improvements in nearby shellfish beds and finfish spawning areas because they are protected from overnutrification. At another location, a wetland with identical capacity to filter nutrients and the same opportunity to filter nutrients might be adjacent to a fast-moving, highly polluted river which empties directly into the open sea, resulting in no watershed-level payoff at all. Differences in the residence time of receiving water adjacent to 2 wetlands, therefore, may be a reasonable index of differences in payoff. Note that these kinds of indices do not require ethical judgments.

And finally, there are *equity* considerations. Society may concern itself with the difference between identical wetlands that generate identical values at 2 different locations if there are significant differences in who gains from them (e.g., rich or poor, urban or rural). Equity considerations involve policy choices, not scientific or eco-

[18] Some widely used wetland assessment methods include "social significance" components that employ terms similar to those used here. However, the socioeconomic components of those methods have never been fully developed or peer reviewed and have never been used to develop relative indicators of wetland values. For a review of how 28 of the most widely used ecosystem-assessment methods deal with issues related to services and values, see King (1997).

nomic criteria, but the nature of the policy choices depend in critical ways on location. Who has access to the wetland or to the different fisheries or waterfowl populations that depend on them? Whose property is protected from flooding? Whose scientific or educational opportunities or aesthetic values are enhanced and diminished? Indicators of who gains and who loses from wetland mitigation trades, for example, can be developed quite reliably without making any ethical decisions or value judgments about whether the group that gains is more or less "deserving" than the one that loses.

Same factors/different criteria

The influence of site and landscape factors on an ecosystem's capacity or opportunity to provide a function and on the resulting services and values will be vastly different for different functions. However, this does not mean that the relevant factors themselves are different or that vastly different data are needed to estimate indicators related to each function. Preliminary field testing of this type of indicator system to evaluate the size, characteristics, and siting of vegetative riparian buffers in the Chesapeake Bay watershed, for example, suggests that a limited number of site and landscape factors related to soil, hydrology, shape, vegetative cover, distance to open water, up-slope land use, accessibility, and so on can be used in different ways to develop indicators for many different ecosystem functions, services, and values.[19] Developing indicators for different ecosystems functions, in other words, does not require collecting different kinds of data for each function.

An illustration

The situation depicted in Figure 5-2a illustrates how the criteria listed above affect the services and values of ecosystems. In the situation depicted, 2 wetland areas are located on either side of a highway. They are being compared on the basis of the values they generate by providing 3 specific functions: nutrient trapping, wildlife habitat, and fishery support. The 2 wetland areas are the same size, the same shape, and have identical biophysical characteristics. However, because of slight differences in their landscape contexts, Site A is shown to generate significantly more benefits in each of the 3 categories than Site B.

In this illustration there are no differences in the capacity of the 2 sites to trap nutrients, support wildlife, or protect and nourish coastal fish habitat. However, Site A has more opportunity to provide all 3 of these functions because of its proximity to upland land uses that generate nutrients, its closeness to the coast and adjacent fish habitat, and its accessibility to wildlife from the upland wildlife refuge area. The payoff from providing functions at Site A is also greater than at site B because of its accessibility to

[19]These initial field trials using the system of indicators described here (but without considering equity impacts) involved prioritizing riparian forest buffer restoration projects in 3 sub-watersheds of the Chesapeake Bay. The application was aimed at ranking each stream reach in terms of its capacity, opportunity, and payoff potential with respect to 8 specific functions that were eventually aggregated into indicators in 3 areas: water quality, in-stream habitats, and terrestrial habitats. For details refer to King et al. (1996) and King and Bohlen (1996).

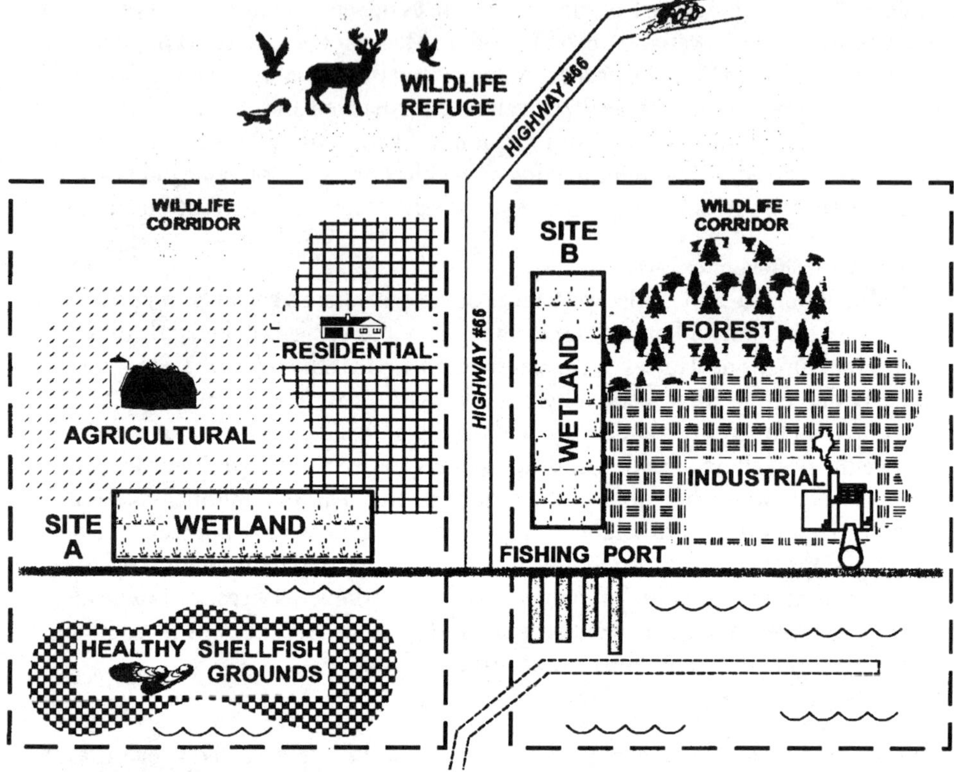

Site characteristics

Wetland Site A and Wetland Site B are identical in size, shape, and biophysical characteristics, and they are located in the same sub-watershed on either side of Highway 66.

Landscape context

Site A

near the coast, downstream is a beach area
adjacent to large healthy shellfish grounds that are accessible to the community
up-slope is agricultural land (nutrient run off)
wildlife corridor open from the north
near residential areas (aesthetics, scenic)
good access, adjacent public lands
access to many urban poor people

Site B

slightly off coast, downstream is industrial site
adjacent to fishing port and small shellfish beds that are contaminated and remote
up-slope is forest (no nutrient runoff)
wildlife corridor is blocked by Highway 66
nearby industrial sites (no proximity to people)
poor access, surrounded by private lands
access to few suburban rich people

Figure 5-2a Effects of wetland location on function, service, and value

	Wildlife Habitat		Fishery Support		Nutrient Trapping	
	Site A	Site B	Site A	Site B	Site A	Site B
Capacity	Identical size, shape, biophysical characteristics Score: Medium	Identical size, shape, biophysical characteristics Score: Medium	Identical size, shape, biophysical characteristics Score: Medium	Identical size, shape, biophysical characteristics Score: Medium	Identical size, shape, biophysical characteristics Score: Medium	Identical size, shape, biophysical characteristics Score: Medium
Opportunity	Wildlife corridor open from the north Score: High	Wildlife corridor blocked from north by Highway 66 Score: Low	Traps agricultural sediment, near coast, adjacent to fishing grounds Score: High	Little sediment to trap, off the coast, adjacent to boat channel Score: Low	Upslope is farm land generating nutrient flow, natural water flow, nonpoint discharge Score: High	Upslope is industrial sites and forests (little nutrients) channelized water flow to point discharge Score: Low
Payoff	Near residential areas, accessible, public land Score: High	Surrounded by industrial sites, inaccessible, private land Score: Low	Adjacent to large healthy shellfish area, public access, nearby parking Score: High	Few shellfish nearby, little access if there were, near point source discharge Score: Low	Adjacent to large healthy shellfish area, public access, nearby parking Score: High	Few shellfish nearby, little access if there were, near point source discharge Score: Low
Equity	Aesthetic, recreational opportunities for many poor Score: High	Access limited to few rich Score: Low	Aesthetic recreational opportunities for many poor Score: High	Access limited to few rich Score: Low	General water quality improvements, but also adjacent to healthy shellfish area accessible to poor Score: High	General water quality improvements only Score: Medium
Overall rating	High	Low	High	Low	High	Low

Figure 5-2b Relative values of Site A and Site B

people and the fact that the fish habitat it protects is larger and less contaminated than the one adjacent to Site B. For sake of argument, Site A and the fish and wildlife resources it supports are also assumed to be located where they provide scarce aesthetic and educational opportunities to a large urban disadvantaged population. Site B, on the other hand, is surrounded by large tracts of private land and forest areas that benefit only a few relatively wealthy families.

Without judging the merits of protecting and restoring wetland capacity at *both* Site A and Site B, the evidence presented in Figure 5-2a leaves little doubt that the expected services and values from Site A exceed those from Site B. Investments in protecting and restoring wetlands at Site A, therefore, would yield greater environmental and economic benefits than protecting and restoring wetlands at Site B. In the situation depicted in Figure 5-2a, the 2 sites are located very near one another, yet are shown to have significant enough landscape contexts to result in different functions, services, and values. This illustrates that the effects of location may be important even when making "on-site" comparisons.[20]

Landscape-level criteria for developing indicators

To make the comparison of Site A and Site B in the illustration even easier, assume that in the county's 10-year land-use plan the area around Site A is designated "environmentally sensitive recreation" and the area around Site B is designated A fast-track-industrial." The environmental and economic values provided by Site A are not only higher than those provided by Site B, they are less likely to be lost due to the future development of adjacent land. The same type of differences in risks might be associated with differences in exposure and vulnerability to risks from water diversion, sea level rise, and other factors. This suggests that the criteria listed above may only be suitable for forecasting ecosystem services and values in the relatively short term as long as site conditions and landscape context are expected to persist. For some purposes it may be important to take a broader and longer perspective that accounts for 1) the likelihood that landscape conditions may change; 2) the fact that different ecosystems may be more or less vulnerable (exposed to change), resistant (able to withstand change), and resilient (able to recover from change); and 3) the fact that the people who benefit from different ecosystems have different capacities to adapt and to respond to change.

The following list of criteria reflect one important set of factors: an ecosystem's ability to generate future values under current landscape conditions. To introduce a more dynamic perspective, they are placed alongside other criteria that reflect differences in

---

[20] Since the 2 sites are adjacent, it might be logical to assume that the same people would gain from investments at either site. However, to illustrate that equity issues can be important even when comparing nearby sites, a few assumptions are made here about the access and proximity of the 2 sites to urban/poor and suburban/rich populations.

the costs and risks associated with the differing effects of change on different ecosystems (see Table 5-2).

Table 5-2 Criteria for leading indicators of ecosystem values

Criteria	Typical question	Typical indicator
Capacity	Does this wetland have the biophysical characteristics to trap nutrients?	soil type, vegetative cover, hydrology (What's the expected nutrient uptake capacity?)
Opportunity	Is this wetland in a location where it can and will trap nutrients?	slope and land use of adjacent land (Does it have a source of nutrients to trap?)
Payoff	Will environmental and natural resources in adjacent water bodies be affected by the reduction of nutrient loading at this location?	residency time of nutrients delivered to receiving water (What changes are expected if nutrients are trapped here?)
	How important are the resources being protected at this location compared to those that would be protected elsewhere?	proximity of wetland to water important for fishing, swimming, and drinking; finfish, or shellfish spawning, and feeding; and waterfowl spawning, feeding and nursing
Equity	Whose recreational, educational, aesthetic opportunities are enhanced?	proximity of wetland to various populations; demographic and land use characteristics

Quality

- Capacity (Do the features of this wetland allow it to trap nutrients?)
- Opportunity (Is it in a location where nutrients will be available to trap?)
- Payoff (What resources are protected by trapping nutrients at this site?)
- Equity (Who gains by having nutrients trapped here rather than elsewhere?)

Scarcity The relationship between current supply and expected demand for services associated with this type of resource.

Critical factors: *Abundance* and *availability* of the resource

Critical questions:

- What is the quantity and quality of existing assets?
- What are the trends in supply and demand for services of these assets?

Vulnerability The extent to which this type of resource is susceptible to being lost to various types of controllable risks (e.g., land-use patterns) and uncontrollable risks (e.g., storm surge, sea level rise).

Critical factors: *Exposure* and *sensitivity*

Critical questions:

- Is resource at this site likely to be lost anyway making it *less* valuable?

- Are other similar sites likely to be lost making this one *more* valuable?

Reversibility The scientific, technical, and economic feasibility of restoring and rehabilitating this type of resource.

Critical factors: Where we are on the learning curve for restoration technologies that can be applied to this resource.

Critical questions:

- Do we know how to restore this resource if we misjudge threats or reconsider priorities later?
- Can restoration depend on natural processes or does it require engineered solutions?
- What would restoration cost, how long would it take, and what are the risks?

Replaceability The capacity to produce perfect or near-perfect substitutes for this resource or the services of this resource.

Critical factors:

- Scarcity of resource at broader ecological scale (e.g., outside the watershed).
- Where we are on the "learning curve" for restoration technologies that can be applied to this resource (e.g., fish spawning habitat) or artificial substitutes (e.g., hatcheries).

Critical questions:

- Do we know how to replace this resource if we misjudge threats or reconsider priorities later?
- Can replacement depend on natural processes or require engineered solutions?
- What would replacement cost, how long would it take, and what are the risks?

Substitutability The capacity to find imperfect but acceptable substitutes for the services of this resource. (e.g., lake fishing versus ocean fishing opportunities)

Critical factors: The uniqueness of this resource and the abundance and availability of similar resources or services of comparable value at a reasonable cost

Critical questions:

- What substitutes are available for the services of this resource?
- What are the differences in quality, costs, and who has access to them?

Developing actual indicators

This section develops general criteria for specifying leading indicators of ecosystem values, but stops short of recommending specific indicators. This is because the appropriate focus, scale, precision, frequency, and reliability of indicators depends on circumstances. The following section illustrates why an indicator system based on the criteria outlined in this section, or something very similar, will be essential to settle natural resource damage claims related to oil spills under a 1996 ruling related to the settlement of damage claims under the Oil Pollution Act of 1990 (OPA). This provides a useful context for exploring applications of the types of indicators being considered here for 2 reasons. First, the 1996 OPA ruling requires comparisons of injured and restored ecosystems based on services and values, not just "functional equivalency." Second, the economic stakes involved in oil spills litigation are high enough, and the frequency of spills is low enough, that the development and testing of site-specific indicators to form a basis for comparing losses from injuries with gains from restoration should be worthwhile.

A separate paper based on this one provides a preliminary profile of 28 of the most widely used ecosystem-assessment methods and evaluates their potential usefulness as a basis for developing indicators of capacity, opportunity, payoff, and equity with respect to various ecosystem functions.[21]

Applications under the Oil Pollution Act of 1990

Background

The Oil Pollution Act of 1990 authorizes public trustees-federal and state governments and some Native American tribes-to seek recovery of damages for injuries to natural resources. The goal of OPA is "to make the environment and the public whole for injuries to natural resources and natural resource services resulting from an incident involving a discharge or substantial threat of discharge of oil."[22] Under a final rule issued in January 1996, this goal is to be achieved "through returning injured natural resources and services to baseline and compensating for interim losses of such natural resources and services through the restoration, rehabilitation, replacement or acquisition of equivalent natural resources and/or services."[23] Efforts to restore the injured resource to baseline conditions are referred to in the 1996 rule as "primary" restoration. Restoration undertaken to compensate the public for interim lost services is referred to as "compensatory" restoration.

[21]This preliminary evaluation of ecosystem assessment methods is presented in King (1997). More detailed evaluations dealing with the development specific indicators and with respect to specific applications under OPA are forthcoming.

[22]"Section 1006 (e)(1) of the Oil Pollution Act of 1990 requires the President, through the Under Secretary of Commerce for Oceans and Atmosphere, to promulgate regulations for the assessment of natural resource damages resulting from a discharge or substantial threat of a discharge of oil" (15 *Federal Register* 990).

[23]"The final rule is for the use of authorized federal, state, Indian tribe, and foreign officials, referred to as 'trustees.' Natural resource damage assessments are not identical to response or remedial actions addressed by the larger statutory scheme of the Oil Pollution Act of 1990. Assessments are not intended to replace response actions, which have as their primary purpose the protection of human health, but to supplement them, by providing a process for restoring natural resources and services injured as a result of an incident involving oil" (15 *Federal Register* 990).

The 1996 final rule specifies that the adequacy of restoration should be determined by the following process:

1) *Compare* the type and quality of lost resources and services with those that result from primary and compensatory restoration,
2) *Determine* if they are of *comparable value*; and, if they are not, and
3) *Implement* scaling procedures that adjust the level of restoration to a size that will compensate the public for the injury.

Guidance for ecosystem comparisons

The rule does not provide specific guidance regarding how the type, quality, and comparable value of lost and replacement resources or services should be compared or how "scaling" should be accomplished. However, under certain circumstances, it does recommend using specific types of analyses. According to the rule, "when the injured resources and/or services are primarily of indirect human use (e.g., species habitat or biological natural resources for which human uses are primarily off-site) the appropriate basis for evaluating and scaling the restoration is *Habitat Equivalency Analysis* (HEA)."

Federal agencies have prepared draft guidance for implementing "scaling" and completing some other tasks required by HEA (15 *Federal Register* 990). The classification system used in these draft guidance documents identifies 4 specific types of comparisons that may need to be made. They include

Type 1: same type, same quality, and comparable value;

Type 2: same type, same or different quality, and *not* of comparable value;

Type 3: different type (and therefore of different quality and not of comparable value), but of comparable type and quality, nonetheless; and

Type 4: different type (and therefore of different quality and not of comparable value) and not of comparable type and quality.

Applying valuation criteria

The draft guidance documents do not discuss specific measurement tools, but it is inferred in these documents that some combination of ecosystem-assessment methods and ecosystem-valuation methods will provide an analytical basis for performing HEA and for addressing issues related to "scaling." Section 1 of this paper provided evidence that neither methods provide an adequate basis for comparing ecosystem services or values. The implication is that they cannot, by themselves, provide an analytical basis for conducting HEA. Section 2 of this paper outlined criteria for developing sets of indicators to compare ecosystems in terms of their relative values. The implication was that such indicators might provide a practical alternative to conventional ecosystem-assessment and valuation methods; and would, in any case, provide a way to link the results of those methods for purposes of comparing ecosystem services and values. This section gives the general framework for conducting HEA and describes why an indicator system similar to the one discussed in the previous section will be needed to carry out HEA and to address "scaling" issues.

The basics of habitat equivalency analysis (HEA)

Consider the simple Type 1 situation listed above where the lost and restored habitats are the same type and the same quality and are of comparable value. Assume that habitat type under OPA can be defined adequately using the widely accepted Cowardin system for classifying wetlands and deep-water habitats shown in Figure 5-3.[24] Habitats within each Cowardin classification-each habitat type under OPA-can be expected to have similar capacity to provide the functions listed in Table 5-1.

Habitats of a given type may have vastly different biophysical characteristics and landscape contexts and, as a result, may have vastly different functions, services, or values. However, for simplicity, assume that they are identical and, also, that a linear relationship exists between measures of the functional capacity of wetlands and the functions it will provide and between these and the services and values it is expected to generate. Under these simplifying assumptions a percentage change in the functional capacity of habitat, as a result of restoration for example, can be expected to result in an identical percentage change in the functions, services, and values provided by the site. These assumptions greatly simplify the task of comparing ecosystems, of course, because functional capacity is relatively easy to measure and responds directly to restoration, whereas the others are relatively difficult to measure and may not respond directly to restoration efforts.[25]

Graphical depiction of habitat equivalency analysis

Under these simplifying assumptions, relative measures of functional capacity can serve as the "currency" for comparing ecosystem values. The values lost at the site of the injury (which is also the primary restoration site) can be expressed in relative terms using the pre-injury capacity of the site as the baseline (100%) (this is depicted in Figure 5-2a. Likewise, the gains in values at the compensatory restoration site can be measured in relative terms using the pre-restoration capacity of the site as a baseline (this is depicted in Figure 5-2b). In both Figure 5-2a and Figure 5-2b the level of functional capacity is expressed in each period as a percent of the baseline level of capacity, which is shown to increase over time after the injury and as a result of primary and compensatory restoration. At both the site of the injury and the compensatory restoration site, the values generated each year on a per acre basis can be expressed as "the percent of baseline value." However, for the relative units of value to be comparable—for the scale of the "y" axis to be the same for both sites—2 additional conditions must exist. The baseline functional capacity and the fixed propor-

[24] The widely used Cowardin system of wetland classification includes 5 types of wetland systems, 11 types of wetland subsystems, and 55 classes of wetlands (Cowardin et al. 1979).

[25] These are the assumptions that are used implicitly whenever differences in the biophysical characteristics of ecosystems (measures of functional capacity) are used to compare ecosystem values.

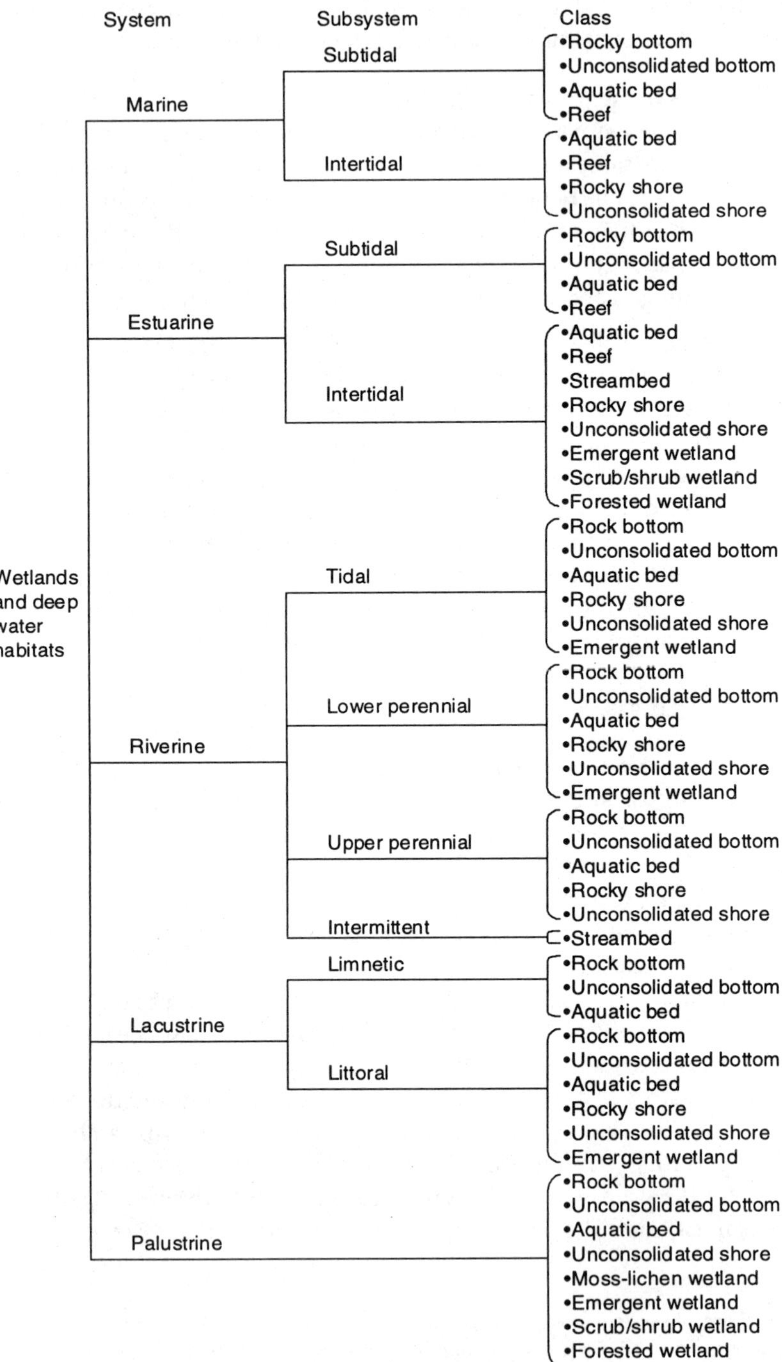

Figure 5-3 Overview of the Cowardian System for Classifying Wetland and Deep Water Habitats

tions between functions, services, and values assumed for the injured site must be identical at the compensatory restoration site.[26]

Criteria for establishing Type I conditions

The first place where the criteria developed in the previous section might be useful would be in determining whether or not a Type 1 situation exists. Based on the logic used in the previous section, determining if the site of the injury and the site of proposed restoration are of similar quality and of comparable value will require comparisons of site-based and landscape-based criteria. Using the terminology developed in the previous section, this could be established on the basis of whether or not the 2 sites have the same capacity and opportunity to provide a certain mix of functions and whether these functions will result in the same levels of services.

Type 2, Type 3, and Type 4 situations

As a practical matter, HEA will need to be performed most often to compare habitats that are not of the same quality and comparable value: Type 2, 3, or 4 situations.[27] Under OPA, the process of "scaling" is intended to equate units (acres) of restored habitat to the quality and value standard of units (acres) of injured habitat.[28] The process of scaling can become very complicated unless specific criteria are established as a basis for comparing ecosystem quality and value. As simplifying assumptions about fixed relationships between site capacity and functions, services, and values are relaxed to reflect real-world conditions, the process of conducting scaling without some type of indicator system may become impossible.

The first problem is one that would be encountered in comparing lost and replacement services and values even in Type 1 situations. Since compensatory restoration projects will be undertaken sometime after the injury, they are likely to provide replacement services and values sometime after those associated with the injured site are lost. Adjusting for differences in the timing of services lost and gained can be accomplished by introducing the concept of discounting into HEA; this has been

---

[26]These are the conditions necessary to conduct HEA using relative measures of restoration success.

[27]Until recently wetland mitigation provisions under Section 404 of the Clean Water Act included a clear preference for "on-site, in-kind" mitigation. This closely resembles the Type 1 situation identified under OPA. This preference, however, resulted in many restoration projects being undertaken at inferior sites and failing to meet environmental goals while diverting restoration funds away from more promising "off-site" projects. As a result, the preference for on-site mitigation has softened and off-site mitigation, including mitigation banking, has gained more acceptance.

[28]"Scaling" under OPA involves adjusting the size of compensatory restoration projects to account for differences in the quality and value of habitat at the injured and restoration sites. Scaling can be based on resource-to-resource, service-to-service, or value-to-value comparisons and usually takes the form of adjusting the size or intensity of restoration projects. The process of "scaling" under OPA is described in draft guidance documents prepared by the NOAA Damage Assessment and Restoration Program (1996).

described fully elsewhere.[29] What is more difficult is determining what unit of measurement the discount factor should be applied to.

The first complication is that differences in quality and value of habitats can be assessed with respect to more than one set of services and values (e.g., fish versus waterfowl habitat, recreational versus aesthetic value). Undertaking the process of scaling to account for each of the ecosystem functions listed in Table 5-1 will be quite challenging unless some prearranged criteria or indicator system is used to compare site and landscape conditions with respect to each functions. Using this approach the scaling factors may be different for different functions and services.[30] Moreover, a mediocre habitat in an exceptionally good location (moderate capacity, high opportunity) may generate the same expected level of service (quality) and comparable value as high quality habitat in a poor location (high capacity, low opportunity).

In the final analysis

In the final analysis, HEA requires that the discounted present value of the expected interim loss of service flows at the site of the injury (Area X in Figure 5-4a) must equal the expected increase in the discounted present value of service flows provided over time at the compensatory restoration site (Area Y in Figure 5-4b). Under very simple assumptions it might be possible to use differences in measures of capacity at the 2 sites to determine an appropriate scaling factor. However, under more realistic conditions all of the issues raised in earlier sections of this paper come into play. In the typical situation, assuming that 2 sites are identical and in identical landscape contexts, what criteria should be used to conduct HEA and perform scaling? The criteria outlined in the previous section that allows ecosystems to be compared and ranked on the basis of differences in biophysical characteristics and landscape contexts is one way. If an indicator system based on these or similar criteria are not used to develop scaling factors, how can alternative compensatory restoration sites be compared, and how can the adequacy of investments in primary and compensatory restoration be evaluated? In practice, scaling restoration projects cannot take place on the basis of service-to-service or value-to-value comparisons but only on the basis of comparisons of *expected* services and values. That is the purpose of the criteria developed in the previous section: to form a basis for making resource-to-resource comparisons.

Conclusions about HEA and scaling

The criteria outlined in the previous section raise more questions about performing HEA and scaling than they answer. Under the simplifying assumptions listed above to

---

[29]For a discussion of how discounting affects the comparison of ecosystem services and values provided at different times see King (1991), King et al. (1993) and Unsworth and Bishop (1994).

[30]Perhaps some type of weighting criteria applied to functions and services on the basis of other factors and abundances and shortages identified in specific landscape contexts could provide an unambiguous basis for scaling restoration at various sites.

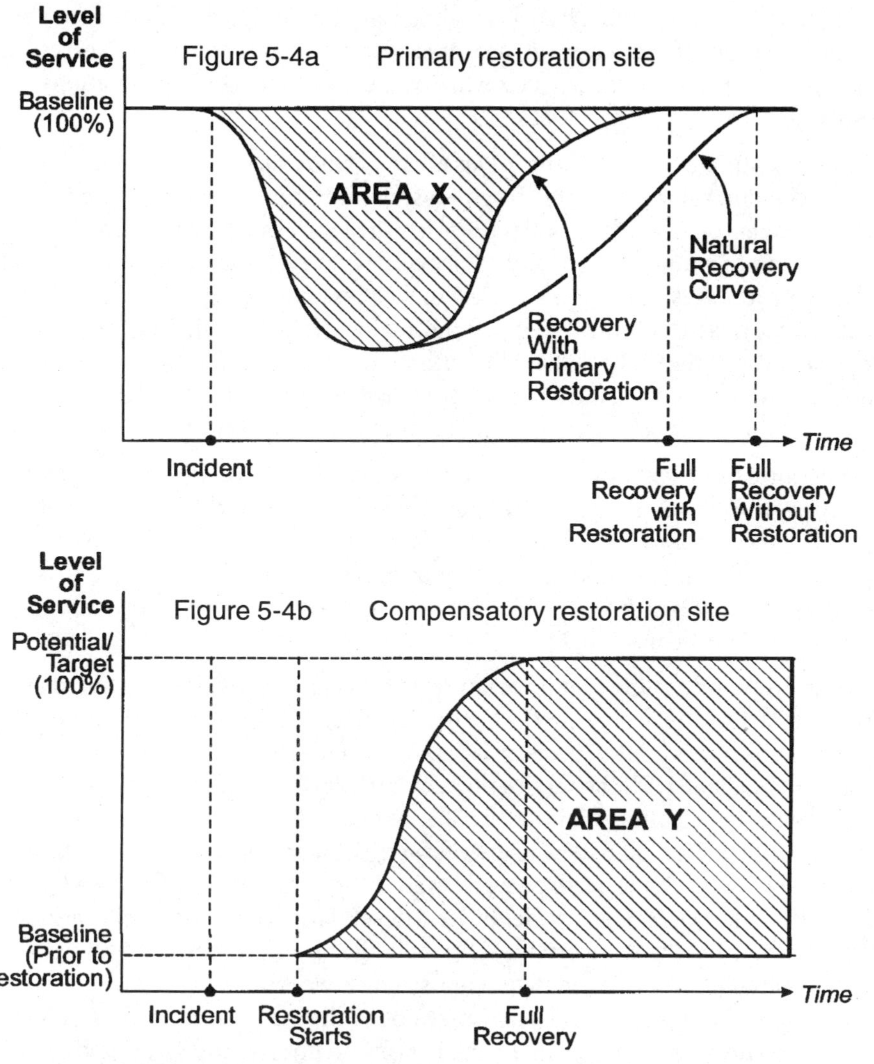

AREA X: Services *lost* at injury site with primary restoration expressed as % of baseline or expected level

AREA Y: Services *gained* at compensatory restoration site expressed as % of potential/target level less baseline (pre-restoration) %

Figure 5-4 Relationship between service flows at primary and compensatory restoration sites

characterize Type 1 situations, HEA and scaling can be accomplished fairly easily by comparing appropriately discounted measures of capacity to represent the success of natural recovery and restoration efforts. However, under more realistic situations there are 4 complicating factors that need to be addressed.

First, and most important, is the enormous effect of landscape context on the functions, services, and values generated by an ecosystem. Where the compensatory restoration being considered takes place off-site, the typical situation under OPA, differences in opportunity, payoff, and equity come into play and need to be factored into scaling procedures. Although the effect of location may be negligible in the case of restoration that is strictly "on-site," opportunities for strictly "on-site" restoration will be rare. Even restoration sites that are identical in physical features to the injured site and are close enough to the injured site to be considered "on-site" (a distance of less than 2 mile for instance) may generate significantly different services and values.

Second, because there will usually be more than one habitat function to consider, using scaling procedures may yield ambiguous results. Performing HEA and applying scaling procedures to individual functions, services, or values may yield conflicting results. Some weighting or ranking of functions or services may be needed to make tradeoffs when applying HEA, especially if several different compensatory restoration possibilities are being considered.

Third, both HEA and scaling require forecasting flows and services from injured and restored habitats relatively far into the future. The uncertainty associated with the outcome of habitat-restoration projects is well-known and is generally higher than the uncertainty associated with the service flows of undisturbed natural habitats or naturally recovering habitats. This uncertainty has several identifiable sources. For example, the restoration plan itself may be flawed, sound restoration plans may not be implemented properly, unexpected natural events (e.g., storms, droughts, sea-level rise) or man-made events (e.g., accidents, land development) may intervene, and so on. Differences in risks and uncertainty and their effects on the "expected values" of service flows are not the same for all functions and services or at all prospective restoration sites. More importantly, they may not be the same at restoration sites as they are at the site of the injury. Differences in risk and uncertainty associated with expected streams of services and values over time need to be factored into HEA and scaling procedures.

Finally, there are the logical bounds of achieving equivalent functions, services, and values by scaling the size and intensity of compensatory restoration projects. A huge quantity of low quality habitat may not be equivalent to a small quantity of high quality habitat. Similarly, the difference in the expected recovery of functions and services with and without investments in restoration may not justify the level of investment necessary to undertake compensatory restoration at the preferred (on-site) location. Stated differently, investments at the extensive margin (more area restored) may not be a reasonable substitute for investments at the intensive margin (more restoration per unit area) and requiring either investment on-site may represent a wasteful use of restoration dollars after more promising off-site alternatives are considered.

Conclusions about indicators and OPA

Section 1 of this paper described how ecosystems generate services and values and identified the factors that influence the level and distribution of those services and values. The conclusion reached on the basis of Section 1 is that the available ecosystem-assessment methods and ecosystem-valuation methods provide only part of the information required to compare ecosystems in terms of the services and values they can be expected to provide.

Section 2 developed a preliminary framework and identified criteria for developing "leading indicators" of ecosystem services and values. The conclusion reached in Section 2 was that it should be possible to integrate the results of ecosystem-assessment and valuation studies with information about landscape context in a practical framework for comparing ecosystems on the basis of expected services and values.

This final section reviewed some of the requirements for conducting HEA and performing scaling procedures under OPA. The conclusion reached here is that performing HEA and scaling requires assessing differences in the *expected* services and values from different ecosystems. As a practical matter these differences need to be assessed on the basis of observable or measurable differences in site and landscape characteristics that influence future services and values. These do not necessarily require the estimation or comparison of current services or values.

Since ecosystem comparisons under OPA must determine if compensatory restoration makes "the environment and the public whole for injuries to natural resources and natural resource services," the use of conventional biophysical ecosystem-assessment methods, by themselves, are not adequate. On the other hand, ecosystem-valuation methods are too expensive to be applied to all ecosystems services at all prospective restoration sites and do not link expected values with specific ecosystem characteristics that change as a result of injuries and restoration efforts. These limitations seem to justify the further development and testing of value-based criteria that draw on both ecosystem-assessment and ecosystem-valuation methodologies to form a practical analytical basis for performing HEA and scaling.

References

[Anonymous]. 1992. Guide to economic indicators: making sense of economics. London: The Economist Books.

Bakkes JA, van den Born GJ, Helder JC, Swart RJ, Hope CW, Parker JDE. 1994. An overview of environmental indicators: state of the art and perspectives. Bilthoven, The Netherlands: National Institute of Public Health and Environmental Protection.

Brinson MM. 1993. A hydrogeomorphic classification for wetlands. Washington DC: U.S. Army Corps of Engineers. Wetlands Research Program Technical Report WRP-DE-4.

Cowardin LM et al. 1979. Classification of wetlands and deep water habitats of the United States. FWS/OBS79/31, Office of Biological Services, Fish and Wildlife Service. Washington DC: Government Printing Office.

Freeman III AM. 1993. The measurement of environmental and resource values: theory and methods. Washington DC: Resources for the Future.

Gunderson LH, Holling CS, Light SS, editors. 1995. Barriers and bridges to the renewal of ecosystems and institutions. New York: Columbia University.

Hammond A, Adriaanse A, Rodenburg E, Bryant D, Woodward R. 1995. Environmental indicators: a systematic approach to measuring and reporting on environmental policy performance in the context of sustainable development. Baltimore MD: WRI Publications.

Karr JR. 1992. Ecological integrity: protecting Earth's life support systems. In: Costanza R, Norton BG, Haskell BD, editors. Ecosystem health: new goals for environmental management. Washington DC: Island. p 223–238.

King DM. 1991. Wetland creation and restoration: an integrated framework for evaluating costs, expected results and compensation ratios. Solomons MD: University of Maryland. System, CEES Technical Contribution No. UMCEES-CBL-91-42 prepared under cooperative agreement with the USEPA, Office of Policy Analysis, Washington, DC.

King DM. 1997. Use of ecosystem assessment methods in natural resource damage assessment. Silver Spring MD: NOAA Damage Assessment and Restoration Program.

King DM, Bohlen CC. 1996. A framework for assessing and comparing the payoff from riparian buffers. University of Maryland System, CEES Technical Contribution No. UMCEES-CBL-96-162 prepared under a Cooperative Agreement between University of Maryland, CEES, and the USEPA, Office of Policy.

King DM, Bohlen CC, Adler KJ. 1993. Watershed management and wetland mitigation: a framework for determining compensation ratios. University of Maryland System Report #UMCEES-CBL-93-098. Solomons MD: University of Maryland.

King DM, Hagan PT, Bohlen CC. 1996. Setting priorities for riparian buffers: A practical framework for comparing the benefits and costs of vegetative buffers. University of Maryland BCEES Technical Contribution No. UMCEES-CBL-96-160. Solomons MD: University of Maryland.

Kopp RJ, Smith VK. 1993. Valuing natural assets: the economics of natural resource damage assessment. Washington DC: Resources for the Future.

Kusler JA, Quammen ML, Brooks G. 1986. National Wetland Symposium: Mitigation of impacts and losses. Berne NY: Association of State Wetland Managers, Inc.

Likens G. 1992. An ecosystem approach: its use and abuse. Excellence in ecology, Book 3. Oldendorf/Luhe, Germany: Ecology Institute.

National Research Council. 1992. Restoration of aquatic ecosystems: Science, technology, and public policy. Washington DC: National Academy.

[NOAA] National Oceanic and Atmospheric Administration. 1992. Report of the NOAA Panel on Contingent Valuation; Damage Assessment and Restoration Program, U.S. Department of Commerce, National Oceanic and Atmospheric Administration. Silver Spring MD: NOAA.

[NOAA] National Oceanic and Atmospheric Administration. 1995. Habitat equivalency analysis: an overview. Damage Assessment and Restoration Program, U.S. Department of Commerce, National Oceanic and Atmospheric Administration. Silver Spring MD: NOAA.

[NOAA] National Oceanic and Atmospheric Administration. 1996. Draft guidance document: scaling compensatory restoration projects *(Oil Pollution Act of 1990)* ; Damage Assessment and Restoration Program, U.S. Department of Commerce, National Oceanic and Atmospheric Administration. Silver Spring MD: NOAA.

[OECD] Organization for Economic Cooperation and Development. 1993a. OECD core set of indicators for environmental performance reviews. Environment Monograph No. 83. Paris, France: OECD.

[OECD] Organization for Economic Cooperation and Development. 1993b. Indicators for the integration of environmental concerns into energy policies. Environment Monograph No. 80. Paris, France: OECD.

Pitelka LF. 1996a. Ecological issues in wetland mitigation [Special issue]. *Ecological Applications* 6(1).

Pitelka LF. 1996b. Forum: perspectives on ecosystem management. *Ecological Applications* 6(3).

Shabman L, Scodari P, King D. 1994. National wetland mitigation banking study. Expanding opportunities for successful mitigation: the private credit market alternative. Alexandria VA: U.S. Army Corps of Engineers. IWR Report 94-WMB-3.

Smith VK. 1996. Estimating economic values for nature: methods for non-market valuation. Cheltenham, UK: Edward Elgar.

Unsworth RE, Bishop RC. 1994. Assessing natural resource damages using environmental annuities. *Ecological Economics* 11(1):35–41.

Wilson EO. 1988. Biodiversity. Washington, DC: National Academy.

5a

Discussion Paper I on Leading Indicators of Ecosystem Services and Values

*Steven J. Cary**

Dennis King addresses implementation of the Oil Pollution Act (OPA) and the National Oceanic and Atmospheric Administration's (NOAA's) damage assessment process through development and use of indicators of ecosystem values. My comments are influenced by the fact that New Mexico has no coastline and relies primarily on Comprehensive Environmental Response, Compensation and Liability Act (CERCLA) authority and the Department of the Interior (DOI) regulations in its natural resource damage assessment (NRDA) activities. Some of my comments can be traced to my perspective from an inland state. Nevertheless, evolution of the NOAA regulations and assessment procedures is of interest because in some ways NOAA is out in front of DOI and is generating new approaches, policies, and techniques that eventually will serve as models for revised DOI regulations.

I found King's concept of "leading indicators of ecosystem values" to be intellectually stimulating, appropriate for the situation, and well-researched. In particular, his point is well taken that landscape context should be one of the criteria for developing indicators. Regrettably, one effect of considering landscape context is to add yet another variable to a matrix that already has too many variables to allow solution at reasonable cost.

The text of the paper did not fulfill the promise of the title. King seems to be in the early stages of mapping out potential criteria that could later be used to develop indicators that could substitute for real measurements of value. We seem to be at least 2 long strides away from implementation: we cannot measure comparative ecosystem values, but we could if we had good indicators, if we had good criteria for indicators.

King's indicators have conceptual appeal. If not carefully constructed, however, they may prove to be nearly as elusive, costly and time-consuming to develop as the actual ecosystem values that are intended to replace. King's caveats strongly hint that workable indicators will not be available for some time, even simply for wetlands. It is sobering to remember that wetlands represent but one, and perhaps the best studied, of numerous ecosystems for which trustees are responsible. King's search for "detailed

*State of New Mexico, Office of the Natural Resources Trustee, Santa Fe, New Mexico

sets of indicators" is not a near-term solution to the problem that resource values cannot be reliably measured at reasonable cost. "General indicators" may be a useful interim step while detailed indicators are being developed.

While ecosystem value indicators are still under development, it is up to stakeholders to devise creative approaches to deal with retroactive, current, and near-future natural resource damage (NRD) situations. For example, we can adapt NRD cases to fit the limitations of the valuation tools. One way to do this is to emphasize acquisition and protection of intact ecosystems, whose values and services are relatively easy to compare. In contrast, attempts to actively restore injured ecosystems are often poor investments because they force awkward comparisons of values and services and because such efforts have unpredictable results. Acquisition of equivalent resources will also help slow the transformation of natural ecosystems by humans, which is occurring at a rate that far exceeds our restoration efforts in most cases.

Arriving at indicators

The title of King's paper, "Leading indicators of ecosystem services and values," contains the implicit acknowledgment that actual measurement and reliable determination of ecosystem services and values are often not reasonable goals. This realization forces stakeholders to open the door to the possibility of surrogates, or indicators, which could facilitate such comparisons.

King identifies features, functions, services, and values as ecosystem attributes that can be compared between baseline, injured, and restored situations. As one proceeds down this list from features to values, measurement becomes more expensive and less reliable. Of these attributes, only ecosystem features (e.g., acres, slope characteristics, species composition) can be reliably measured. The remaining attributes can be quantified, calculated, or estimated, but only with increasing amounts of professional judgment and at increasing cost. Ecosystem functions, for example, are best quantified in mathematical equations and models that approximate processes and interactions that take place within an ecosystem.

For ecosystem services and values, measurement becomes orders of magnitude more difficult because they involve aspects of human thought and behavior. The scientific and economic communities may agree that such services and values exist, and they may agree on theoretical approaches for ascertaining those values. Perhaps some day we will even agree on techniques that can be employed to obtain the data necessary to calculate ecological services and to determine ecosystem values. Currently, however, these techniques are prohibitively expensive and most ongoing NRD cases will not benefit from development of these techniques.

It is important to identify the attributes of good indicators. Although what follows is not necessarily a comprehensive list, the attributes of good indicators should include

1) strong correlation with ecosystem services and values;
2) independence from human value systems; and

3) measurable with a reasonable trade-off of reliability for cost in injured ecosystems, at baseline conditions and in restored, replaced, or acquired equivalent ecosystems.

King seeks to arrive at indicators via the criteria they should meet, but his criteria all address attribute 1 above. His proposed criteria relate primarily to ecosystem characteristics that affect value and service, i.e., quality, scarcity, vulnerability, reversibility, replaceability, substitutability. These are essential considerations, although the last 2 may be duplicative. Attributes 2 and 3, however, above are not addressed by King. This is not necessarily a criticism of King, but someone needs to examine the logistical considerations raised by 2 and 3 so it can be determined whether workable indicators are even a theoretical possibility.

Good indicators should be independent from human value systems (Attribute 2) because we already know that direct measurement of human value systems is a costly endeavor. We ought to be certain that the indicators themselves can be developed without going through controversial valuation gauntlets. If indicators cannot be measured independently from value systems, then they are destined to engender the same controversy as contingent valuation in a passive-use scenario. That would defeat their very purpose. A good indicator should be highly correlated with, yet independent of (or at least measurable independently from) human value systems.

Indicators that have Attribute 3 will be practical. We have several valuation tools that are reasonable under idealized, simplified scenarios. Unfortunately these scenarios are not encountered very often in real life, so the tools are of limited value. A good indicator should be usable in the variety of baseline, injured, and restored systems likely to be encountered in natural resource damage contexts. Application of this criterion may have the result that the indicators will be simple functions of easily measured ecosystem characteristics.

The timing problem

A discussion of "Lessons from Wall Street" provides useful context, but despite an intriguing and informative beginning, King's conclusions are sobering. He suggests that there will always be an information gap and that uncertainty about ecological values will always be a large factor in value comparisons. What Wall Street does in the face of uncertainty is to develop indicators, and it makes a certain amount of sense to establish indicators of natural resource value for use in NRD contexts. King suggests that for some purposes, such as wetlands mitigation, all that may be necessary is "general purpose" indicators based on "limited, on-site testing." King contrasts that situation with an NRD context for which it may be necessary to "develop detailed sets of indicators to evaluate each type of injury, base them on documented statistical relationships, and apply them carefully using biophysical profiles of specific sites." This sounds good, but excessive time will be needed to develop indicators having this degree of rigor and sophistication.

King proceeds to address development of general criteria for designing indicators of ecosystem values. The design seems sound. Unfortunately, he confides that the criteria "are not used here, and probably cannot be used, to develop a general set of leading indicators of ecosystem values that can be used in all circumstances." For trustees, it was distressing to acknowledge that real resource values may be too costly and too complicated to derive and compare in the majority of cases. To make matters worse, King is now suggesting that indicators themselves also will be costly and time-consuming to develop. I hope it does not have to be this way.

For indicators to be workable, they must be simple and affordable. He cannot have the most desirable option (a Lexus), so I fear that King is working toward a less desirable option (a Cadillac). Many trustees have neither the time to wait for this Cadillac to come off the assembly line nor the funds to gas-up or buy insurance for the Cadillac should it even come on the market. Trustees need an even less desirable option, a Chevrolet or Toyota. After we can handle the Chevrolet or Toyota, we an work toward the fancier version. I am skeptical that King's "detailed sets of indicators" will ever result in anything useful to trustees for inland, non-coastal resources. The situation is reminiscent of DOI's Type A and Type B regulations. Despite the regulatory capability and the passage of time, there seems to be little chance that expedited DOI Type A assessments will ever be possible for non-aquatic, nonmarine natural resources. King should investigate opportunities for scaled-down indicators based on the most easily measured ecosystem features. They may be more practical.

The long developmental period for King's indicators is less of a shortcoming for NRD claims under OPA because that statute is directed toward future incidents, includes no retroactive liability, and the OPA statute of limitations does not start to run on an incident until the NRDA is completed. Even if it takes 20 years to get good indicators, I suppose that there will be new incidents to which these indicators could then be applied.

The same cannot be said for NRD claims under CERCLA. Improved hazardous waste management pursuant to the federal Resource Conservation and Recovery Act should minimize the number of future sites with hazardous substance releases and with CERCLA NRD liability. In addition, much of CERCLA's effectiveness relies on its retroactive liability provisions. Thus, CERCLA NRD liability may be most influential for preexisting sites rather than new incidents. This leverage is counterbalanced by the 3-year statute of limitations that starts to run upon a trustee learning of the release and connecting it with the damage, whether or not an NRDA is performed. The long intervals needed to develop criteria for indicators and then the indicators themselves are inconvenient in view of these timing constraints. Most CERCLA NRD claims will either lapse or be settled before the first legitimate indicator is available for use. Trustees clearly are looking for help, but these detailed sets of indicators seem to be a long time from realization.

One might also inquire about the regulatory standing or status of these indicators. Will they have to be approved by NOAA or DOI before they can be used by trustees? Will they have to become part of the regulations through standard public participation procedures? Will trustees be able to get a rebuttable presumption by using these indicators? Indicators may be useful even if they simply made intellectual sense. My experience has been that the regulations are not carefully followed in most cases. Creative application of available tools and regulations contributes to reasonable settlement of many cases without litigation. Indicators may contribute to settlement of cases whether or not they were part of the regulations. This brings me back to "general purpose" indicators, which King may have dismissed prematurely. They may not be ideal for NRD situations, but they may be easy to use and cost effective while the more sophisticated "detailed sets of indicators" are still on the drawing board.

Future directions

King often had to simplify situations in order to make a point or to use a tool. For example, comparing Sites A and B was easier if they were similar (same size, same shape, same biophysical characteristics, etc.) than if they were different. If they are similar, one may not even need to know their actual values or capacities in order to develop an appropriate restoration plan. The fact that they are the same in all important, measurable ways means they provide the same ecological or human-use services and have the same value. The more different 2 sites are, on the other hand, the greater the likelihood of substantial error in the resulting comparison of values and services, and the greater the uncertainty that the restoration plan is adequate.

King asks the reader to consider the simplest type of comparison, Type 1, for sites of the same type, same quality, and comparable value. This comparison first hinges on the (presumed) ability of the Cowardin classification system to adequately define habitat. King then asks the reader to assume:

1) that habitats of a given type have the same biophysical characteristics and landscape contexts;
2) that as a result they generate the same functions, services, and values; and
3) that linear relationships exists between:
   a) measures of functional capacity and actual function;
   b) function and services; and
   c) function and value.

One also must assume that the 2 sites share the same baseline functional capacity and the same fixed ratios between functions, services, and values. But given these assumptions (a long list, but sadly reasonable under the circumstances), King implies that value comparisons are manageable in Type 1 situations. But what does one do in other situations, which King admits will include the majority of cases? "As simplifying assumptions about fixed relations between site capacity and functions, services and values are relaxed to reflect real-world conditions, the process of conducting scaling without some type of indicator system may become impossible." It may also become impossible even with a sophisticated indicator system.

King recognizes that value comparisons and habitat equivalency analysis (HEA), even with indicators, will entail considerable uncertainty except in the most simplistic situations. King then identifies one path for us to follow. That path is improvement and elucidation of the comparison machinery to improve its performance in more realistic situations. This is no easy task, so King identifies "4 complicating factors" that need to be addressed. This is the path that King intends to follow.

It may not be the only path, however. There is a short-term strategy that may be useful in the absence of more powerful tools. Specifically, NRD stakeholders could manage cases in ways that steer them toward Type 1 comparisons that are relatively easy to make. For example, consider King's third complication. He observes that "uncertainty associated with the outcome of habitat restoration projects is well-known and is generally higher than the uncertainty associated with the service flows of undisturbed natural habitats or naturally recovering habitats." Perhaps active restoration should not be the prime directive in all cases because HEA and scaling results will be highly suspect. NRD stakeholders may wish to reexamine the program's emphasis on active restoration and consider, in lieu thereof, acquisition of equivalent resources. Comparisons will be more reliable when using stable, undisturbed ecosystems of the same type, rather than manipulated ecosystems that are prone to instability. Analytical reliability, in turn, will contribute to predictable results and greater assurances that the public will be made "whole." Until HEA and scaling become more meaningful for Type 2, 3, and 4 comparisons, perhaps via King's indicators, we should embrace acquisition of equivalent resources as a surer way to make the public whole.

The merit of this approach can be appreciated when we consider that undisturbed ecosystems are disappearing at a much faster rate, due to urbanization and expansion of human habitats, than we are restoring injured ecosystems. Why focus on restoration projects with a low likelihood of success when a much larger eco-volume is being consumed by inexorable population growth and habitat alteration? Would it not be better to focus on protection or preservation of ecosystems that already exist in a reasonable condition? If these systems are never injured in a CERCLA or OPA sense, then we have won a major victory by preventing future losses of human uses.

Physical restoration should be the action of last resort. Instead of restoring lost human uses, we should be protecting those human uses where they currently exist, or could exist in the future, and are under threat; call it "preventing future losses."

Superfund brownfield initiatives may illuminate a path for us. Development is gobbling up greenfields and altering natural ecosystems at an alarming rate. Meanwhile, NRD stakeholders are trying to figure out how to spend millions of dollars to make brownfields less brown by emphasizing projects with limited hopes of fully restoring lost uses. We could use those same funds and same authorities to protect and preserve uncontaminated natural resources and unaltered ecosystems before they become brownfields. Cleanup and restoration are more expensive and less effective than prevention of pollution in the first place. It comes down to prevention versus restoration, and stakeholders should be selling NRD as a prevention program.

Summary

My main points can be summarized as follows:

1) King presents a thoughtful framework for developing detailed sets of indicators of ecosystem values.
2) Landscape context is an important feature that merits proper consideration in the value comparison process.
3) King's paper places all the emphasis on the need for indicators to accurately predict services and values, while not adequately recognizing that indicators also should be convenient and cost-effective. Useful indicators will balance the 2 countervailing forces of sophistication and practicality.
4) "General indicators" that are dismissed in this paper should be investigated by King and developed for use in NRD situations because they may be timely and cost-effective. These indicators may have more of a future than "detailed sets of indicators."
5) Many NRD cases are being, and will be, resolved while sophisticated tools are developed to address current analytical shortcomings. Meanwhile, stakeholders should find ways to steer their cases in ways that capitalize on the strengths of existing valuation tools.
6) Stakeholders should reexamine "acquisition of equivalent" as a means to minimize the weaknesses of existing valuation tools, the unpredictability of restoration plans, the instability of restored ecosystems, and the inexorable alteration of natural systems by human inhabitants.

5b

Discussion Paper 2 on Leading Indicators of Ecosystem Services and Values

*Robert D. Rowe**

This paper provides information to improve the use of the habitat equivalency approach (HEA) in natural resource damage assessments (NRDA) under The Oil Pollution Act of 1990 (OPA). My observation on the initial HEA illustrations and applications in recent years is that the problem of resource and service equivalency has been oversimplified. Often, ecologic and social values are represented by simplistic proxy measures such as acre-years of injured habitat based on little more than simple measurements and reasoned judgment. The early work illustrated the convenient use of the HEA tool for settlement and to avoid monetization of damages, but this early work often lacked the rigor that would be required if the work were taken to court. NOAA is investing in developing literature and guidelines for the HEA approach. Other work by King for NOAA provides a much needed synthesis of the literature available to increase the rigor and defensibility of the ecologic assessment portion of HEA analyses (King 1997).

King's presentation of ecosystem basics provides beneficial background on ecosystem features, functions, services, and values. The identification of capacity, opportunity, payoff, and equity, and other criteria provide useful ideas for the characterization and evaluation of restoration alternatives and are well illustrated through the wetlands case study example provided. But, one must be careful to simply consider these as suggested criteria to consider among others, rather than prescriptive requirements because their general applicability is not well established, and because trustees and resource managers often will have entirely different criteria that should be considered.

King's mention of uncertainties in the assessment is of significance for trustees. If trustees are to reflect the public values, and given that the public is often risk adverse, uncertainty needs to be factored into the computation of both injuries and restoration and appropriately compensated.

Much of King's focus is on the concept of "leading indicators" of ecosystem and public services and value. This is a useful and simple concept: we may not know the level of actual ecologic and public-use services that a compensatory resource project will

*Hagler Bailly Services, Inc.

provide, but we can use characteristics, or indices of characteristics, of the resources as indicators of the types and levels of services that can be expected to be provided. For example, if we restore vegetation, we may get more wildlife habitat and other environmental services and more public direct-use and passive-use services.

Because the concept of leading indicators is already embedded in many, or most, habitat and public-benefit evaluations, although not always so explicitly, King overplays it. Given the significance of improving HEA procedures in general, I found the extended discussions of Wall Street and of leading and lagging indicators to be distracting. Further, whether we call them resource characteristics, characteristic indices, or leading indicators has little impact on the underlying objective of selecting characteristics of resources that can be reasonably expected to produce (or at least to be highly correlated with the production of) desired environmental and public-use services.

The paper needs more focus. It is a mixture of background information on ecologic characterization, the concept of leading indicators, and a specific case study that is not always clearly woven together. Two of my continuing questions while reading the paper were, "Where does this work fit in?" and "Where does it contribute to extending the development of a unified and consistent approach (an approach that can be generally followed regardless of the resource and public use services injured) to using HEA in NRDAs?"

The paper would be greatly enhanced if King first put into perspective what part of the HEA problem is being addressed, related the terms used from the ecology literature to the terms used in the NOAA NRDA regulations, and gave more thought to what in the presentation is truly generalizable to other applications. Much the discussion in Sections 1 and 2 could be traded for more insight on other problems such as how to address uncertainty and nonlinearities and how to address more, different, and complex habitats and conflicting resource services flows. King seems to struggle with this in his third, and least developed, section on applying this work in HEA. He states that "the previous sections raise more questions about performing HEA and scaling than they answer." He is right, except that the questions about HEA have been there for some time. The task at hand is to work toward better documentation of how to conduct HEA for a broad range of circumstances.

It may be difficult to expect to have an accepted unified approach to HEA applications for NRDA, even for a subset of resources or public-use services. Even after decades of research on resource-valuation methods, we still have major battles about fundamental strategies and methods to value natural resource service flows. We should expect no less of a debate with HEA when it is brought forth as the cornerstone of large scale, complex NRDAs rather than when it is used in relatively simplistic cases (or portions of a case). NOAA has made progress toward the goal of a unifying approach that will enhance the acceptability and rigor of the methods, and I encourage King and NOAA to continue this work.

Finally, I plead that we move away from the generic use of the term "habitat equivalency analysis" to refer to the NOAA compensatory restoration scaling process. While habitats are often a critical link to providing ecologic and public services, the concept of equivalency presented in the NOAA regulations is much broader than just habitats. Consider, for example, contaminated ground water and surface water used for consumptive purposes, or oil on a beach where the primary or perhaps the only significant impact is to recreational services. We should call it "services equivalency analysis" or, with a broader view that restoration of resources will provide ecologic and public services, to "resource equivalency analysis."

Minor comments

King should reconsider several of his comments regarding economic-valuation methods. I cannot agree with some of them, and most are simply unnecessary to the theme of the paper. Some economic methods do give consideration to specific biophysical or landscape features of the problems they address. Not all economic methods or applications of these methods are "extremely expensive," and issues of reliability are not so firmly established as is suggested.

King suggests that "no generally accepted methodology exists for conducting benefits transfer studies," and the work here may provide a reasonable basis for this activity. He overstates issues concerning benefits transfer procedures and, while it is possible that some of the concepts in the paper could also be used in benefits transfer, this is not thought through in the paper and it should be. In fact, many of the criteria suggested by King are frequently identified in the benefits transfer literature (e.g., quality, scarcity, reversibility, replacability/uniqueness, and substitutability).

5c

Discussion Paper 3 on Leading Indicators of Ecosystem Services and Values, or Putting "Leading Indicators" into a Restoration Framework Based on Impaired Human Use

*James L. Connaughton**

I would like to focus on one concrete aspect of Dennis King's paper that is of direct significance and ready application to the natural resource damages (NRD) liability regime. King proposes 4 definitional building blocks to guide restoration decision-making: "ecosystem features," "ecosystem functions," "ecosystem services," and "ecosystem values." While these concepts are not necessarily new to the NRD liability regime, King's specific definitions and analytical framework offer a particularly useful variation on the theme. Most important is King's definition of ecosystem services:

> The beneficial outcomes that result from ecosystem functions (e.g., better fishing and hunting, cleaner water, better views). These require some interaction with, or at least some appreciation by, humans. However, they can be measured in physical terms (e.g., catch rates, water quality, aesthetics).

This human-use-focused definition of "services" critically differs from the ambiguous definition of services currently found in both the Comprehensive Environmental Response, Compensation, and Liability Act (CERCLA) and Oil Pollution Act of 1990 (OPA) rules, which meld the terms by defining services as the "functions" that an ecosystem provides. King stresses the importance of maintaining clear definitional distinctions, offering a series of cogent reasons for why such distinction is analytically necessary. My take on his fundamental insight is that treating "functions" and "services" as distinct analytical concepts, with "services" rooted in human use, provides a critical missing link (King calls it the "critical science-policy gap") upon which restoration decision-making depends and practical resolution of NRD cases can be achieved.

King constructively describes the missing link in the context of 2 complementary problems that frequently emerge in NRD policy discussions. On the one hand, King

*Sidley & Austin, Washington, DC

identifies problems in ecosystem-valuation methods developed by economists that attempt to assign values without much regard for specific ecosystem features or functions that generated them. This view echoes concerns about incomplete or inaccurate market-based measures of value raised by the D.C. Circuit in the *Ohio*[1] case. Policy and technical dissatisfaction with valuation is similarly reflected in NOAA's semantically interesting pronouncements that, under the OPA natural resource damage assessment (NRDA) rule, NRD is no longer about assessing "damages," but is about "restoration." On the other hand, King also notes problems in the methods developed by scientists of assessing ecosystem functions that strive to "objectively" identify features and functions but ignore services and values. Such "value-free" scientific assessments provide only the "front-end part," but they cannot serve as the complete analytical basis for judicial determinations of injury and reasonable damages for restoration. From the perspective of an NRD litigant, the OPA NRDA rules—which would impose liability based on "any measurable adverse change" to a resource—and to a slightly lesser degree the CERCLA NRDA rules, inappropriately emphasize the ecosystem function side of the equation to the exclusion of considering cost/benefit and socioeconomic trade-offs through valuation measures. At the end of the day, a trustee must add up how much restoration will cost and must justify that the costs are worth the benefits in order to compel a liable party to pay money (i.e., "damages") to accomplish the restoration.

Accordingly, I agree with King that tools are necessary to bridge the apparent divide between the scientists and economists, particularly in the NRD litigation context where, to grossly overstate the dynamic, the scientists tend to dominate the trustee plaintiff's perspective, whereas the economists tend to dominate the federal facility/industrial defendant's perspective. "Objective" consideration of functions divorced from "rational" consideration of social value spawns litigation to the detriment of commitments to reasonable restoration.

Unfortunately, when he explores "leading indicators" as a methodological tool for linking assessment of ecosystem function with ecosystem valuation, and when he considers its application under OPA NRDA, King does not focus on the critical conceptual link he describes between ecosystem function and ecosystem valuation—his human-use-based definition of "ecosystem services." For some of the reasons described below, consideration of ecosystem services in the context of a particular NRD case is one of the most productive areas for further exploration of criteria for leading indicators. Human-use-based leading indicators appear promising as a potentially useful tool for guiding restoration decisions and for settling NRD cases

The advantage of King's leading indicators approach in the context of NRD is that it might promote the use of "rough justice" measures as a means of exploring mutually agreeable resolution of NRD litigation without compelling the defendants to sacrifice their right to an independent judicial determination of their liability and restoration

[1]See *State of Ohio v. U.S. Department of the Interior*, 880 F.2d 432, at 445 fn.9 (D.C. Cir. 1989).

obligations. One fundamental problem giving rise to seemingly endless litigation over the OPA and CERCLA Type B NRDA rulemaking has been the failure of the rules to specify appropriate benchmarks and tools that bring some measure of discipline to the complex process of injury determination and restoration decision-making. King provides his own example of this problem with respect to the lack of specific guidance concerning how to determine the adequacy of alternative restoration measures. Conversely, through proposed compensation formulas and Type A models, NOAA and DOI have initiated a countervailing approach that would, based on elemental information about an incident, assume losses in ecosystem function and human-use services, select a presumably adequate and effective restoration option, and generate the presumptive cost of such an action. Trustees would be bound to implement such action without any confidence that the plan will accomplish an ecologically and socially beneficial result. This approach inflexibly takes evaluation and decision-making out of the hands of all parties. A leading-indicators approach would appear capable of bridging these extremes, enabling plaintiff trustees and defendants alike to agree on evaluation shortcuts based on mutually accepted criteria.

For the purposes of developing criteria for selecting indicators, King usefully distills and reinforces a number of considerations that percolate through discussions about injury determination and the adequacy of proposed restoration measures. I would highlight the following, which are directly relevant to an approach geared toward reinstatement of human services:

- Ecosystems should be viewed "not as life-support systems, but as collections of assets with specific values" in order to effectively compare ecosystems.
- Most decisions involving ecosystems do not involve total losses of ecosystems or the elimination of ecosystem functions without perfect or near-perfect substitutes elsewhere in nature.
- Important and often overlooked questions involve the scarcity of services (resources) provided, the availability of perfect or near-perfect substitutes for them, the ability of the ecosystem to recover or to be restored or replaced, and the capacity of humans to adjust and adapt to temporary or even permanent ecosystem changes.

Indicators that operationalize these considerations could be very useful in deciding whether and the extent to which a reduction in ecosystem services has occurred and whether cost-reasonable restoration alternatives can be found to reinstate such services. In both instances, the availability of substitutes, both temporary and permanent, is a critical consideration.

Distributional concerns are best resolved through human-use framework for restoration decisions

At several points in his paper, King identifies certain distributional concerns that might have to be taken into account in restoration decision-making, e.g., intragenerational and intergenerational equity, ethical decisions in context of developing indicators of equity considerations, example of trade-off between benefits to large urban disadvantaged population or few relatively wealthy families on rural area. King translates these concerns into the following "equity" questions in his "criteria for leading indicators of ecosystem values," "Whose recreational, educational, and/or aesthetic opportunities are enhanced?" In the context of NRD, however, these concerns are minimized to the extent that restoration options are bounded by conceptual limits of liability. The NRD schemes under both OPA and CERCLA base damages liability on injury caused by releases of oil or hazardous substances at specific locations at specific points in time. As representatives of the public, trustees are obligated to sue to recoup the costs of redressing, through restoration, the impairment of the public services provided by those injured natural resources. Although the liability scheme affords some measure of flexibility in the types of restoration options a trustee may select, that selection is bounded by obtaining at least rough equivalence in service benefits to those that were actually impaired. In this context, King's "equity" question is incomplete and should be supplemented to ask, "Whose recreational, educational, aesthetic opportunities were impaired as a result of the resource injuries; did those people have a public right to enjoyment of those opportunities?" In terminology borrowed from the CERCLA NRDA rules, the question might be framed, "What was the nature and extent of the 'committed public use' (i.e., ecosystem service dedicated to the public) of an injured resource at the time of injury?" As long as the objective of restoration is reinstatement of ecosystem services (defined in human terms), the NRD scheme affords a ready benchmark for distributional equity.

Difficulties with HEA and scaling may be minimized and the asserted distinction between primary and compensatory distinction falls away when the leading indicator approach is applied through a human-use framework for restoration decisions.

Not surprisingly, by approaching the issue in terms of developing a practical, unified evaluation of restoration requirements based on reinstating tangible services to society, King encounters inherent conflicts and technical difficulties in some of the current concepts recommended for use in NRDA under OPA (but not currently under CERCLA). For example, with respect to the "scaling" and "habitat equivalency analysis," King reinforces a common view that these applications "raise more questions... than they answer." Although King's analysis does not explicitly reference the missing link of evaluation of ecosystem services, it appears that some of the central difficulties that he identifies with scaling and HEA are most dramatic when the applications are not linked to human-use-based services and values as benchmarks, but instead are considered only in relation to ecosystem features and functions per se. Most importantly, in the absence of a link to human-use-based services and values, it becomes virtually impossible, even with the most developed assessment techniques, to make the determination that law and public policy require in damages actions: a showing that the costs of the desired restoration alternative is proportionate to its benefits. Further, a particular resource hypothetically may serve a variety of different ecosystem functions and may provide numerous and sometimes competing services to humans (e.g., consumption versus preservation) and certainly to other resources under a "resource-to-resource" analysis. When divorced from indicators of the actual human services a resource provided to the public prior to injury and the value of those services, the scaling and habitat equivalency exercises become wholly arbitrary, subject to the particular preferences of whomever is performing the scientific aspects of an assessment. No established, principled means exist to address inherent trade-off or to weigh priorities among functions to produce the most socially beneficial outcome.

King also inevitably blurs or glosses over the supposed distinction between "primary restoration" and "compensatory restoration" under the OPA NRD regulations ("restoration" and "compensable value" in CERCLA parlance). To simplify, the bifurcated scheme in the OPA regulations requires selection of primary restoration purely in terms of reversing changes in ecosystem features and functions, whereas compensatory restoration is evaluated separately in terms of implementing additional, potentially overlapping restoration measures based on the temporary reduction in ecosystem features and functions, as well as the temporary reduction in ecosystem services pending completion of primary restoration. This dichotomy becomes meaningless when decision-making appropriately links the evaluation of changes in ecosystem features and functions with the human services and values to produce a unified plan to reinstate the services through restoration. Primary restoration is compensatory restoration. To his credit, King does not attempt to rationalize the primary/compensatory distinction, but neither does he explicitly acknowledge that such a scheme is incompatible with his framework of linkages from ecosystem features, to functions, to services, to values.

Uncertainty points in direction of replacement/acquisition alternatives

King highlights a number of areas of uncertainty in the assessment and decision-making process. Among the most intriguing is his assertion that "the uncertainty associated with the outcome of habitat restoration projects is well-known and is generally higher than the uncertainty associated with the service flows of undisturbed natural habitats or naturally recovering habitats." This asserted fact actually is not well-known in NRDA policy context and deserves much more attention and discussion. Although the federal government in the *Kennecott* case successfully defended the proposition that CERCLA does not create a presumption in favor of on-site restoration measures versus replacement or acquisition measures, many trustees engaged in NRD policy discussions, particularly when it comes to King's example of wetlands, proceed with great faith and a strong preference not only for on-site habitat restoration measures, but also for so-called compensatory measures predicted on habitat restoration. King's assertion is particularly unsettling when one considers that the CERCLA Type A regulations are based on computer-generated assumptions about the efficacy of on-site resource restoration measures and ignore replacement or acquisitions alternatives. Yet King's comment plainly points in the direction of replacement and acquisition-based restoration alternatives as the more viable and presumably more cost-effective solutions. Amplification and further policy development of this subject is plainly warranted.

Conclusions

King's proposed leading indicators approach for evaluating resource-restoration decisions appears to be a promising tool for facilitating cooperative discussion among trustees and responsible parties about mutually agreeable courses of action. The application of tools such as HEA and scaling in the context of NRD deserves much closer scrutiny than it has received to date and likely warrants significant policy reformulation. I would recommend that King further develop his analysis on how to appropriately distinguish between and ultimately link his concepts of ecosystem functions and ecosystem services as the focal point for the next stage development of leading indicators.

6

Restoring Human Services: The Experience of the *Exxon Valdez* Oil Spill Trustee Council

*Molly McCammon**

The *Exxon Valdez* Trustee Council was formed in 1991 following an out-of-court settlement of the federal and State of Alaska claims against Exxon Corporation for injuries resulting from the 1989 oil spill, the largest in U.S. history. The $900 million settlement for civil claims was (and remains) the largest recovery in the U.S. for natural resource damages settled under the Clean Water Act (32 U.S.C. sec 1321) and the Comprehensive Environmental Response, Compensation, and Liability Act (CERCLA) (42 U.S.C. 9601 *et seq.*).

With the exception of reimbursement of certain funds to the state and federal governments, the settlement agreement requires that restoration funds be used for "restoring, replacing, enhancing, or acquiring the equivalent of natural resources injured as a result of the oil spill and the reduced or lost services provided by such resources." The term "enhancement" was unique to this settlement and its inclusion was insisted upon by the State of Alaska. This term underscores the parties' intent that uses of the settlement not be limited to restoration to pre-spill conditions.

To oversee the funds and restoration program, an August 1991 memorandum of agreement between the state and federal governments affirmed the continued role of 3 state and 3 federal trustees, all of whom are public officials, to act as co-trustees. All actions by the 6-member Trustee Council must be unanimous.

Management and staff functions are centralized in a single Restoration Office, with the Executive Director reporting directly to the Trustee Council under a federal-state cooperative agreement. This organizational structure has proven to be an effective mechanism for garnering agency input and expertise, incorporating public input from a 17-member Public Advisory Group and the general public, and enabling the Trustee Council to fashion a restoration program that can be supported unanimously by 6 trustees.

The following 3 issues will be covered in this paper: 1) the decision-making framework of the Trustee Council, particularly as it relates to restoration of human services; 2) the actions to date that the Council has taken to restore human services; and 3) some

*Exxon Valdez Trustee Council, Anchorage, AK

observations based on these experiences that will relate to restoration of services under the OPA regulations.

Decision-making process

The Trustee Council adopted the following mission statement in November 1993: "The mission of the Trustee Council is to efficiently restore the environment injured by the *Exxon Valdez* oil spill to a healthy, productive, world-renowned ecosystem, while taking into account the importance of the quality of life and the need for viable opportunities to establish and sustain a reasonable standard of living." In adopting this mission statement, the Council made it very clear that humans were to be considered a part of the spill-area ecosystem.

Soon after the 1991 settlement, the Trustee Council began planning its restoration program. Two differing approaches were considered. One approach was to identify all possible restoration projects that might be accomplished over time and package them as an overall plan. Another was to use the restoration plan as a more generic policy document, with general policies, recovery objectives, and strategies. Decisions on actual projects would be made through the annual work plan process. The Council adopted the latter approach in its formal *Restoration Plan* in November 1994. This plan laid out a number of policies to guide the use of settlement funds. Several of these are especially pertinent to the Council's decision-making process for the restoration of human services, including

- Restoration will focus upon injured resources and services and will emphasize resources and services that have not recovered. Resources and services may be enhanced, as appropriate, to promote restoration. Restoration actions may address resources for which there was no documented injury if these activities will benefit an injured resource or service.
- Priority will be given to restoring injured resources and services that have economic, cultural, and subsistence value to people living in the oil spill area, as long as this is consistent with other policies.
- Possible negative effects on resources or services must be assessed in considering restoration projects.
- Projects designed to restore or enhance an injured service must have a sufficient relationship to an injured resource, must benefit the same user group that was injured, and should be compatible with the character and public uses of the area.

In addition, the *Restoration Plan* identified recovery objectives and strategies for the various resources and human services injured by the spill. The status of injury and recovery and the recovery objectives were most recently updated in September 1996. Restoration strategies are updated annually in the *Invitation to Submit Restoration Proposals*.

The federal government views the *Exxon Valdez* Oil Spill (EVOS) trust funds as federal funds, even if expended by a state agency. Therefore, all expenditures are subject to the requirements of the National Environmental Policy Act (NEPA). In fact, the Council's *Restoration Plan* was subject to a full, programmatic Environmental Impact Statement prior to its adoption.

The annual work-plan cycle begins in January with a workshop for all principal investigators and the core scientific review team. Based on information received from the prior season's field results, an invitation for project proposals is issued in mid-February, allowing 60 days for submission of proposals. Project proposals are then subjected to multiple reviews, first by the Restoration Office staff:

- Does the proposal have a link to restoration of an injured resource or service?
- How does it relate to the recovery objectives in the *Restoration Plan* and strategies in the annual *Invitation to Submit Restoration Proposals*?
- Is it consistent with restoration policies in the *Restoration Plan*?
- Is the budget reasonable, given the work proposed?

The Trustee Council also relies heavily on advice from an independently contracted Chief Scientist who provides peer review and quality control for the research, monitoring, and general restoration work funded under the program. Five additional scientists of national caliber review the entire program twice each year, and they and other from a large cadre of peer reviewers provide ongoing oversight for individual projects and overall program direction. Proposals are evaluated by this scientific team according to the following criteria:

- The scientific merits of the proposal as demonstrated through 1) understanding of the problem, 2) soundness of the technical approach, 3) innovation and uniqueness of the proposal, and 4) feasibility (i.e., prospects for the proposal's success).
- The extent to which the proposal will help achieve the restoration objectives identified for a given resource or service.
- The proposer's capabilities, experience, and record of past performance, as well as the experience and qualifications of key personnel and whether facilities or other factors integral to the proposal's success are available to support the proposal.
- The cost-effectiveness of the proposal.

The Public Advisory Group, a 17-member group representing a cross-section of interest groups affected by the oil spill, also reviews the proposals individually and provides comments on the overall program.

Attorneys for both the federal and state trustees review restoration proposals for their legal permissibility under terms of the settlement. The Alaska Department of Law provides the review for the state trustees. Individual agency solicitors and the Department of Justice provide the review for the federal trustees. In general, the attorneys review whether the proposals are in fact designed to restore, replace, enhance, or acquire the equivalent of natural resources injured as a result of the oil spill or the reduced or lost services provided by such resources.

Following these reviews, a draft plan is then developed by the Executive Director in consultation with the trustee agencies and issued for review and comment by the general public and the Public Advisory Group. Based on these comments, the Trustee Council takes action on restoration projects. Only those that are unanimously agreed to by the trustees can go forward. Even then they must have the agreement of the Alaska Department of Law and the U.S. Department of Justice, who are authorized to request release of the funds from the federal district court.

Restoration of human services by the EVOS Trustee Council

The Trustee Council has worked to restore human services since the settlement was reached in the fall of 1991. Under the settlement, injured human services were identified as commercial fishing, subsistence, recreational, and tourism (including sport fishing, sport hunting, and other recreation uses), and passive uses.

In its chapter on injury, the *Restoration Plan* provides that services were reduced or lost if the *Exxon Valdez* oil spill or cleanup

- reduced the physical or biological functions performed by natural resources that support services,
- reduced aesthetic and intrinsic values or other indirect uses provided by natural resources, or
- reduced the desire of people to use a natural resource or area.

Commercial fishing was reduced as a result of the oil spill through injury to commercial fish species and also through fishing season closures. In 1989, fisheries were closed in Prince William Sound, lower Cook Inlet, upper Cook Inlet, the outer Kenai coast, Kodiak, and Chignik. Most of these fisheries opened again in 1990. Since then, there have been no spill-related district-wide closures, except for the Prince William Sound herring fishery, which was closed from 1993 until this spring because of the collapse of the herring population. These closures harmed the livelihoods and home communities of persons who fish for a living.

For commercial fishing, the Trustee Council's recovery objective provides that this service will have been restored "when the commercially important fish species have recovered and opportunities to catch these species are not lost or reduced because of the effects of the oil spill." On this basis, the Trustee Council has made major investments in projects to understand and restore commercially important fish species that were injured by the spill, especially pink and sockeye salmon and Pacific herring. Restoration techniques include supplementation and creation of new, alternative commercial fisheries; development of new fishery management tools such as stock assessment techniques and thermal mass marking of hatchery-reared fish; and research to enhance the ability to predict and manage fisheries over the long term.

Millions of dollars have been spent on these efforts, many of which are anticipated to continue for at least the next 5 years.

Has commercial fishing been restored through these actions? Using "the functions performed by a natural resource for the benefit of another natural resource or for the public" as the definition of services, the answer is that progress has clearly been made. Pink salmon and sockeye salmon are now considered to be "recovering" biological resources. Estimates of Pacific herring biomass for 1997 in Prince William Sound are sufficient to allow for a roe fishery this spring for the first time since 1993, a promising sign that this species too may be on its way to recovery. Accordingly, if one approaches the question of whether the commercial fishing service has been restored from the perspective of whether there are now salmon and herring to catch, one can argue that the commercial fishing service is also "recovering."

However, the problem the Council has in explaining its restoration program to the public is that defining the commercial fishing service narrowly in terms of the resource conditions capable of providing the opportunities for commercial fishing, it is very confusing to the public. The public wants to know whether commercial fishing itself has recovered, the answer to which is complicated in the Council's experience by several factors, including:

- At about the same time as the 1989 oil spill, the salmon fishing industry began an economic downturn largely due to the increase in farmed salmon worldwide. The industry is still reeling from this, and with prices for pink salmon at 8 to 10¢ per pound (with some processors unwilling even to take pinks) and the price of Prince William Sound seine permits extremely depressed, the salmon industry in Prince William Sound is still in disarray. The key point is that merely providing opportunity to harvest previously injured fish stocks will not necessarily assure recovery of the industry.
- With the herring roe fishery in Prince William Sound closed for 4 straight years, once the fish have returned and the fishery reopens, it is unclear whether markets and processors will be available as they have been in the past. Again, the fish may come back, but it does not directly follow that the fishing industry will also be made whole. It is very difficult to convince a near-bankrupt commercial fisherman that the Trustee Council program is successfully restoring the commercial fishing service.
- The Council's efforts are targeted toward restoration of wild fish stocks, yet the largest hatchery program in North America exists in Prince William Sound. The effects of the hatchery program on wild fish stocks and the health of the overall ecosystem, as well as on the commercial fishing industry, clouds the ability to precisely assess the benefits of some restoration activities.

Some commercial fishermen have argued that the fishing industry itself should be more directly aided in recovery, through such means as the purchase of commercial fishing limited-entry permits in order to reduce the size of the fishing fleet; direct financial support of the hatchery programs, which are currently burdened by both operating and capital construction loans; or by direct payments to individual fishermen. These kinds of projects have not been viewed favorably for use of public settlement funds, primarily because they appear to benefit individual fishermen rather than the resource itself. In addition, commercial fishermen and seafood processors have been able to seek individual and class action relief from economic injuries through private litigation still pending in the courts nearly a decade after the spill. In short, the public continues to be confused whenever we talk about the commercial fishing service, which they define as the industry itself, and they continue to believe that the Council is not doing enough to restore it.

Restoration of the subsistence service has been particularly challenging under the terms of the settlement. Fifteen predominantly Alaska Native communities (numbering about 2200 people) in the oil spill area rely heavily on harvests of subsistence resources such as fish, shellfish, seals, deer, ducks, and geese. Subsistence harvests in most of these villages declined substantially following the oil spill. Reasons for the declines include reduced availability of fish and wildlife to harvest, concern about possible health effects of eating contaminated or injured fish and wildlife, and disruption of lifestyles due to cleanup and other activities.

The recovery objective for subsistence provides that this service will have been restored "when injured resources used for subsistence are healthy and productive and exist at pre-spill levels." In addition, it is recognized that people must be confident that the resources are safe to eat and that the cultural values provided by gathering, preparing, and sharing food need to be reintegrated into community life.

The Council's primary restoration strategy for subsistence has been first to focus on restoring those injured resources used for subsistence, such as herring, salmon, and seals. Protection of subsistence uses has been a prime justification for the major investments made in the Council's habitat protection and acquisition program. The Council has then focused on enhancing or replacing these resources with alternative resources to be used for subsistence. Some examples are remote releases of hatchery fish to be used for subsistence purposes, supplementation of existing wild fish populations, and fishery habitat improvements to increase natural production. The Council continues to test the safety of any abnormal fish or wildlife found by subsistence users. Lastly, the Council has funded projects to increase the involvement of subsistence users in the restoration process. These efforts include a local network of community facilitators tasked with providing local information on restoration and recovery to the Council and also acting as a conduit back to the village with information gained from the Council's research projects; a project to involve spill area students in ongoing research projects; 2 spill area-wide conferences on subsistence and the oil spill, especially aimed toward village elders and youth; and financial support for the Alaska Native Harbor Seal Commission, which involves subsistence hunters in harbor seal management and research. In addition, the Council has just embarked on a new effort to incorporate traditional ecological knowledge (TEK) into the restoration program.

While the estimated size of the subsistence harvest in pounds per person now appears to have returned to pre-spill levels in some communities, the relative contribution of certain important subsistence resources, such as seals and herring, remains unusually low. Different types of resources have varied cultural and nutritional importance, and the change in diet composition remains a serious concern to subsistence users. Subsistence users report that they still have to travel farther and expend more time and effort to harvest the same amount as they did before the spill, especially in Prince William Sound.

Subsistence users argue that the value of subsistence cannot be measured in pounds alone. This measure does not include the cultural value of tradition and customary use of natural resources, which is dependent on uninterrupted use of fish and wildlife resources. The more time users spend away from subsistence activities, the less likely they will return to these practices. Continuing injury for natural resources used for subsistence may affect ways of life of entire communities well into the future, if not permanently.

The socioeconomic dislocation and disruption of subsistence harvests following the spill were severe and extended. These impacts, although difficult to measure, cannot be overemphasized. The lives of Alaska Natives and their subsistence lifestyle were severely disrupted in 1964 by the Alaska Earthquake. The village of Chenega Bay in Prince William Sound, for example, was all but destroyed. In time, the village finally was relocated and rebuilt, and people once again began to live off the land and the sea, only to have the 1989 oil spill cause another disruption in their lives, not the least of which was another break in the traditional handing-down of knowledge from elders to youth. How are the young people to learn the traditional subsistence lifestyle and practices when there are no herring to catch and prepare, when the once boundless resources of the intertidal zone have either disappeared or are so suspicious of taint that they simply go unused?

Subsistence users further argue that subsistence cannot be fully restored by just focusing on the resources alone. However, it has been difficult to fund projects specifically aimed at rebuilding the cultural ties that subsistence users view as vital to their way of life and to the perpetuation of that way of life. For example, proposed projects such as spirit camps, cultural centers, and community fish and game processing centers have not been viewed favorably by federal legal counsel, although they have been funded to some extent through funds from the state's criminal settlement with Exxon.

These legal interpretations and the Council's resulting unwillingness to fund these projects have been particularly distressing to Alaska Natives, who attempted to press for compensatory damages for injury to the subsistence way of life and culture as part of the private plaintiffs' claims against Exxon. In March 1994, their claims were rejected by the federal district court judge who stated that "the plaintiffs must find recompense for interference with their culture from the public recoveries that have been demanded of and received from Exxon.

Recreation and tourism were obviously disrupted immediately following the spill, and some effects still linger. Resources important to wildlife viewing such as killer whales and marine birds were injured, residual oil still exists on some popular recreation beaches; some sport fishing and hunting and trapping closures still remain in effect, and the displacement of human use from oiled to unoiled areas has increased management problems. The prime restoration activity for recreation has been the purchase of thousands of acres of privately owned lands that are now in public ownership and are available for public use, although the primary justification for purchase of most of these lands is protection of fish and wildlife habitat and subsistence uses. Other potential restoration activities such as enhancement of a sports fishing area and construction of such recreational amenities such as cabins, mooring buoys, etc., have not been viewed favorably by the federal side because of the lack of a direct link to an injured resource, although again they have been funded somewhat through state criminal funds from Exxon.

Passive use of resources includes the appreciation of the aesthetic and intrinsic values of undisturbed areas, the value derived from simply knowing that a resource exists, and other nonuse values. Injuries to passive uses are tied to public perceptions of injured resources. The Council's recovery objective for passive uses is that recovery will occur "when people perceive that aesthetic and intrinsic values associated with the spill area are no longer diminished by the oil spill." The Council's primary strategy in this regard has been restoration of the natural resources injured by the spill. Additionally, the Council has funded monitoring activities for some resources, e.g., killer whales, even if the monitoring may not lead to actual restoration activities, so that the public will know what is happening with these resources. Another important strategy has been public information and education about the current status of restoration and recovery efforts. The Council has greatly expanded its public outreach efforts in the past 3 years; the Council now publishes an annual report and bimonthly newsletter, produces a weekly radio program and newspaper columns, and has created a web site on the Internet.

Observations

Based on these experiences, the following observations on the issue of restoring human services may be of use in deciding how best to restore human services in the event of future spills:

- The definition of "service" is very confusing to the public. In fact, in the Council's experience, most members of the public view the human use or service more as an extension of an economic injury than as merely a function or opportunity. This is not simply an arcane matter; it has resulted in very real (and continuing) frustration, disappointment, and tension among members of the public and the spill-area residents.

- Restoration of human services injured as a result of the 1989 *Exxon Valdez* oil spill has been attempted primarily through restoration of the natural resources upon which those services depend. However, this prioritization is not totally accepted by the State of Alaska trustees, by the public, or by the service user groups. They believe that restoration of services, and especially the relationship between the proposed restoration activity and an injured resource, should be viewed more expansively than it currently is.
- Determining what is or is not restoration is not always clear-cut, and what constitutes restoration for human services is even less clear than what constitutes restoration for natural resources. This lack of clarity has often left the public confused and frustrated.
- Restoration of services has been more challenging than restoration of natural resources because the human, i.e., public, element is more closely tied to services. Service restoration is also more closely related to the private claims against Exxon that have yet to reach final settlement. The *Exxon Valdez* oil spill civil funds are not intended to supplant private recoveries for spill injuries, but the line between the two is not always clear.
- It would not have been possible at the time of the settlement in 1991 (day 1 of the restoration effort) to decide how best to spend all the EVOS civil settlement funds. The information and knowledge gained from past and current research and restoration activities are critical to making informed decisions concerning future restoration activities. A major element of the Council's *Restoration Plan* is restoration using an adaptive management approach: "restoration should be guided and reevaluated as information is obtained from damage assessment studies and restoration activities." Under this approach, information on recovery is reviewed by the Trustee Council at least on an annual basis and is used to guide the development or modification of future restoration activities.

Using the Council's recovery objectives, services will be restored once the natural resources are restored. On this basis, progress in restoring human services cannot be adequately assessed until substantive progress in restoring the resources has been made. Only then can you analyze whether the restoration activities are working or even be in a position to decide which are the most appropriate.

The Trustee Council believes that full recovery from the effects of the 1989 *Exxon Valdez* oil spill will not have occurred within the 10 years of payments from Exxon—more than 12 years after the event itself. That belief is the major reason for the Council's decision to set aside funds in a Restoration Reserve account, with the funds intended for restoration activities after the last payment is received from Exxon in September 2001. Planning for future use of the Restoration Reserve funds has just begun and will continue to make strong use of the adaptive management approach.

The *Exxon Valdez* Oil Spill Trustee Council is currently overseeing the largest restoration program in the country. Based on the Council's experience, the following recommendations are offered:

- clarify up front, to the extent possible, both the definition of human use or service and what type of activities qualify as restoration for human services in order to reduce public confusion and frustration, and
- build into the process of restoring human services some means to ensure that the process can adapt to changing information as restoration proceeds, thus allowing restoration activities and priorities to be modified accordingly.

6a

Discussion Paper I on Restoring Human Services: The Experience of the *Exxon Valdez* Oil Spill Trustee Council

*Keith Eastin**

The Oil Pollution Act of 1990 and the Comprehensive Environmental Response, Compensation, and Liability Act codified society's interest in the recovery of damages to natural resources arising from the discharge of oil or the release of hazardous substances into the environment. Natural resource damage assessments (NRDAs) under the law have been performed since the mid-1980s.

Since the passage of the CERCLA, more than 30,000 hazardous waste sites have been catalogued in the U.S. Much of this inventory is composed of sites at which significant damages to natural resources have occurred. The inventory of sites has not declined in any significant way. Ways must be found to deal with this large number of sites, returning services to the public, while protecting the public's purse and imposing liability and costs expeditiously and fairly onto the responsible parties. The challenge to the trustee community is to find a way to return lost services so that the public might enjoy them in the foreseeable future.

Molly McCammon discusses experience in disposing of trust funds obtained in the settlement of the *Exxon Valdez* litigation. In a way, this Mother of All Spills is a matter unto itself. A great number of studies have been completed analyzing the most significant effects of the incident. By virtue of the trust funds, the Trustees do not suffer from a significant lack of funding. While many other natural resource trustees attempt to find funds with which to do rudimentary NRDAs, the *Exxon Valdez* Oil Spill Trustee Council can now concern itself with sorting through worthy projects that might help replace their lost services.

The author discusses the Council's problems in dealing with a populace that confuses public human uses with economic opportunities lost to private profit-making activities. While the line here is far from bright, these are problems that most other trustees likely will not face.

---

*Deloitte & Touche LLP, Wilmington, DE

6b

Discussion Paper 2 on Restoring Human Services: The Experience of the *Exxon Valdez* Oil Spill Trustee Council

*Pierre H. duVair**[1]

Molly McCammon raises several difficult issues that she and the Trustee Council administering the *Exxon Valdez* restoration trust fund have had to wrestle with to date. The most potent theme throughout her paper is the fact that restoring the ecological and human-use impacts due to a pollution event can be a very complex process facing trustee agencies and the public. A key message provided is that when possible, lessons learned should be shared and used to inform future efforts towards restoration.

McCammon has observed that what constitutes "restoration" is often unclear, at least to many but select trustee attorneys. This is especially true for the general public, whom she claims has difficulty understanding the concept of natural resources as a flow of "services." I would emphasize that people have difficulty understanding the law and vocabulary used to explain the law. In general, I think people understand that natural resources provide services, but may understand less how one restores services without restoring the actual resources. Based upon McCammon's description of what has been done to date that is focused on "restoring" the lost human uses resulting from the spill, I too seem to share many of the same questions being asked by the Alaskan public.

I believe there is a potential for some trustees to apply a double standard toward projects that are aimed primarily at ecological restoration versus those aimed at compensating for lost human uses of resources. Clearly projects that restore the ecological resources can simultaneously compensate for certain types of human-use losses. Based on several factors that can be extracted from her paper, one could suggest that compensation for lost human uses of injured resources is somewhat poorly represented for the *Exxon Valdez* case.

McCammon suggests that restoration of lost human uses is reflected in the Council's mission statement. One could interpret the reference to human uses in this statement

---

*California Department of Fish and Game, Sacramento, California

[1]The opinions presented herein are expressly those of the author and do not necessarily reflect the views of the Department of Fish and Game. Thanks go to Larry Espinosa and Steve Turek for their helpful insights.

more as a constraint on ecologically focused restoration than as a directive to provide some compensation for use losses. In addition, the Trustee Council crafted statements that describe when commercial and subsistence uses have been "restored," and these statements appear not to include compensation for interim losses incurred by the public.

The restoration guidance cited by McCammon seems to provide relatively limited explicit language on the compensation of lost human uses. One item mentions people, culture, and economics, but references only a subset of the injured public. Another item requires that "the same" user group be restored, a standard that is stricter than that for ecologically focused restoration.

Many would agree that the intent of Congress, when passing the Oil Pollution Act into law, was to have trustees both restore injured natural resources and compensate the public for lost uses of injured natural resources. Some people view accomplishment of the former as innately superior to that of the latter. I believe these views are, in large part, based on the perception that ecological injuries tend to take longer to recover and need greater assistance in that process. A quick review of her description of the broad public socioeconomic losses directly resulting from the injuries to natural resources, one can argue that view may not be an entirely accurate one.

I agree that what constitutes restoration "is not always clear-cut," but I have to disagree that restoring lost human uses is always "even less clear" than what constitutes restoration within a complex ecosystem. I also disagree with McCammon's contention that restoration of services is inherently more challenging than restoring actual resources because of the human element of services. Estimation of baseline and the various confounding influences on recovery, as well as imprecise or differing criteria for evaluating recovery success, often can lead to equal challenges for restoration of resources and services.

I contest McCammon's view that compensation for lost human uses must wait until resources are restored and the interim losses fully quantified. The same logic could be applied to restoration of specific types of ecological injuries. Emergency restoration of human-use losses could "minimize" some of the spill impacts, but more often may be "compensatory" rather than "interdictory" of such losses (see Birdsall et al., this volume).

As McCammon points out, it is the timely primary restoration of injured resources that will minimize interim human-use losses. A point not made is that this fact does not imply that compensatory human-use-focused alternatives inherently deserve a backseat to the ecological primary restoration-focused alternatives. Trustees have a responsibility to restore and compensate. It is a combination of factors like restoration policies, strategies, evaluation criteria, national caliber "scientists," attorneys, and occasionally politics that drives which alternatives control the issues. Most could agree that good natural and social science should be driving the restoration and compensation process.

6c

Discussion Paper 3 on Restoring Human Services: The Experience of the *Exxon Valdez* Oil Spill Trustee Council, or Natural Resource Damage Assessment: A Texas Perspective

*Diane B. Hyatt**

Purpose

Although this paper was reviewed by all Texas trustees, I am not speaking for the other trustees, and there may be differing opinions on some of the points discussed. Overall, it is the trustees' duty to restore the resources and their services. It is difficult for me to isolate the narrow interim lost human use from the whole. The human uses and other service flows from our natural resources are directly correlated to the health and diversity of the ecosystem from which the services flow. The trustees endeavor to work as a team to restore the whole. It is the goal to restore with no net losses to the system or to the users that are, in fact, part of the same system.

The Alaska experience

Alaska was the first state to create a trustee council. In Texas, the Federal-State MOA incorporates the "Trustee Council" philosophy. However, our cases have not reached the magnitude of injuries that were assessed in the *Valdez* spill. As of April 1997, the state trustees are working on 29 active cases: 13 oil-spill related, 16 Superfund cases, and 3 under preliminary investigation. Our limited resources do not permit assigning specific personnel to restricted cases. Local governments and local advisory committees may serve as a resource for the trustees particularly with regard to restoration planning. We are working in some areas of the coast on initiation of an "equivalent resource plan," taking a watershed management approach. This form of regional restoration involves outreach to the state Coastal Management Program, National Estuary Programs, as well as local environmental groups, foundations, academia, and government.

The Texas state trustees focus on restoration of the injured resources and the services that flow from those resources. As codified in the state NRDA rule (30 Texas Adminis-

*Director, Natural Resource Damage Assessment, Texas General Land Office, Austin, TX

trative Code, Chapter 20), the restoration must be tied to the resource that was injured. In cases where natural recovery or direct restoration is accomplished, lost human uses are regained in part by the restoration of the injured resource from which the human-use service flows. Compensatory restoration is for interim lost use and can involve off-site substitution and enhancement projects.

The state trustees have a policy for immediate response to oil spills of magnitude or threat to resources. It is our duty to fulfill the mandate to protect the resources in advising the on-scene coordinator and to mitigate whatever injury possible, as well as to document the ephemeral conditions of an oil spill (nature and extent of exposure). Resource recovery is monitored over time to scale the injuries and the restoration necessary.

According to statute and by rule, the state trustees issue an invitation to the responsible party in an oil spill to participate with the trustees in data collection and to share these data in order to have a more cost-effective and efficient assessment. The generic MOA provides for this process and clearly defines the roles of the parties. Early participation of the trustees in the remedial investigations (RI) at hazardous waste sites provides the same sort of cost-effective participation by using shared RI data and by scaling of injury and restoration contemporaneously with the decisions for remedy.

In Texas, we have some cases that involve only the state trustees. These cases are not considered to fall under the National Environmental Policy Act (NEPA), however, our process includes public participation and public comment on each case. When the federal trustees are partners, we comply with NEPA.

The criteria utilized by the Alaska Council for selection of restoration proposals is similar to those used in Texas in the Apex Oil Spill case. The trustees utilized the information provided by project proponents, best professional judgment, interviews of restoration proposal managers, and literature sources as guides to answer the initial and detailed screening criteria. This process includes applicable requirements under NEPA. Because the trustees received a lump sum settlement, rather than resource-to-resource compensation, it is necessary to meet specific criteria for restoration. This process defines the boundaries and reduces the possibility of political maneuvering for "pet projects."

The trustees first considered an initial screen to evaluate all the proposals. From this primary screen several proposals were eliminated from further detailed review. The primary screen consisted of the following questions:

- Is the project within the Galveston Bay tidal system impacted by the spill?
- Does the project address the injured natural resources and the services they provide?
- Is the project cost $1.3 million or less? (Amount of total settlement for NRDA.)

The first question reflects the concern of the trustees to address impacts within the tidal system of Galveston Bay as well as the area directly impacted by the spill. The second question reflects the legal requirements that the restoration undertaken address the injuries sustained by natural resources as a result of the Apex oil spill. The trustees believe that the most significant injuries occurred to aquatic and emergent wetland natural resources. The third question addressed the trustees' limit of available funds.

The trustees considered a secondary screen to evaluate all the remaining proposals. From this secondary screen the trustees' preferred alternatives were decided. The secondary screen consisted of the following area of questions:

- Environmental factors: 1) What is the proposed habitat productivity for natural resources injured by the spill? 2) What is the proposed habitat type? 3) What amount of habitat will be acquired, protected, enhanced, or constructed? 4) Does the proposed location have the proper hydrology, salinity regime, and a tidal connection? 5) Is the soil type adequate for the success of the proposal? 6) Does the proposal have any conflicts with endangered species? 7) What is the current site use? 8) Does the proposed location have any known contamination problems? 9) What is the level of compatibility with the surrounding land use?
- Economic factors: 1) What is the cost per acre of habitat? 2) What is the timing if the funding is secured? 3) What is the accessibility for construction of the habitat? 4) Is monitoring included in the proposal? 5) What is the total project cost?
- Public acceptance factors: 1) What is the local community support level? 2) What is the Houston Galveston area community support level? 3) What is the local, state, and federal government support level? 4) What is the level of community benefits associated with the proposal? 5) What is the level of educational opportunities associated with the proposal for the local area schools and universities?
- Legal factors: 1) What will be the future ownership and/or management of the proposal site? 2) Are state and/or federal permits required? 3) If the proposal involves acquisition, are the existing owners willing sellers? 4) Are there any identified liability problems associated with the proposal? 5) Are there any archeological/historical issues that need to be considered?
- Risk factors: 1) Is the subsidence rate in the proposal area high, medium, or low? 2) Is the proposal area susceptible to future degradation or loss through erosion, oil spills, or contamination? 3) Is there concern with the proposal's technological approach or difficulty of success of the proposal? 4) Is there associated maintenance required for the success of the proposal?

Texas monitors restoration projects to meet success criteria. A typical example of a monitoring plan that describes success criteria and the frequency and method of monitoring is that of the Gum Hollow Oil Spill, October 1994. Primary restoration for this case is planting of emergent estuarine vegetation (smooth cordgrass). In this monitoring plan that is implemented by the responsible party, the general criteria which define an overall positive trend are the 100% survival and stabilization of the plant plugs and a positive trend in plant recruitment from seeds. Surveys are conducted at 180 days, 1 year, and 2 years. If the success criteria have been achieved after 2 years, then a 3-year maintenance plan with semiannual site evaluations is implemented. A maintenance and restoration fund is established for corrective measures during the 3-year period. This enables the trustees to make mid-course corrections and to initiate planting should a "force majeure" event take place within that finite period. Any surplus from the maintenance fund is refunded to the responsible party at the end.

Texas agrees with Alaska that "services" are confusing to the public and to the responsible parties. In Texas, we see these services flowing from the direct restoration of resources when feasible, through preservation, acquisition, enhancement, and reconstruction of essential habitats. The goal of direct restoration of habitats is one that can lead to gains in production in habitat-limited resources. We seek to restore diversity and natural systems that can support multiple resource recoveries. We feel service flows are best restored in the long term by this simple philosophy. The strictly lost interim human uses such as beach-days, recreational fishing, or boating, swimming, snorkeling, and scuba diving, or bird watching, hiking, wildlife viewing, etc., can be reduced only by substitution or enhancement projects that promote more or better experiences in the future. The restoration must provide both components: direct and compensatory restoration.

The Texas trustees have experienced the conflict between the commercial interests that depend upon public trust resources. There have been third-party suits in these instances. Other private, third-party claims are often made as a result of direct injury to private property. Texas is careful to distinguish between legitimate private claims and injury to natural resource service flows which belong to the public trust.

Acknowledgment—I wish to thank my colleagues who provided comments and critical review of this paper: Ingrid K. Hansen, Texas General Land Office, David Chapman, National Oceanographic and Atmospheric Administration, David Sager, Texas Parks and Wildlife, and my staff, Patricia M. Rives and Peter A. H. Samuels.

6d

Discussion Paper 4
Restoring Human Services: The Experience of the *Exxon Valdez* Oil Spill Trustee Council

*Bruce Peacock**

McCammon provides a "progress report" on the status of natural resource restoration in the *Exxon Valdez* oil spill case. The reported efforts of the Trustee Council are very interesting and encouraging. However, 2 important issues are raised with implications for other natural resource restoration cases. These issues are summarized below.

Natural resource restoration versus human use restoration

The author describes 2 situations in which efforts to restore lost human uses have been less than fully successful. The first situation deals with commercial fishing. From a biological standpoint, progress is being made, and the salmon and herring fisheries are recovering. However, progress has been less than encouraging from a human standpoint. Human use has not fully recovered because, in part, the market for naturally harvested salmon has been depressed by an increase in aquaculture worldwide. Additionally, because the fishery has been closed for a significant period of time, it is not clear that the markets and processors will be available to support a viable commercial catch.

These problems have led commercial fishermen to argue for more direct aid such as purchasing commercial fishing permits to reduce the size of the fishing fleet and financial support for hatchery programs. However, these projects have been denied since they do not fit a more narrow definition of natural resource restoration.

The second situation in which the restoration of human use has been less than complete deals with subsistence hunting and fishing by Native Alaskan communities. Subsistence harvesting by these communities declined substantially as a result of the oil spill. While the size of the subsistence harvest (measured in pounds per person) has substantially recovered, the required level of effort and the resulting harvest composition have not recovered. Subsistence users argue that the cultural values of traditional and customary use have not recovered. Nevertheless, projects focused on these cultural values have apparently been denied since they are not strictly natural resource restoration.

---

*Department of Interior, Washington, DC

The problem identified by the author is that while natural resource restoration may be a necessary condition for the recovery of lost human uses, it is not sufficient. The "build it and they will come" approach fails to restore lost human use in some situations. The relevant question, then, is can the public be made whole if human uses cannot be restored? If the answer is no, then the resolution of this issue may require reconsideration by regulatory agencies or even legislative action to authorize appropriate restoration actions.

Adaptive management

The second issue is raised by the author's statement that an adaptive management approach is being employed by the *Exxon Valdez* Oil Spill Trustee Council to guide restoration decisions. This approach to restoration management is laudable. Adaptive management is an approach for managing resources while simultaneously reducing uncertainty with respect to management alternatives. The premise of adaptive management is that the best management policy cannot be determined ex-ante, but rather ex-post through a sequential reassessment of management responses. As the author states, "It would not have been possible at the time of the settlement . . . to decide how best to spend all of the EVOS civil settlement funds."

The issue is how such a realistic approach can be applied to other cases where the restoration plan *is* the settlement? Under the Oil Pollution Act, the claim presented to responsible parties is a restoration plan. Even in CERCLA cases, responsible parties demand certain closure in settlements, often in terms of specific restoration actions. Recognizing that neither trustees nor responsible parties have a crystal ball into the future regarding the use of evolving sciences to restore inherently variable ecological systems, adaptive management would seem to be a reasonable approach.

Summary

This paper raises 2 questions with important implications for other natural resource restoration cases. The first question asks how the recovery of lost human uses can be assured from natural resource restoration. The second question asks how can an adaptive management approach be implemented to guide natural resource restoration decisions. It is beyond the scope of these comments to offer solutions to these complex questions. Rather, these questions require thoughtful consideration and public debate if the public is to be truly made whole.

6e

Discussion Paper 5 on Restoring Human Services: The Experience of the *Exxon Valdez* Oil Spill Trustee Council

*Neal S. Brody**

I approached each of my critiques with a focus on 2 distinct components. First, I examined the overall approach to restoration in each of the cases described by the authors. These approaches were as varied as the underlying facts in each of the cases. Second, in addition to an overall assessment, I studied the specific recommendations proposed as a result of the authors' experiences. Without exception, each author offered valuable considerations for future cases involving restoration of lost human uses.

The McCammon paper

General response

I had 2 reactions following my reading of the McCammon paper. On the one hand, it is an illuminating presentation, describing the culmination of an exceptionally complex environmental matter. Without question, the *Valdez* spill presented a unique event with dramatic images and descriptions of injury to natural resources, and the restoration processes outlined in the paper reflect those circumstances. Despite the complexities involved and threat of extraordinary lost human uses of resources, the trustees appear to be making tremendous progress in addressing the injuries through an inclusive decision-making process.

On the other hand, the *Valdez* experience describes a utilization of the natural resource damage assessment (NRDA) process that probably would not be optimal for most cases. Following the *Valdez* spill, trustees and the responsible party negotiated a dollar settlement, seemingly even before restoration was ever considered. The actual restoration of lost human uses described in the paper seems to have been initiated *following* settlement. In other words, the trustees collected money from the responsible party long before they had any idea what to do with it. This process, developing restoration projects after a settlement has been negotiated, is less favorable than the alternative case, as adopted in the Cantara Loop case, of negotiating a settlement following determination of the appropriate restoration. While in the *Valdez* case it may

*ARCO, Los Angeles, CA

not have been practicable for any number of reasons, developing restoration plans before you collect money damages should be the preferred model for prompt, cost-effective restoration of lost human uses following natural resource damage incidents.

Recommendations

McCammon makes 2 specific recommendations following the *Valdez* experience. The first is that the definition of human uses or services should be clarified to the fullest extent possible. This suggestion holds true for the *Valdez* case and should be generally considered a top priority in natural resource damage cases. Too often trustees are torn between physical restoration projects which, while relatively easy to determine, make no sense from a cost-effectiveness perspective, and projects that, although they cost-effectively restore lost human uses, do not restore the same uses that were lost as a result of the resource injuries. For this reason, any opportunity to define committed uses to natural resources would be extremely valuable. This is noted following the *Valdez* case, and it is equally evident in the Lavaca Bay and Cantara Loop cases.

McCammon's second major conclusion is that the NRDA process should be flexible enough to change as the restoration proceeds. While this suggestion is extremely reasonable, my concern with the recommendation is that it should not unduly complicate restoration cases that would otherwise proceed relatively directly. Not every case will involve the complexities of the *Valdez* situation. For most other cases, including perhaps, the Lavaca Bay, Cantara Loop, and Idarado mine cases, restoration of lost human uses of natural resources may be achieved more quickly and efficiently without the cumbersome process as described by McCammon.

Conclusion

Each of the papers (Chapters 6, 7, and 8) offers valuable lessons in restoring lost human uses of the environment. These lessons include clarifying the definition of human uses or services, maintaining flexibility throughout the NRDA process, considering the restoration of lost identifiable human uses early on in the NRDA process, improving the integration of economic and biological sciences, considering substitutes in the restoration decision-making process, accepting imperfect solutions, and the importance of trustees and responsible parties working together.

In addition to the specific lessons detailed previously, an overall lesson to be learned from these papers is that the approach taken to restoration really does matter. If trustees and responsible parties follow, understand, and heed the experiences of the *Valdez*, Lavaca Bay, Cantara Loop, and Idarado cases, as thoughtfully presented in these papers, win-win situations can be developed, and most importantly, the public will benefit from expedited and effective restoration of lost human uses of the environment. Finally, I propose a challenge to everyone concerned with lost human uses of natural resources to develop a process through which this occurs as a rule rather than as an exception.

7

Measuring and Restoring Lost Human Uses: Two Real-World Case Studies, or Substitutes Really Do Matter[1]

Thomas H. Birdsall, Ralph C. d'Arge, Edward J. McGrath

Compared to the proliferation of case law addressing important issues under environmental statutes such as the Clean Water Act, the Clean Air Act, and the Comprehensive Environmental Response, Compensation, and Liability Act (CERCLA or Superfund), there is very little case law addressing important issues in natural resource damage (NRD) cases. To our knowledge, only one case to date has been tried to judgment.[2] This is not because of a lack of activity in the NRD area but because all cases except one have been resolved through settlements rather than court decisions.[3]

Aside from case law, it is possible to look for guidance on important NRD issues in cases that have been settled, of which there have been at least 125.[4] Most, if not all, of the analyses performed by natural resource trustees and defendants are considered confidential (e.g., protected by the attorney-client privilege or by attorney work product immunity), making it difficult to research. Even after settlement, parties are frequently reluctant to reveal or discuss in any detail the work that was conducted on such issues as injury determination, injury quantification, and damages determination. This reluctance is understandable but unfortunate, since much can be learned from these efforts. There is a particular need to learn about efforts to quickly and efficiently restore the human uses of the environment that are interrupted due to spills of oil or hazardous substances, in order to minimize the losses from future spills.[5]

---

[1] Valuable assistance in preparing this paper was provided by Deborah Jay, president of Field Research Corporation in San Francisco, CA and by Wayne Lifton, an aquatic ecologist at Entrix, Inc. in Walnut Creek, CA. The views expressed herein are solely those of the authors.

[2] *State of Idaho v. Southern Refrigerated Transport, Inc. et al.*, U.S. District Court for Idaho, Memorandum Opinion and Order, January 24, 1991. The total damages awarded in the case were $45,453.37.

[3] One motivation for settlements may be the extra uncertainty created by the lack of legal precedents on key issues, particularly with respect to how damages should be determined.

[4] Natural Resource Damage Case Database, Barbara J. Goldsmith and Company and Ropes & Gray.

[5] While prevention of spills and other injurious events should generally be the highest priority, it is unlikely that all such spills and events will be prevented during the foreseeable future. Therefore, efforts to minimize and mitigate the damages that stem from those spills and events also need to be given very high priority.

Here, we intend to counteract the tendency not to reveal confidential information, in small part, by discussing several aspects of 2 NRD cases in which claims were made, partially litigated, and ultimately settled. In particular, we'll focus on the important role that substitutes for injured resources can play in both the measurement of NRDs and the restoration of lost human uses of the injured resources. The first case will discuss the use of man-made resources to restore successfully lost human uses of an injured fishery. The context is the July 1991 derailment of a tank car from a Southern Pacific Transportation Company (Southern Pacific) train and subsequent spill of metam sodium into the Upper Sacramento River (USR) in northern California. The spill killed most of the fish and other aquatic life along a 40-mile stretch of the USR, which was subsequently closed to fishing for several years. The second case will discuss the role and measurement of substitution in determining the required scale of restoration efforts. The context is the Idarado Mine case in southwest Colorado, which involved acid mine drainage into a reservoir from multiple sources near the mine site. Much of the information provided in this paper has not previously been discussed or revealed in any public forum.

This paper is organized into 4 sections. The first section lays a foundation for the 2 case studies by discussing the economic theory of substitution and the restoration of lost human uses through substitution. The second section discusses the USR case, particularly the success of a man-made fishing area in restoring a significant amount of the lost fishing use of the USR. The third section discusses the evaluation of substitutes in the assessment of recreational damages in the Idarado case. The final sections summarizes the lessons learned from the 2 case studies and the implications for the future measurement and restoration of lost human uses of the environment.

Economic substitution and restoration through substitution

From an economic perspective, the goal of resource restoration is to cost-effectively reinstate human uses (consumptive and non-consumptive services to the public) that have been lost as a result of environmental releases notwithstanding cleanup remedies. The extent of lost uses, if any, and the appropriate extent and means of restoration should be determined in welfare economic terms. The economic concept of substitutes has a vital role in both of these elements of the restoration decision-making process.

Restoration decisions must first determine whether releases into the environment have resulted in any reductions of human uses and the extent of any such reductions. If, for example, existing substitute resources are readily available for the injured resource and provide the same or similar public uses, there may be no need for restoration measures because the substitute resources can support relevant uses pending natural recovery of the injured resource. If the substitute resources cannot fully compensate for uses that would otherwise be lost as a result of resource injury, they can substantially reduce the level of lost uses. Accordingly, the availability of substitutes must be examined in determining the need for and extent of use-based restoration.

If lost uses occur, taking into account the availability of existing substitute resources, decision-makers should consider and evaluate a variety of restoration options, both temporary and permanent and select the combination that will reinstate the lost uses in the most cost-effective manner. Under the NRD statutes, these options include natural recovery, on-site rehabilitation, and replacement and acquisition of equivalent resources. In many instances, injured resources will recover naturally following cleanup, although this process may take a number of years. In such situations, either permanent or temporary acquisition of substitute resources may be the preferred restoration option, possibly in combination with other measures. They may provide the public with resource uses that offset those lost, pending eventual restoration of the resource injured, at less cost than other alternatives. Once again, the availability of substitutes must be considered and integrated into the restoration decision-making process.

Many of the lost human uses in oil or hazard substance spills involve recreation or other outdoor activities. Perhaps the most extensively studied substitution process for outdoor activities in resource economics is for recreational fishing. There is substantial literature on various models describing the fishing experience and potential substitution processes that can occur. Substitution effects have also been examined in empirical studies. Anglers can substitute different fishing sites, fish for alternative species, vary the time committed to fishing, pursue other types of fishing, and use other activities to substitute for fishing (e.g., bowling, boating, hiking, movie-going, etc.). Some of these substitution possibilities are examined later in this paper.

In economics, the typical expectation is that substitute activities induced by lost human uses of the environment are less desirable and thereby less valuable to those engaging in them. It is assumed that at current prices and given the current menu of recreational activities, each individual will select the combination of activities that makes them as well off as possible. If their preferred activity becomes unavailable and they are forced to substitute, they will have to select less desirable activities, locations, fish species, etc. and thus be made worse off. However, this need not be the case for "lost human-use values." With sufficient payments or subsidies, a "superior" set of activities may emerge, in fact making the individual better off.[6] To cite one hypothetical example, an angler loses one or more of his normal fishing sites for a time period. The angler is then given access to a closer or more convenient site with better fishing opportunities in which all other aspects of the fishing experience are superior to the normal experience. This angler is made better off, and human-use loss becomes human-use gain.

[6] Provision of a superior substitute for a period can be viewed as one way to offset net habitat equivalency losses as envisioned by NOAA and as discussed by Unsworth and Bishop (1994).

There is another conceptual possibility in which a perfect substitute is provided for the lost use. This is unlikely, since either every attribute of the lost use including cost has to be identical, or the total experience must otherwise be viewed by the recipient as of exactly equal value.

The final case is one in which a substitute does not provide equivalent services to the lost use. In this case, there may be additional services required.

The various economic measures of willingness to pay and compensation for superior, perfect, and imperfect substitutes are recorded in Table 7-1. These measures assess the net effect of natural or augmented provision of substitutes.

Because a spill is typically accidental and inadvertent, its consequences cannot be adequately assessed until it occurs. Likewise, substitution possibilities are often only dimly perceived by the affected users until they become necessary. Thus, reliable evaluations of substitution possibilities must be constructed after a spill has occurred. Prior to a spill, observation about human responses can provide information on values lost, the cost of substitutes, and individual substitution possibilities. But they will not provide very much information on augmented or subsidized substitution possibilities. These will require careful case studies and documentation of actual augmented substitution. One such case study follows.

Table 7-1 Provision of substitutes for lost human uses

	Economic value measure	
Type of substitute provided	Compensation	Willingness to pay
Superior substitute	Minimum compensation necessary to offset not having the superior substitute	Maximum willingness to pay for the superior substitute less the maximum willingness to pay for the lost use
"Perfect" substitute	None	None
Inferior substitute	Minimum compensation necessary to offset the value difference between the lost use and the actual substitute	Maximum willingness to pay to avoid the loss in the future less the maximum willingness to pay for the substitute

Restoration of lost fishing use in the Upper Sacramento River case

Upper Sacramento River region

The Upper Sacramento River (USR) flows north to south for approximately 47 miles. It starts at the outlet of Box Canyon Dam, which forms Lake Siskiyou near the city of Mt. Shasta in northernmost California, approximately 70 miles south of the Oregon border. The river ends at Shasta Lake, a large man-made reservoir created by the Shasta Dam just north of Redding. The region around USR includes Mt. Shasta, a snow-capped mountain 14,162 feet high, along with extensive national forests and recreational areas and numerous lakes, rivers, and streams. These include the Shasta-Trinity National Forest, the Klamath National Forest, the Wiskeytown-Shasta-Trinity National Recreation Area , the Salmon Trinity Wilderness Area, the Marble Mountain Wilderness Area, and the Castle Crags State Park.

Bordered by Interstate 5, the major north-south highway in northern California, the USR is very accessible to anglers and other recreational users. At the time of the spill, the USR was considered one of the 14 "blue ribbon" trout streams in California due to its excellent trout fishing, ease of access, and a 14-mile designated catch-and-release section for rainbow trout (Sunderland and Lackey 1991; CDFG 1991). No hatchery-raised fish were planted by the California Department of Fish and Game (CDFG) in this section, and the limit was 2 rainbow trout per person rather than the normal 5 per person. But the USR was not the only blue ribbon stream in the region. Both the McCloud River and the Pit River, located to the east of the USR, were and continue to be top locations for trout fishing, as are Hat Creek, the Lower Sacramento River, the Trinity River, the Fall River, Lake Siskiyou, and Shasta Lake (Sunderland and Lackey 1991). There are also other rivers and lakes in the region that provide good trout fishing opportunities.

Spill and closure of USR to fishing

On the night of July 14, 1991, several cars of a Southern Pacific train derailed while the train was crossing a bridge across the USR at what is called the Cantara Loop, just north of the town of Dunsmuir. One of the tank cars ruptured and spilled approximately 19,000 gallons of metam sodium, a broad-spectrum soil sterilizer.[7] Over the next 2 weeks, the metam sodium and its breakdown compounds flowed down the USR and into Shasta Lake. In the process, it killed most of the fish and other aquatic life in the main stem of the USR between the Cantara Loop and Shasta Lake. Once the metam sodium reached Shasta Lake, it dissipated through natural breakdown processes and by aeration of the plume, a cleanup measure devised and undertaken by Southern Pacific with oversight from state and federal government officials. Once it comes into contact with water, metal sodium quickly breaks down principally into hydrogen sulfide and methyl isothiocyanate (MITC); therefore, within 2 weeks of the spill, essentially all of the chemical compound and its derivatives had dissipated.[8] Unlike oil or hazardous substances such as heavy metals, which tend to persist in the environment for months or years, the metam sodium disappeared relatively quickly. As a result, one of the major challenges facing the natural resource trustees and

[7] Metam sodium is an agricultural product that is applied to fields several weeks prior to planting crops. It acts as a soil fumigant, herbicide, and pesticide to kill nematodes, insect larvae, fungi, and weed seeds in the soil. Given this intended use, the compound is designed to work relatively quickly once it is applied to soil. It then dissipates into innocuous components, allowing crops to grow and leaving no toxic residuals.

[8] On July 28, 1991, the natural resource trustees authorized Southern Pacific to discontinue its response actions.

potentially responsible parties (PRPs) was not how to rid the environment of the contaminant (it was already gone) but rather how best to mitigate and restore the lost human uses of the injured resources.

The primary lost use was fishing because of the large number of fish killed and the closure of the USR to fishing. The CDFG closed the USR to fishing immediately following the spill and kept it closed until the 1994 fishing season, when fishing was again allowed on a restricted basis. In addition, the relatively rapid dissipation of the metam sodium meant that other uses of the USR, such as swimming and boating, could resume quickly following the spill.

Character and magnitude of lost fishing use prior to consideration of substitutes

Prior to the spill, the 40-mile stretch of the USR between the Cantara Loop and Shasta Lake was popular with anglers from the surrounding region as well as with anglers from other parts of California and other states. It was also a popular river because of its ease of access. While recognized as a blue ribbon trout stream based largely on its wild trout population,[9] the popularity of the USR was based on or enhanced for many anglers by the large number of hatchery-raised trout added to the river each season since the 1930s. Some anglers on the USR preferred the challenge of fishing for wild trout using fly fishing gear, but many others preferred the typically far easier task of fishing for hatchery-raised trout using bait or lures (CDFG 1993).[10]

Between 1980 and 1990, the CDFG stocked an average of 78,853 hatchery-raised trout per year in the USR. As shown in Figure 7-1, the per year average for this period includes one unusually low year, 1988, when only 40,817 trout were added to the river. Without this year, the per year average rises to approximately 82,600 stocked trout[11].

The exact magnitude of fishing activity on the USR prior to the July 1991 spill was difficult to estimate given the paucity of available data on such use levels. However, various data became available after the spill that allowed development of a rough estimate of the likely use levels. Using the available data, together with assumptions based on experience with key parameters, a probabilistic approach was used to estimate both an expected value and probability distribution of the baseline use levels. This approach yielded an expected value estimate of approximately 92,000 angling hours per year, absent the spill and the closure of the USR to fishing. Based on a 200-day fishing season,[12] this translates to an average of approximately 460 angling hours

[9] Wild trout are spawned and grow to maturity in the wild (as opposed to hatchery-raised trout).

[10] The CDFG recognized the importance of hatchery trout to the USR fishery when it stated that "hatchery trout were a significant component of the prespill fishery."

[11] The reasons for the low value in 1988 are unknown. Potential explanations include disease at the hatchery, budgetary constraints, and stocking needs at other rivers and lakes. The average stocking levels were higher from the late 1950s through the late 1970s. From 1956 through 1979, an average of approximately 100,000 catchable rainbow trout were added to the USR each year.

[12] The fishing season opens on the last Saturday in April and closes on November 15.

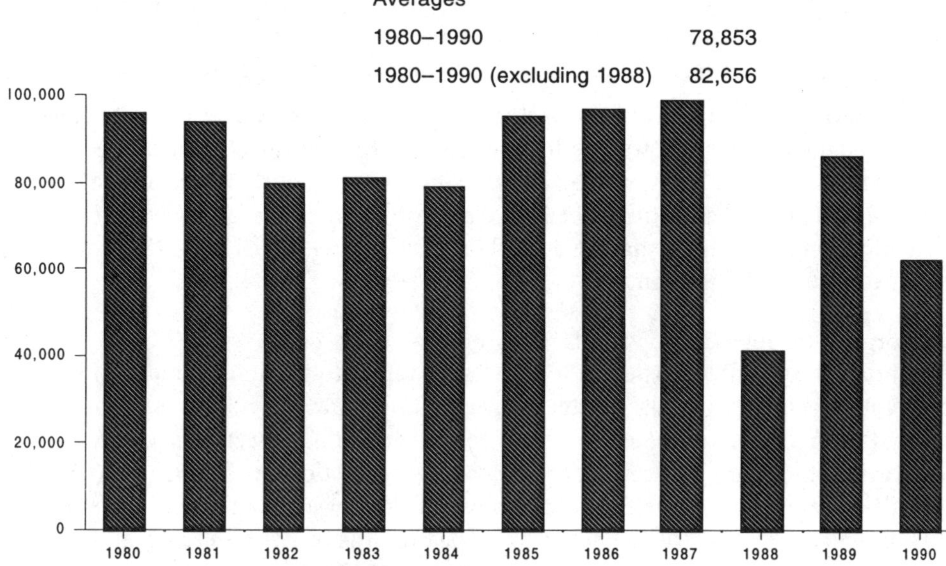

Figure 7-1 Number of catchable fish stocked in USR
Source: California Department of Fish and Game

per day.[13] This analysis also indicated that the 10th and 90th percentiles were at 62,000 and 108,000 hours per year, respectively.[14]

Using the same data sources, rough estimates were also developed for the types of fishing on the USR prior to the spill. Creel surveys conducted in 1980 and 1986 indicated that in terms of hours fished, bait and/or lure (hereafter just bait) fishing was 3 to 5 times more prevalent than fly fishing. In other words, bait fishing hours comprised 75 to 83% of all angling hours on the USR, while fly fishing accounted for the remaining 17 to 25%. Using the best estimate of annual angling hours of 92,000, these proportions indicate that bait anglers accounted for approximately 69,000 to 76,000 hours per year, and fly anglers accounted for approximately 16,000 to 23,000 per year.

From the perspective of restoring the lost fishing use of the USR during the period that the river was closed, these are the estimated losses of baseline angling hours prior to any consideration of substitution effects or migration efforts. Based on the nature of the data available to develop them, these estimates were necessarily rough, but, at the

[13]If the average angler spent 3 hours per day, this estimate of total angling hours translates to an average of approximately 153 anglers fishing on the USR every day from late April through mid-November. Over the distance of approximately 40 miles, this further translates to 4 anglers per river mile per day.

[14]These percentiles indicate that there was only a 10% likelihood that the number of baseline angling hours per year was greater than 108,000 and only a 10% chance that the number was smaller than 62,000 angling hours per year. Therefore, there was an estimated 80% likelihood that the annual angling hours lay between 62,000 and 108,000 hours.

same time, they provided an appropriate basis for comparing various restoration alternatives. Now they provide a basis for evaluating the success of the restoration alternatives that were actually implemented while the USR was closed to fishing.

Based on various data sources, the likely ranges for the hourly values for bait anglers and fly anglers on the USR were estimated. These estimates, together with the relative proportions of angler types, yielded an estimated average hourly valuation of $11 to $14.[15] Based on the best estimate of 92,000 angling hours per year, this average valuation range suggested that the annual baseline fishing value for the USR was in the range of $1.0 to $1.2 million.

Restoration through Castle View fishing area

Potentially responsible parties in NRD cases are rarely able to initiate independent restoration activities because trustees typically control most, if not all, of the actions related to an injured resource and nearby resources that might serve as replacements or provide equivalent services to people.[16] While the Castle View fishing area (CVFA) described below was ultimately a cooperative effort between Southern Pacific, the CDFG, and a private recreational business operator, the concept, funding, and enthusiasm to create the area came from Southern Pacific.[17]

Objectives for the area

The primary objective for the CVFA was to provide a place for fishing near the USR that licensed anglers could use for no charge while the USR was closed to fishing. Put in economic terms, the objective was to provide an attractive substitute for the primary service provided by the injured resource for use during the period required to restore the original service.[18] To help meet this objective, Southern Pacific sought to make the area attractive to a broad range of anglers; to make it convenient through on-site sale of fishing licenses, bait, and other fishing equipment; to make the area accessible to anglers in wheelchairs; to provide a stock of hatchery-raised trout sufficient to produce attractive catch rates; and to take whatever reasonable steps necessary to maximize the enjoyment of anglers using the area.

---

[15]Assuming 3 hours of angling per day, this translates to $33 to $42 per day.

[16]"Restoration" is used herein as a shorthand for "restoration, replacement, or acquisition of the equivalent resource" consistent with *State of Ohio v. United States Department of the Interior*, 980 F. 2d 432 (D.C. Dir. 1989), at 441.

[17]The idea originated with Edward McGrath, outside counsel for Southern Pacific.

[18]Consistent with common law tort principles and economic theory, injured parties (trustees in the case of NRDs) must take or accept measures which interdict lost uses. Such measures will have the greatest chance of success if they are cooperative between the trustees and the PRPs. Trustees typically control actions regarding the resources at issue, while PRPs are often in the best position to finance and to implement such actions cost-effectively. Successful cooperation in this area, however, will require that both sides agree to work together and not quickly retreat to the shelter of litigation positions at the first sign of discord.

Cooperative development of the Castle View fishing area

In the spring of 1992, Southern Pacific negotiated an agreement with the owner of the Railroad Park Resort in Dunsmuir to rehabilitate and use 2 neglected ponds on the resort property, including the option to renew for 1993 and 1994. Southern Pacific Engineering Group designed and renovated the ponds; the surrounding area was cleared of debris and nuisance vegetation, and additional renovations, including wheelchair access for the handicapped, improved access. A new lot provided ample parking.

The ponds opened in the summer of 1992 under the new name of the Castle View Fishing Area. They provided free put-and-take trout fishing throughout the regular trout seasons of 1992, 1993, and 1994. The trout were supplied through a contract with CDFG for the first 2 summers and through a private source for the 1994 season, the final year of the program. The CVFA was gradually phased out of operation when the CDFG reopened and stocked (and maintained hatchery stocks in) 6 miles of the USR in the vicinity of Dunsmuir for put-and-take fishing with a 5-fish daily limit beginning in 1994. This program is still in effect today. The remainder of the river above and below the town was also reopened in 1994 but remains restricted to catch-and-release fishing.

By the end of 1994, the CVFA had hosted approximately 70,000 anglers from every state in the U.S. and 16 foreign countries and had been stocked with nearly 60,000 pounds of trout.

Use of the area

Approximately 1 year after the spill, the CVFA opened to anglers on July 11, 1992 and remained open through the end of the 1992 fishing season. It then reopened for the entire length of the 1993 and 1994 fishing seasons. By the end of the partial 1992 season, more than 26,000 visitor hours had been logged at the area, and during the full 1993 season, almost 65,000 visitor hours were logged at the area. Since anglers accounted for 83% of the total hours in 1993, total angling hours exceeded 54,000 in that year. This clearly represents a sizable portion, 59%, of the estimated baseline angling hours for the USR of 92,000 per year. If compared to just the estimated number of baseline angling hours for bait and lure fishing of 69,000 to 76,000 hours per year, the proportion rises to 71 to 78%. Below we discuss the various efforts that were undertaken to collect these and other data on the visitors to the CVFA and the results of those efforts.

Data collection efforts - A 2-stage process was used to collect data on the visitors to the CVFA. In Stage 1, data were collected from every visitor to the area. In Stage 2, a telephone survey was conducted of a sample of the visitors to assist in assessing their satisfaction. This section will focus on the Stage 1 process and its results. The following section will discuss Stage 2 and its results.

Stage 1 data collection process and results - Stage 1 data were collected during the 1992 and 1993 seasons using a standard log-in and log-out process at the entry gate to the

CVFA.[19] Visitors to the area were logged in when they entered the area and then logged out when they left. This allowed precise tracking of the number of hours each visitor spent at the area. Photocopies of anglers' fishing licenses were made on the log-in form, providing information on their home address, age and gender, and whether they were an adult or junior angler.[20] Anglers were also asked to provide the number of fish they caught, the number they kept, the type of gear they used (i.e., bait, fly, spinner, or other type of lure), and whether they had fished the USR within the last 3 years. All visitors, including non-anglers,[21] were asked how they had learned about the area, how many children were accompanying them, and, for those with a nonlocal address, where they were staying. Stage 1 data permitted a very accurate and complete picture of the visitor population. The Stage 1 data also revealed that in both 1992 and 1993, anglers accounted for over two-thirds of the visits (see Table 7-2) and over 80% of the hours spent at the area (see Table 7-3).

Table 7-2 Distribution of visits by type of visitor

	1992 (partial) season		1993 season	
Type of visitor	Visits	Percentage of total visits	Visits	Percentage of total visits
Adult anglers	5125	35.7	12,926	41.6
Junior anglers	4766	33.2	10,534	33.9
Subtotal anglers	9891	68.9	23,460	75.5
Non-anglers	4464	31.1	7613	24.5
Total	14,355	100.0	31,073	100.0

Table 7-3 Distribution of hours by type of visitor

	1992 (partial) season		1993 season	
Type of visitor	Hours	Percentage of total hours	Hours	Percentage of total hours
Adult anglers	11,790	43.9	30,115	46.3
Junior anglers	10,487	39.0	23,909	36.8
Subtotal anglers	22,277	82.9	54,024	83.1
Non-anglers	4599	17.1	10,959	16.9
Total	26,876	100.0	64,983	100.0

[19]Stage 1 data collection efforts in 1994 were conducted using a more streamlined approach than the one described herein. The 1994 process will be described when the data become available.

[20]An adult angler is a person over 16 years old, and a junior angler (also referred to as an underage angler) is a person 16 years or younger.

[21]Non-anglers frequently accompanied anglers during their visits to CVFA, but some non-anglers also simply enjoyed visiting the area.

Not surprising for an area that emphasized fishing, anglers stayed longer at the CVFA per visit than did non-anglers. Both adult and junior anglers stayed an average of about 2.30 hours per visit in both years, while non-anglers stayed about 1 hour per visit in 1992 and 1.44 hours per visit in 1993 (see Table 7-4).

Table 7-4 Average length of visit by type of visitor

	1992 (partial) season	1993 season
Type of visitor	Average length of visit (hours)	Average length of visit (hours)
Adult anglers	2.30	2.33
Junior anglers	2.20	2.27
All anglers	2.25	2.30
Non-anglers	1.03	1.44
All visitors	1.87	2.09

The average duration of visits to the CVFA is one potential indicator of satisfaction with the area, since satisfied visitors will presumably stay longer and dissatisfied visitors will presumably stay shorter periods of time. The fact that the average length of visits increased slightly for anglers and increased significantly for non-anglers suggests that the visitors to the area were at least as satisfied, on average, in 1993 as in 1992 in spite of the 29% increase in the average visits per day from 117 to 151. The increased visitation levels do not appear to have caused the ill effects of congestion (at least not for the average visitor).

While Stage 1 produced enough information regarding the visitors to the CVFA and their visits to keep analysts busy for days, we will highlight a few more results before moving to Stage 2:

- Anglers who had recently fished the USR prior to the spill accounted for more than 13,000 of the visits to the area in 1992 and 1993, representing 29% of all visits during these years and about one-third of the anglers visiting the CVFA. Since anglers who had fished the USR prior to 1990 were not included in this total, this percentage likely understates the proportion of CVFA users who had previously fished the USR.
- Adult anglers caught an average of 1.3 fish per hour and kept an average of about 1 fish per hour. Junior anglers' catch and keep rates were approximately 60 to 70% of these numbers.
- Approximately one-third of all visits to the area in 1993 were made by individuals who had visited in 1992. Many of these individuals may have lived in the surrounding Dunsmuir/Redding region, since visitors from this region accounted for 45% of the visits to the area in both 1992 and 1993.[22]

[22]The Dunsmuir/Redding region includes the communities of Dunsmuir, Mt. Shasta, Redding, Weed, Castella, McCloud, Anderson, and Central Valley.

- Repeat visitors, those who visited the CVFA more than once in a season, comprised 20% of all visitors in both 1992 and 1993.

In sum, the CVFA attracted a large number of visitors in 1992 and 1993. The visitors were predominantly anglers who stayed an average of more than 2 hours and caught an average of 2 to 3 fish and kept 2 of them per visit. About 1/3 of the anglers visiting the CVFA had fished the USR in the 2 years prior to the spill. Over the 1992 to 1993 period of CVFA operations, anglers who had recently fished the USR prior to the spill accounted for more than 13,000 of the visits to the area, or 29% of all visits during these years. As mentioned, this percentage likely understates the proportion of the CVFA users who had previously fished the USR.

Evaluation of the area in restoring lost fishing use

How successfully did the CVFA restore lost fishing use during the period that the USR was closed to fishing? To answer this question, we will first discuss the Stage 2 data collection effort and some of its results. We will then use these data and the Stage 1 data to evaluate the use of the CVFA relative to the estimated baseline level of fishing on the USR discussed above.

Stage 2 data collection effort and results - The Stage 2 data collection effort involved a telephone survey of a random sample of visitors to the area in 1992.[23] The objectives of the survey were 1) to collect quantitative data for estimating the economic value of the CVFA, specifically as a substitute for fishing on the USR and 2) to collect data useful for understanding attributes of high value fishing experiences and to perhaps design a follow-on survey of potential baseline users of the USR.[24] The survey was conducted in 2 phases. In the first phase, a random sample of households was selected from those with at least 1 angler who had visited the CVFA between 15 July 1992 and 15 September 1992; households with multiple visits to the area within this period were oversampled. A total of 405 interviews were completed between 23 October 1992 and 18 November 1992; the average duration of the interviews was 17 minutes. In the second phase, a random sample was selected, using the same criteria, from visitors to the CVFA between 16 September 1992 and 15 November 1992. A total of 163 interviews were completed from this sample during early 1993.[25]

---

[23]A similar survey of visitors from the 1993 season was not conducted because the natural resource damages litigation settled.

[24]This latter survey was never conducted due to settlement of the natural resource damages litigation.

[25]The telephone survey questionnaire was designed and drafted by Southern Pacific's economic consultants, Thomas Birdsall and Ralph d'Arge, together with Deborah Jay of Field Research Corporation (FRC). After the questionnaire was drafted, it was pretested to ensure that respondents understood the questions as intended and were able to recall the information necessary to answer the survey questions. Based on the pretest, the questionnaire was revised as needed, and a program was developed that would allow the survey to be administered using computer-assisted-telephone interviewing (CATI) from FRC's central interviewing facility. Only skilled interviewers were used to conduct the interviews. Before commencing data collection, interviewers participated in a training session that included a review of interviewing techniques, question-by-question review of the questionnaire, and interviewing practice. Interviewers were monitored throughout data collection to ensure that quality was maintained.

The survey results were compiled and analyzed to detect any biases or other problems that might limit their usefulness. No evidence was found of nonresponse bias, strategic behavior, context bias, or other problems identified in the literature (Biemer et al. 1991; Tanur 1992). The results were also examined to determine if they were internally consistent, consistent with economic principles, and otherwise reliable for purposes of assessing the value people derived from their visits to the CVFA. All of the response relationships analyzed were sensible and consistent with economic principles. Also, 2 tests of the respondents' knowledge and ability to provide accurate responses yielded acceptable results.[26]

The survey covered a number of topics related both to the CVFA and other aspects of the household's fishing activities. The survey was specifically designed to collect information potentially useful in investigating the following 4 approaches to evaluating the CVFA's substitution effect:

- Evaluate the extent to which the CVFA satisfies the characteristics that anglers seek in selecting fishing locations.
- Ask anglers with past fishing experience on the USR to compare their fishing experience at the CVFA with their prior USR fishing experiences.
- Ask anglers their willingness to pay to fish on the USR, assuming controlled access to the river.
- Estimate anglers' net willingness to pay for visits to the CVFA based on travel costs, demographic, and trip characteristics.

The telephone interview began with questions about the household's general fishing activities, including detailed questions regarding the level of annual fishing activity per angler in the household, the type of fishing gear used, and the importance of various factors in selecting fishing locations (e.g., ease of getting to the location, ease

---

To enhance completion rates for the telephone interviews and to minimize the potential for nonresponse bias, multiple attempts were made to complete an interview with each person selected for the sample. Initial contact attempts were made during the evenings and on weekends. However, if a sample member was reached but preferred to be interviewed at another time, an interview was scheduled according to the convenience of the respondent. The refusal rate for the survey was very low; only about 13% of the eligible respondents who were reached refused to participate in the survey. A greater difficulty was in locating eligible respondents. We were unable to locate approximately half of the visitors to the CVFA because their telephone numbers were unlisted, they had moved, or their numbers were disconnected.

[26] In the first test, respondents in households that had fished on the USR in the last 5 years were asked the following question: "To the best of your knowledge, is the Upper Sacramento River—that is, the part of the river between Box Canyon Dam at Lake Siskiyou and Lake Shasta—currently open or closed to fishing?" A total of 84% of the respondents replied correctly that the USR was then closed to fishing. In the second test, respondents were asked to estimate the distance in miles that the CVFA was from their home. These responses were then compared with actual distances based on the estimated driving distances from the respondents' home addresses to the area. Expecting for some outliers, these responses also yielded an acceptable level of accuracy given the objectives of the survey and how the results were expected to be used.

of catching fish). The respondent was then asked about the household's trips to the CVFA and the particular visit used to randomly select the household for the survey. If that visit was just part of a single-day trip, the respondent was asked questions to determine travel costs for the trip. They were also asked if they fished at any locations other than the CVFA and whether they engaged in other recreational activities. Respondents who visited the CVFA as part of a multiday trip were asked a similar set of questions as well as questions regarding their lodging costs.

The respondents were then asked how satisfied they were with the CVFA with respect to various factors. Since these were the same factors they were asked about earlier in terms of selecting fishing locations, the 2 sets of answers could be compared to determine how well the CVFA satisfied the anglers. Table 7-5 shows the ranking of the factors in response to the first question, and Table 7-6 shows how well the CVFA satisfied the household's selection criteria.

Table 7-5 Most important characteristics in the household's choice of fishing location[1]

Rank	Characteristic	Mean score (5-point scale)
1	Attractiveness of location	3.81
2	Opportunity to catch any type trout	3.73
3	Opportunity to catch large trout	3.66
3	Ease of taking children fishing	3.66
5	Ease of catching fish	3.49
6	Ease of getting to location	3.46
7	Opportunity to catch many fish	3.42
8	Opportunity to catch wild trout	3.39
9	Comfort of location	3.20
10	Closeness to angler's home	3.05
10	Remoteness of location	3.05
12	Closeness to campgrounds	2.95

[1]The respondents were asked the following question: "Next, I would like to read you a list of characteristics that may or may not be important in your household's choice of a fishing location. Please indicate the importance of each using a 5-point scale, where '1' means 'not at all important' and '5' means 'very important.'"
Source: *Castle View Fishing Area Visitor Survey*

Table 7-6 shows that the CVFA was most satisfying with respect to a number of convenience factors (e.g., ease of getting to location, ease of taking children fishing, comfort of location). Also, these 3 factors, along with the attractiveness of the location and the opportunity to catch many fish, all received relatively high average scores. The CVFA was predictably least satisfying on factors such as the opportunity to catch large trout, the opportunity to catch wild trout, and the remoteness of the location.

Table 7-6 How well the CVFA satisfied the households' selection criteria

Households' selection criteria[1]			Satisfaction with CVFA[2]	
Rank	Characteristic	Mean score (5-point scale)	Rank	Mean score
1	Attractiveness of location	3.81	4	4.34
2	Opportunity to catch any type trout	3.73	8	3.71
3	Opportunity to catch large trout	3.66	10	3.35
3	Ease of taking children fishing	3.66	2	4.73
5	Ease of catching fish	3.49	7	3.96
6	Ease of getting to location	3.46	1	4.77
7	Opportunity to catch many fish	3.42	5	4.09
8	Opportunity to catch wild trout	3.39	12	2.32
9	Comfort of location	3.20	3	4.38
10	Closeness to angler's home	3.05	9	3.54
10	Remoteness of location	3.05	11	2.98
12	Closeness to campgrounds	2.95	6	3.99

[1]From Table 7-5

[2]The respondents were asked the following question: "Next, I would like to read you a list of characteristics you may or may not have been satisfied with when you visited the Castle View Fishing Area. For each, please indicate how satisfied you (and other members of your household) were with the Castle View Fishing Area by using a 5-point scale, where '1' means 'not at all satisfied' and '5' means 'very satisfied.'"

Source: *Castle View Fishing Area Visitor Survey*

The respondents were then asked if any member of their household had fished on the USR during the past 5 years, and 50% of the respondents answered "yes." These respondents were then asked "Does your household enjoy fishing more at the Castle View Fishing Area, more on the Upper Sacramento River, or are both locations equally enjoyable?" If the respondents indicated that they preferred one location over another, they were then asked if they enjoyed their preferred location "a little bit more, somewhat more, or a great deal more?" Figure 7-2 shows the responses to these 2 questions.

The strong preference of more than half of the respondents for fishing on the USR is not surprising, given that the CVFA is man-made and small in addition to other differences between the 2 locations. The more interesting result is that 31% of the respondents found the 2 locations to be equally enjoyable, and 10% favored the CVFA over the USR. In other words, when asked to directly compare the 2 experiences, over 40% of the respondents found that fishing at the CVFA was at least as enjoyable as fishing on the USR. While one can and should ask whether these responses can be believed, they are consistent with the high visitation rates for the CVFA, the similarity between the typical visitors to the area and many of the anglers along the USR, and the anecdotal evidence that many anglers were highly satisfied with their visits to the area. These responses are strong evidence that in the eyes of more than 40% of the anglers with experience fishing at both locations, the CVFA provided, in economic terms, a

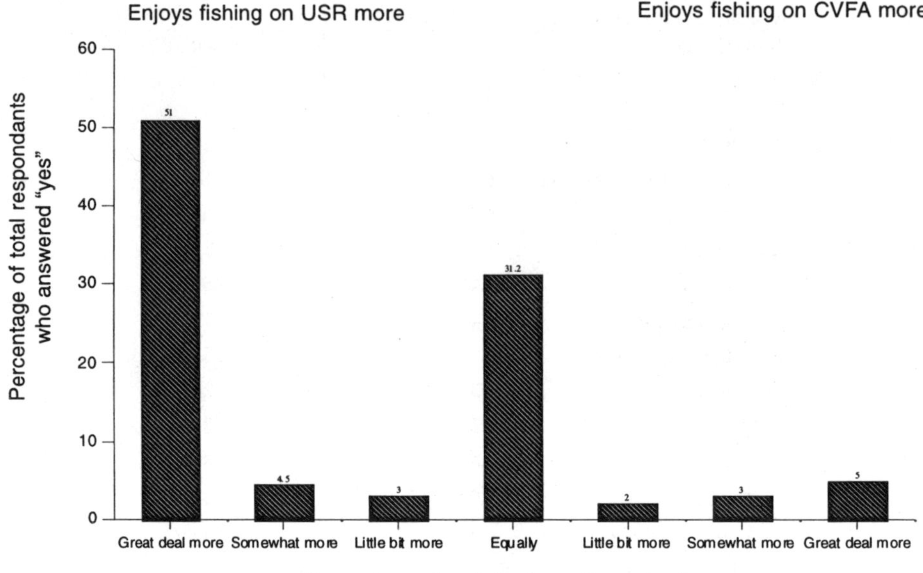

Figure 7-2 Respondents' comparison of fishing at CVFA with fishing on the USR (values = percentage of respondants) Source: Castle View Fishing Area Visitor Survey

very good or even superior substitute for the USR. This result has important implications for future cases, as discussed below.

The third approach to evaluating the substitution effect of the CVFA involved asking the CVFA anglers their willingness to pay to fish on the USR, assuming controlled access to the river. Only those CVFA anglers who had fished on the USR during the previous 5 years were asked about this hypothetical scenario; they represented approximately 50% of the respondents. These respondents were asked the following question:

Now suppose the State of California decides to permit limited fishing on the Upper Sacramento River. In order to limit use of the River, the State may consider issuing 1-day permits. Each permit that is purchased can be used by 1 person to catch the fishing limit on 1 day during this season or next. Would you or any other member of your household consider purchasing at least 1 of these 1-day permits?

Slightly more than half of the respondents answered "yes" to this question. For those who answered "no," they were asked "why not?" Those who answered "yes" were then asked a series of questions regarding the number of 1-day permits that their household would purchase and how much they would be willing to pay on average for each permit. They reported an average willingness to buy 6.3 permits at an average of $4.98 per permit. The median values were 4.0 permits and $5.00, respectively. The average willingness to pay per permit values ranged from $0 to $25 (for a single permit), with the 90th percentile falling at $9 to $10 per day. Figure 7-3 shows the distribution of the average willingness to pay per permit values.

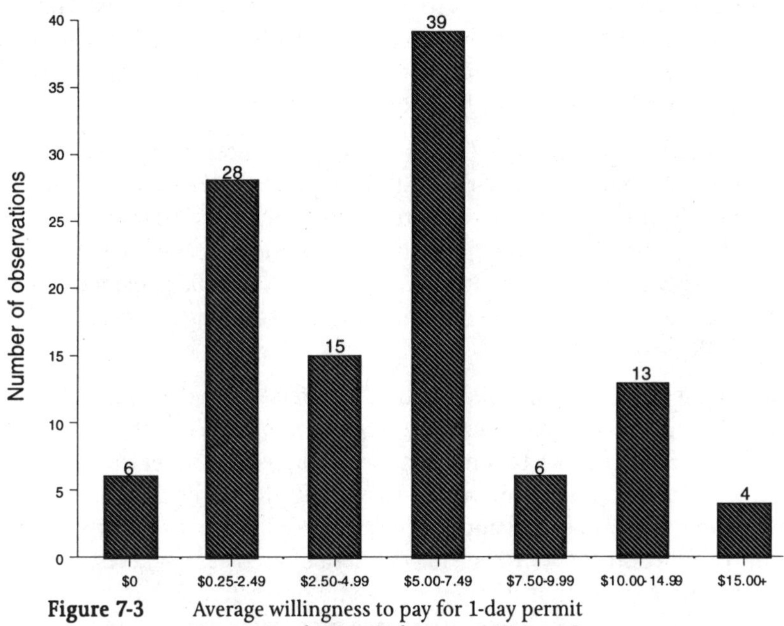

Figure 7-3 Average willingness to pay for 1-day permit
Source: Castle View Fishing Area Visitors Survey

The verbatim responses for the households that would not consider purchasing at least 1 permit indicated that at least some of these households had a 0 willingness to pay.

The average willingness to pay value of $5 per day translates to about $1.70 to $2 per hour of fishing, and the high-end values of $9 to $10 per day translate to about $3 or $4 per hour of fishing (assuming an average of about 2.5 to 3 hours of fishing per day). While we need to be cautious in interpreting these data, they imply relatively high mitigation of fishing-related losses associated with closure of the USR. Many anglers at the CVFA—previously USR anglers—indicated that they were not willing to pay very much extra for access to the river (which, at the time of the survey, was closed to fishing).[27] Recall that the estimated average hourly values for baseline fishing on the

[27] Caution is advised in interpreting these data given the hypothetical scenario to which the respondents were asked to respond. Some respondents might have actually valued fishing on the USR but chose to give a willingness to pay 0 out of "protest." These individuals might have felt that they had already paid enough for their existing fishing license or that a daily permit would be too constraining. The verbatim responses provided some evidence of these sentiments among some respondents. These responses will tend to result in underestimation of true willingness to pay. On the other hand, since this type of hypothetical question does not require that people actually pay, it tends to overestimate true willingness to pay. The precise net effect is unclear in this case.

USR were in the range of $11 to $14. The high mitigation result is also consistent with the anecdotal evidence that many anglers found the CVFA to be very satisfying.

The fourth approach to evaluating the substitution effect of the CVFA involved estimating the anglers' net willingness to pay for visits to the CVFA based on travel costs and demographic and trip characteristics. While this estimation process was begun using standard regression techniques, it did not progress to the stage of providing useful results prior to the litigation settlement.

Restoration of lost fishing use through CVFA - What do all these data tell us regarding the restoration of the lost fishing use of the USR through the CVFA? Clearly, the CVFA provided a heavily used and valuable substitute for many prior users of the USR. It also provided a resource that was enjoyed by anglers and others who had not previously fished the USR. On a pure hourly basis, the CVFA in 1993 provided more than 54,000 angling hours, or 59% of the estimated baseline angling hours of 92,000 per year for the USR.

What is the value of the angling hours at the CVFA relative to the angling hours on the USR? For some anglers, the value may have been the same. While this might seem heretical for those who believe that man-made resources can never provide the same enjoyment as natural resources (even those like the USR that have been heavily affected by man), both anecdotal and survey evidence indicates that this was the case for a sizable proportion of CVFA anglers. The area offered ease of access for both adults and children, freedom from poison oak and other natural hazards, ready access to fishing supplies, friendly informal assistance for anglers in need, and attractive catch rates. For other anglers, the value may have been significantly lower than for the USR. If we conservatively assume that the angling hours at the CVFA were only half as valuable as those on the USR, then the CVFA still restored about 30% of the USR baseline fishing use (59% * 50%). Alternatively, if we assume that 40% of the CVFA anglers found the CVFA angling experience to be at least as enjoyable as the USR angling experience, consistent with our Stage 2 survey findings, and that the other 60% of the CVFA anglers found it to be worth only half as much as the USR experience, then the CVFA restored over 40% of the USR baseline fishing use (59% * [(40% * 100%) + (60% * 50%)]).[28]

We therefore conclude that the area was very successful in replacing a substantial amount of the lost fishing use on the USR. We suspect that the anglers who benefitted the most from the CVFA were those living closest to the spill site and those with the least ability to travel far to substitute sites. This type of benefit to the local users of injured resources should not be overlooked in developing restoration plans.

---

[28] Since the average of these 2 values, or 35%, would imply an annual value of about $385,000 for CVFA anglers (35% * $1.1 million), dividing this by the 54,000 angling hours at the CVFA during 1993 yields an average value of a little over $7 per hour. This value was found to be consistent with research conducted on both privately and publicly operated ponds and lakes that require payment of daily fees to fish.

Restoration through increased stocking of substitute areas

In another effort to restore the lost fishing use of the USR, the natural resource trustees transferred the hatchery-raised trout scheduled to be put into the USR to other nearby rivers and lakes. Some of the trout were put into the CVFA. While the exact magnitude and location of the additional stocking efforts is not known, the CDFG announced plans to plant up to 120,000 more trout than usual in 1992 in waters within easy reach of the spill location. The plan was to continue the additional planting as long as the water temperature remained favorable (which was expected to occur). Fourteen locations were included in the plan (Anonymous 1992).

In 1993 the CDFG announced plans to continue its increased off-river stocking "to provide nearby fishing opportunities (CDFG 1993)." In addition to stocking fish at the CVFA, the CDFG indicated that it would continue these efforts at locations that "may include but will not be limited to" 14 locations within either 15 miles or 50 miles of the Mt. Shasta City/Dunsmuir area (CDFG 1993).[29] The CDFG's announcement did not include any indication of the quantities of fish to be stocked at locations other than the CVFA.

If the CDFG followed through with its 1992 plan to stock 120,000 additional trout in the region, how successful was it in helping to restore lost fishing use on the USR? Without more information on the locations and numbers of additional trout that were actually stocked in 1992 or 1993, we can provide only a rough evaluation of the likely benefits of this program. For simplicity, we can assume that these additional trout produced the same number of fishing hours as those fish historically stocked in the USR. As discussed above, our analysis of USR fishing use indicated that the approximately 80,000 fish stocked in the USR helped produce a baseline value of 92,000 hours per year of angling use. With this ratio of 1.15 angling hours per stocked fish, a total of 120,000 stocked fish would produce 138,000 angling hours. Even 50% of this number, to account for fewer stocked fish or less value in terms of providing angling hours, would yield 69,000 hours. The lower figure is essentially equivalent to the estimated baseline fishing level of 69,000 to 76,000 hours per year for bait anglers on the USR. While this increased stocking plan had the clear potential to restore much if not all of the lost fishing use of the USR, particularly for the bait and lure anglers who were more likely to fish for stocked trout, it is not possible to draw any firm conclusions without more data on the implementation and success of the stocking program.

Other restoration efforts

Two other restoration projects were also planned following the 1991 spill—a river trash cleanup project and 2 hiking trail construction projects. The trash cleanup project was successfully implemented, while the trail construction projects fell victim to the inability to secure necessary easements from land owners.

---

[29] The locations listed included Lake Siskiyou, Castle Lake, the upper McCloud River, the south fork of the Sacramento River, Cold Creek, Wagon Creek, Gunboot Lake, Lake Shasta, Lake Shastina, Juanita Lake, Kangaroo Lake, McCloud River, McCloud Reservoir, and Iron Canyon Reservoir.

The Upper Sacramento River Trash Cleanup Project removed the trash and debris that had accumulated over more than 100 years of heavy human use along the 40-mile stretch of the river affected by the spill. The project, with the theme "Forty Miles in a Summer," was a cooperative effort sponsored by Southern Pacific and CalTrout to stimulate the economic and recreational recovery of the USR canyon and its surrounding communities.

The project attracted 150 volunteers, took over 2 months to complete, and ultimately cost approximately $150,000. Volunteers walking the banks, together with divers and kayakers working on the river itself, collected 120 tons of trash including scrap metal, glass, television sets, mattresses, appliances, giant blocks of concrete, carpeting, and everyday household trash. Southern Pacific crews provided a crane that picked up the heavy items and removed all of the materials recovered from the river and its banks. The project was very successful, generated goodwill, and enhanced available uses of the USR other than fishing, such as swimming, kayaking, and hiking.

Two trail projects were also proposed. The first was intended to follow along a portion of the river between Box Canyon Dam and the town of Dunsmuir and to provide access to the river for hikers, kayakers, and anglers once the river was reopened. Unfortunately, due to the inability to negotiate various easements, the project had to be abandoned. The other project, called the Symbol Rocks Trail, proposed to reopen an old 1-mile U.S. Forest Service trail and extend it an additional half mile. The project would have included trailside picnic areas, benches, and an interpretive program. The purpose of reopening the trail was to provide scenic hiking for local residents and to enhance recreational opportunities for tourists in the Dunsmuir area. This project also ran into easement difficulties and was never completed.

Implications for future cases

What lessons can we learn from the USR case, particularly for the restoration of lost human uses in future cases? First, man-made or man-augmented resources that are temporary in nature can restore substantial portions of lost human uses of the environment that are themselves temporary. In the USR case, both the CVFA and the increased stocking of nearby rivers and lakes are likely to have restored a substantial amount of the temporary lost use of the USR; together, these measures probably restored at least one-half to two-thirds of the lost use, and possibly more.

Second, as in this case, restoration measures should seek to restore uses for major segments of the user population, not just the elite users. In the USR case, the majority of the baseline anglers on the USR were bait and lure anglers interested in catching fish at a convenient location. A minority of the baseline users were fly anglers primarily interested in catching wild trout.

Third, in a variant on the adage "the perfect is the enemy of the good," a good or very good restoration measure such as the CVFA is better than no restoration measure or waiting to design the perfect measure. Restoration alternatives like the CVFA, which restore use levels for a substantial portion of the baseline user population while doing no harm to natural resources, need to be identified as early as possible and implemented aggressively in order to minimize continuing lost uses after a spill. The focus should be on the users, not on deciding the most dazzling or innovative measure that will take years to implement and may not be successful even then.

Fourth, a diversified portfolio of restoration measures can often provide an attractive and robust means of restoring lost human uses in the most cost-effective manner. In this case, the portfolio included a set of man-made fishing ponds close to the spill site, increased stocking of nearby rivers and lakes, and a trash cleanup project along the affected segment of the river. While these measures may have had different values to different segments of the user population, together they likely helped to restore the temporary lost uses to broad segments of the baseline user population. The trash cleanup project will also have value to future users of the USR—essentially a form of compensatory restoration.

Fifth, cooperative efforts between PRPs and trustees can work, but both have to be willing to work together and put aside their litigation interests. The trustees in the USR case must be commended for cooperating with Southern Pacific to make the CVFA a success, even though the area's success reduced the amount of damages that the trustees would have been able to claim if the case ever went to trial. The public's overriding interest in quickly and cost-effectively restoring the lost human uses of the environment after spills must motivate both PRPs and trustees to identify and implement appropriate restoration measures as quickly as possible.

Finally, collecting data on the users of restoration alternatives and substitutes can be very valuable in both assessing their impact and fine-tuning their implementation. In the case of the CVFA, the area's operators learned that providing a few larger trout was an excellent way to promote the area and increase its popularity.

An evaluation of substitution in the Idarado case

Introduction and economic setting

Several counties in southwestern Colorado, including Ouray and San Miguel, contain ore deposits of gold, silver, copper, and other valuable mineral resources. One 10-mile stretch of the mountain road between the communities of Ouray and Silverton was called the "Million Dollar Highway" because of all of the 19th-century prospectors who became millionaires from exploitation of the rich mineral lode. By the middle of the 20th century, much of the mining activity in that area had been consolidated into a single entity called the Idarado Mining and Milling Complex (Idarado Complex). Most of the land area within 20 miles of the Idarado Complex site is contained in the Uncompahgre National Forest, with vast outdoor recreational opportunities. The popular ski resort Telluride is adjacent to the Idarado Complex.

In 1983 the state of Colorado filed a suit against the owners of the Idarado Complex alleging NRDs under CERCLA. The Colorado legislature authorized the expenditure of

$8 million to fund the litigation costs of a set of CERCLA-related lawsuits, including the Idarado case. This case illustrates the important role that substitutes play in measuring lost human uses.

Natural resource damage calculations

In 1986 Drs. Boland and Milliman prepared a report alleging NRDs associated with the Idarado Complex totaling $149.1 million (Boland and Milliman 1986). This claim was based on extrapolation from a state-wide contingent valuation survey regarding hazardous waste sites. In an attempt to provide corroboration for this claim, Drs. Boland and Milliman catalogued 12 distinct categories or alleged NRDs related to human uses of the environment, ranging from lost creek and river fisheries to diminished community reputation. However, they quantified only 3 such categories of alleged use-related damages. One of these categories related to an asserted loss of angler days at Ridgeway Reservoir, a small flood-control-based reservoir located along the Uncompahgre River about 10 miles north of the town of Ouray. In an area with scenic lakes and rivers with large boulders and forests, the Ridgeway Reservoir stands out. Because of substantial seasonal variations in the height of the reservoir, there are few trees around it and the shoreline is primarily mud. Within 12 miles are small pristine lakes with an abundance of fish and related wildlife. There are more than 60 substantially superior fishing sites within a radius of 25 miles, some of which are closer to the population centers of Montrose, Ouray, and Telluride. For the most part, these superior substitutes sites were uncongested and rarely had more than 2 to 3 anglers present at any one of them during the period of interest. Because of natural and man-made contamination of the Red Mountain Creek above it and the Uncompahgre River below it, the Ridgeway Reservoir sustains only a very small fishery.

Drs. Boland and Milliman estimated that from 1989 to 1996, 16,000 angler days were lost at Ridgeway Reservoir. They claimed that no one fished at the reservoir allegedly due to contamination from the Idarado Complex. However, ordinarily no one would fish there anyway because of the availability of superior substitute sites. Better and uncongested fishing in much more scenic surroundings existed at shorter travel distances and thereby lower travel costs than that of Ridgeway Reservoir, even if its fishery were unaffected. Drs. Boland and Milliman asserted that if concentrations of zinc, cadmium, copper, and other substances were lower, "habitat analyses indicate that viable trout populations could exist" in Ridgeway Reservoir. A check every 2 hours for recreational activity for a continuous 21-day period in July and August 1986 found only 1 family using the reservoir for a picnic (they did not fish). They spoke no English and were traveling to eastern Colorado to harvest vegetables. The reservoir offered no amenities besides picnic tables and primitive restrooms.

As long as the reservoir is operated as a committed use for flood control with muddy banks and a high variable shoreline, with little or no vegetation and attendant wildlife, it cannot attain the status of more than a strongly inferior substitute. In consequence, angler visitor days cannot be 16,000 or even 16 in the baseline scenario.

Drs. Boland and Milliman used standard angler day values for Rocky Mountain fishing experiences recommended by the U.S. Forest Service of $21 per day and $14 per day to calculate NRD. These are recorded in Table 7-7. However, these values are clearly for fishing areas that are or can be enjoyed by anglers.

Table 7-7 Estimated natural resource damages for Ridgeway Reservoir, Ouray County, Colorado

Type of damage	Boland-Milliman	d'Arge
Average value of lost angler day	$14.56-$21.84[1]	$0-$0.07
Total damage[2]	$933,900-$1,400,500	$0-$4494

[1] Boland and Milliman's average values for angler days in 1985 dollars are inflated to 1986 dollars using the consumer price index
[2] Estimates are for 16,000 lost angler days per year for the period 1989 through 1996, converted to present value in 1986 dollars using a 10% discount rate.

This case raises a larger question. If no one currently uses a site for fishing and would not use it if it were cleaned up, are there any NRDs? That is, do strongly inferior recreational sites have any economic value? The answer is that it depends. If the site is cleaned up, it becomes less inferior. Does this have value to anglers? From an economic perspective, it does because now the angler has both a greater number and greater variety of sites to fish. The hypothesis was tested by d'Arge using a direct contact questionnaire on a sample of 90 anglers who were then currently fishing creeks, lakes, and rivers in the immediate area. The average angler contacted was willing to spend $0.07 per day to be able to fish one more site in the immediate area, where the site contained the characteristics of Ridgeway Reservoir (d'Arge 1986). An estimate of NRDs based on the addition of a fishing site is recorded in Table 7-7. Note that the estimated damages have been reduced from more than $1 million to less than $5000 by the inclusion of substitute fishing sites. In this case, those substitute sites were superior to the site at issue.

The correct specification of actual substitution possibilities for Ridgeway Reservoir yielded a very marked reduction in NRDs. Further, unless reservoir operations are changed to avoid the radical seasonal adjustments in reservoir height, NRDs will not occur at this site in the future.

Lesson learned

Assumptions with regard to the availability and quality of substitute resources have a significant effect on measurement of the value of lost human uses. In this case, lost human uses were very limited, if not 0. Direct interviews with potentially harmed parties revealed the true nature of actual lost uses. Relying on the common economic practice of calculating lost human uses from standard reference works on use rates and fishing values can be very misleading. Where substitutes are plentiful, it should not be automatically assumed that restoration of physical resources, such as trout populations, will necessarily lead to significant increases in human uses of those resources.

Conclusions

Substitutes need to be given their due. They are important in 2 major respects. First, their existence can vastly reduce the magnitude of lost human uses of the environment caused by oil or hazardous substance spills. This is a basic principle of economics. If a town loses its only movie theater due to a fire, it will suffer a much greater loss than a town that loses one of 10 such theaters. Second, trustees and PRPs who create or augment substitutes, such as the increased stocking of fish or refurbishment and stocking of old fishing ponds in the USR case, can greatly reduce the lost uses or even quickly restore most if not all of the lost uses.

To maximize effectiveness, substitutes must be augmented or created as soon as possible following a spill. This requires the cooperation of trustees and PRPs—the public suffers when appropriate restoration measures are unnecessarily delayed by tactics designed to promote or protect litigation interests over the minimization of damages due to the spill.

References

[Anonymous]. 1992. D-U-N-S-M-U-I-R spells trout. *California Game & Fish* (August 1992):25–53.

Boland JJ, Milliman JW. 1986. Economic damage report: Idarado Mining and Milling Complex.

Biemer PP, Groves RM, Lyberg LE, Mathiowetz NA, Sudman S. 1991. Measurement errors in surveys. New York NY: Wiley.

[CDFG] California Department of Fish and Game. 1991. Final satellite environmental document regarding sport fishing for trout. Table 7: designated wild trout and catch-and-release waters, 1990.

[CDFG] California Department of Fish and Game. 1993. 1993 fishery management plan for the Upper Sacramento River (Box Canyon Dam to Shasta Lake).

d'Arge R. 1986. A review of the economic damage report: Idarado Mining and Milling Complex. Laramie WY: University of Wyoming, Department of Economics. p 1–37.

Sunderland B, Lackey D. 1991. California blue ribbon trout streams. Portland OR: Frank Amato Publications.

Tanur JM. 1992. Questions about questions: inquiries into the cognitive bases of surveys. New York NY: Russell Sage Foundation.

Unsworth RE, Bishop RC. 1994. Assessing natural resource damages using environmental annuities. *Ecolog Econ* 11:35–41.

7a

Discussion Paper I on Measuring and Restoring Lost Human Uses: Two Real-World Case Studies, or Substitutes Really Do Matter

*Keith Eastin**

The Birdsall et al. discussion as well as the approach to services in the Lavaca Bay contamination yields optimism in providing a method by which services can be returned to the public quickly and in a form the public desires.

Dunsmuir case study

Here the authors largely limit themselves to analyzing the values resulting from the creation of 2 enhanced fishing ponds as a replacement of a contaminated blue ribbon trout stream, the Upper Sacramento River (USR). The USR was closed to fishing after the spill and did not reopen for nearly 3 years, then only on a restricted basis. The ponds were enhanced, stocked with hatchery-raised trout, and opened approximately 1 year after fishing on the USR was closed. The ponds were intended as a partial substitute for the fishing experience in the USR.

The authors conclude that the ponds provided angling hours approximating 60% of the hours previously spent on the USR. When considered with the plans of Fish & Game to stock other nearby streams with trout, they presume the entire lost fishing experience may have been temporarily replaced.

When the study discusses the "quality" of the fishing experience at the ponds, a significant divergence appears. To make the experiences of the USR and the ponds reasonably comparable, anglers at the ponds should be expected to be the same as those formerly using the USR. More specifically, one would need to find anglers that lost a valuable fishing experience at the USR now fishing at the temporary site.

The study finds that, on a per-hour basis, of the anglers fishing at the ponds, only half had fished in the USR within the last 5 years. This was a new fishing area and actually brought the experience to a new group of people. Perhaps more significant, half of those who fished in the USR within the last 5 years said that they were not willing to

*Deloitte & Touche LLP, Wilmington, DE

pay for the experience of having USR reopened. Thus, while a large number of people enjoyed the experience of fishing at the ponds, three-quarters of them either had not fished the USR or placed a low value on that experience. It would appear that "serious" anglers were staying away from the new ponds.

Opening of the ponds brought some grumbling that the experience just was not the same (or more cynically, "no serious angler," would ever spend time at the ponds). While no panacea, opening of the ponds brought a fishing experience to a large number of people who either did not use or did not value the USR. Presumably they enjoyed themselves. While no one seriously has claimed that the ponds provided the quality of the experience of the USR, opening them provided a usable substitute and brought out a large number of people.

Rather than analyze the issue for a lengthy period, the substitute experience was made available reasonably quickly. The ponds did not replace the USR with a highly comparable resource, and USR anglers may have been deprived. However, from the point of view of society as a whole, many members of the public enjoyed a resource that would not have been in place but for the accelerated action on the part of the trustees and the responsible party.

Conclusion

Both the Dunsmir and Lavaca Bay scenarios may help in the expeditious return of services of damaged resources to the people. While the ponds in Dunsmuir may not mirror the quality experience of the River, the services were returned to the public quickly. At Lavaca Bay, services of the natural resources might be returned in a form that might maximize their value to the public. Both methods may herald a small step to more efficient handling of damaged natural resources.

7b

Discussion Paper 2 on Measuring and Restoring Lost Human Uses: Two Real-World Case Studies, or Substitutes Really Do Matter

Pierre H. duVair[*1]

Economists have recognized for some time that the number and quality of substitutes can influence an individual's demand for recreation at a particular site. While this is not new information, the title of this paper suggests that recognition of this concept has not made its way into the arena of natural resource damages. The paper would be much stronger if the authors cited more than one 11-year-old case study to make their point. In the other real-world example presented, the authors cited numerous "blue ribbon" substitutes for the Upper Sacramento River (USR) fishery, but then provided no information as to levels of substitution that occurred at these locations or how their existence influenced the Southern Pacific Railroad damage case.

There are 2 important points regarding substitutes that are worth keeping in mind relative to damage assessments. First, a valid and reliable assessment of the role of substitutes in determination of human-use damages can be very expensive and time consuming. A second key point to consider is that while the existence of substitutes may lessen human-use damages, the existence of substitutes for compensatory restoration actions also lessens the value of such compensation.

The authors focus on the economic perspective of restoring lost human-use values and suggest that "welfare economics" should determine the types and levels of cost-efficient compensatory restoration. While true in large part, maximizing utility of the resource users is clearly not the only challenge facing trustees. Whether or not settlements distinguish public-use losses from the cost of restoring the resources and/or services, compensatory human-use projects are inextricably tied to the overall restoration process. Settlements are just that, and from the trustees' perspective primary and compensatory projects can be viewed as competing for a limited source of funding.

---

*California Department of Fish and Game, Sacramento, California

[1]The opinions presented herein are expressly those of the author and do not necessarily reflect the views of the Department of Fish and Game. Thanks go to Larry Espinosa and Steve Turek for their helpful insights.

The authors argue that not only are substitutes important to natural resource damage assessment (NRDA), but also that the mitigation of human-use losses is worthy of much focus by responsible parties (RPs) and trustees of the natural resources. I find this point particularly true following completion of the emergency cleanup and that all parties should be cognizant of conditions that lend themselves to such mitigation actions. As the authors point out, cooperative relations between the RPs and trustees is one such condition. On this topic aptly described as "emergency human-use restoration," all parties should recognize that costs of interdicting losses can exceed the reduced liability from such actions. This type of outcome is more likely when the actions are planned in hast and the human-use injuries not well identified (i.e., project misses the mark).

I believe the authors are accurate in stating that assessment of human-use losses and the use of values in the literature must be done carefully, with a significant amount of thought given to substitutes and transferability of the literature studies. In this regard, academic resource economists are continuing to make contributions on the subject of valid benefit transfers.

I found the authors discussion of the Idarado case to be very poor and will comment only briefly. It appears that the authors' assumptions about baseline recreation at Ridgeway Reservoir had more to do with the disparity shown in Table 7-7, than did the lack of Boland and Milliman's consideration of substitutes. The authors assume zero baseline losses in human uses due to contamination and present only an "option value" derived from a survey of 90 local anglers. Based upon the brief presentation in this paper, I question the objectivity of their description of a healthy Ridgeway Reservoir that led to a $0.07 per fishing day average benefit to local fisherman. Without more details, little can be said.

I found numerous problems with the authors' evaluation of the degree to which the Castle View Fishing Area (CVFA) mitigated human-use losses resulting from Southern Pacific's release of metam sodium into the USR. The authors provide no calculations or sources for their estimation of 92,000 lost fish hours per year, nor for the $11 to $14 per hour fishing values. The reader begrudgingly must accept these at face value.

The authors are mistaken about the degree to which fishing on the USR is a function of hatchery fish. They assume that fly fisherman alone predominantly fish for wild trout and that bait and lure fisherman fish for convenience and hatchery fish. California regulations combine flies and lures as a category of gear, and lures are allowed along all stretches of the USR. Creel census data from 1994 to 1996 show that well over half the hours fished on the USR are in areas with no hatchery stocked fish. Budget constraints at the Department of Fish and Game (DFG) led to significant declines in stocking of the USR over the last 3 years (12,500 to 16,000 fish), yet no significant drop in angling hours accompanied this change. Many anglers recognize the USR as a "world-class" wild trout fishery. I believe the authors overstate the benefit of stocking and catching hatchery fish at the USR.

A related problem to the labeling of lure anglers as "put-n-take" fisherman is the presumption that anglers at CVFA actually represent 75% to 83% of anglers on the USR. Another significantly mistaken assumption is that the USR fishery can be characterized as an easy access fishery. In fact the opposite is more accurate. Much of the access on the USR should be characterized as difficult. The authors claim they found no biases in responses to their telephone survey, yet they fail to recognize the overriding sample frame bias. I am also unclear as to why the authors made no attempt to eliminate the "over sampling" of return visitors, which serves to exasperate the sample bias problem. The results presented in Table 7-6 are, as the authors note, largely reflective of local and convenience-oriented fisherman.

Characteristics of CVFA visitors were not presented but likely reflect high participation by: 1) local residents, 2) parents, 3) children, 4) elderly, and 5) physically challenged fisherman because the convenience factor is important to many individuals in these user groups. An interesting test of the quality of CVFA as a substitute for fishing on the USR would have been to keep the CVFA open following the reopening of fishing on the USR. If nearly 40% of visitors were indifferent between the two, attendance would have remained at a relatively high level. The fact that only 1 in 5 visitors returned to CVFA, while nearly 1 in 2 visitors were from the region suggests to me the experience was less valuable than portrayed by the authors. The fact that 51% of those interviewed by telephone said they preferred fishing on the USR a "great deal more" also points to the CVFA as a significantly inferior substitute.

The authors suggest that the CVFA may have mitigated between 71 to 78% of lost bait and lure angling on the USR for 1993. The authors fail to recognize 1) the half-year of angling lost in 1991, 2) only a portion of 1992 was mitigated (28 to 31% using their numbers), and 3) losses that have been occurring and continue to occur today. Examples of the ongoing human-use impacts include the fish release requirements, gear restrictions, and smaller and fewer fish per mile of the USR.

The authors caution readers about the interpretation of telephone survey willingness-to-pay results, largely because of the potential for hypothetical bias. I would argue for caution more due to sample frame biases, non-response biases, and protest response biases. In short, my guess is that the NOAA Blue Ribbon Panel would be somewhat critical of the $5 per day average USR fishing value derived by the authors for a blue-ribbon fishery.

In summary, I have a comment and a concern. My comment relates to the injured segment of the public and the focus of human-use restoration. I agree with the authors' contention that segments of injured public should not be overlooked during restoration planning and that trustees should strive to "restore uses for major segments of the user population, not just the elite users," however subjectively "elite" may be defined.

I raise a concern about the authors' criteria used to judge the degree of "success" in replacing lost fishing use on the USR. The authors focused on generic "hours of fishing" and deemed the CVFA successful because it did generate hours. Trustees may want to focus on projects providing high quality/low quantity services, while RPs may focus on projects providing high quantity/low quality services. Clearly this presents a potential for conflict during cooperative discussions of emergency human-use restoration. My personal concern stems from the real-world example where DFG could have heavily stocked the USR immediately following the spill with hatchery fish. This emergency human-use restoration project would potentially have provided high quantity/lower quality services, but only at the expense of ecosystem restoration and long-term human-use losses associated with delayed recovery or collapse of a wild trout fishery.

7c

Discussion Paper 3 on Measuring and Restoring Lost Human Uses: Two Real-World Case Studies, or Substitutes Really Do Matter, or Natural Resource Damage Assessment: A Texas Perspective

*Diane B. Hyatt**

Purpose

Although this paper was reviewed by all Texas trustees, I am not speaking for the other trustees, and there may be differing opinions on some of the points discussed. Overall, it is the trustees' duty to restore the resources and their services. It is difficult for me to isolate the narrow interim lost human use from the whole. The human uses and other service flows from our natural resources are directly correlated to the health and diversity of the ecosystem from which the services flow. The trustees endeavor to work as a team to restore the whole. It is the goal to restore with no net losses to the system or to the users that are, in fact, part of the same system.

Measuring and restoring lost human uses

In consideration of this paper's statement that certain information regarding injury determination and restoration decisions are unavailable, the Texas trustees regard injury determination and injury quantification as an open process. Natural resource case settlements should not be kept confidential because

- recovery is made on behalf of the public, and the public should be able to view and comment on the data used to determine the extent of the injury;
- keeping these matters confidential inhibits the growth of the "learning curve" for all trustees and the public;
- NOAA, DOI, and state trustees should establish and maintain a database of techniques used to determine and quantify injury and scale restoration; and,
- the trustees should not have an interest in keeping such information confidential and should oppose such efforts.

*Director, Natural Resource Damage Assessment, Texas General Land Office, Austin, Texas

The Texas NRDA rule provides for establishment of an administrative record for public review and for public comment on the assessment and restoration plans.

The author's stated intent to disclose how substitutes may affect the outcome of an NRD settlement is worthy. However, the statement "*if substitute resources are readily available. . .then there may be no need for restoration measures because the substitute resources can be used. . .pending natural recovery*" is contested. This statement ignores the net loss suffered when resources are injured; even though substitute resources are available, there is still a net loss. Resources that are already being used are not an equal substitute for injured resources.

Restoration of the lost human use component certainly can be augmented through creative substitution. Timely restoration is what the Texas trustees seek as a goal. However, there are several problems that seem to be glossed over in this paper's quick-substitution approach. First, the State of Texas believes that restoration in terms of economic welfare must incorporate biological health and diversity to be a success in the long term. Readily available substitutes are good and lessen the impact on interim lost use, but do not promote the future viability and sustainability of the resource that was lost or injured. In the fishery example, the "greater good" was considered and a valuable substitution was implemented that satisfied the majority of users. However, within this substitution, there was no component for non-consumptive (aesthetic) value associated with the existence of wild populations of fish species in an ecosystem that could support and sustain these populations. Second, fly-fishermen, 25% of the users, were not compensated. Third, the impact on a natural fish population's genetic diversity by the *increased* dilution of the gene pool with additional "stocked fish" was not considered. The adaptability of future generations of these fish ultimately affects human use and becomes a limiting factor even though stocking has been a practice in all the streams for many decades.

Given the circumstance, the Texas trustees recognize that any improvements to minimize the loss to the public trust is worth pursuing; however, caution must be taken that we do not substitute ourselves out of viable sustainable resources. We should also bear in mind that fishing is not the only use of this valuable river system. Also, the unique attributes associated with the existence of wild populations constitute both a consumptive and a non-consumptive human use. Quick-fix management can have irreversible effects, especially on genetics and diversity.

It is noted that the highest ranking characteristics of the substitute created are not directly related to the "fishing" itself, but to ancillary components. For example, one is "ease of access"; the second is "ease of taking children to the location"; the third is "comfort of the location." The lowest ranking characteristics are the ones related to the "fishing"; last is "opportunity to catch wild trout"; eleventh is "remoteness of the location" (fishing is generally a relatively solitary activity; the less congestion, the greater likelihood of catching a fish); and, tenth is "opportunity to catch large trout." This raises the question of how good a substitute this was in real terms of satisfaction.

Over 58% of the respondents in the survey, when asked to compare the substitute experience with the experience associated with the lost resource (river fishing), chose the river experience. In the majority of responses, it was enjoyed " a great deal more." Almost one-third responded "equal" and only 10% said the substitute was "superior." How then could the authors conclude that in economic terms, the substitute provided a very good or "*even superior*" substitute for the river experience? It is clear that the substitute had value, but I dispute that it was a superior condition. The respondents polled were not considered to be "elite users," and they clearly preferred the river experience.

The substitute fishing experience was an attractive vehicle for certain recreational users and a positive benefit to them; however, it would be hard to justify that this was compensation for the 25% who were fly fishers of wild trout. The fact that approximately one-fourth of the users estimated was in this category is significant.

The restoration of aesthetic values through trash removal is a positive benefit for all human-use categories, consumptive and non-consumptive. Goodwill is also received by the responsible party in making this effort. A real and significant form of human-use (abuse) restoration is made in addressing the trash problem associated with our wild places.

Conclusions

1) We agree that temporary measures can be taken for good, and we expect that there would be a cooperative effort to have the RPs and trustees initiate a substitute together. The trustees recognize that it is difficult to scale the amount of restoration created by substitutes.
2) While substituting what is expedient and practical, the trustees must still evaluate other aspects of the resources that are unique and uncompensated for by the substitute and restore, when possible, or be compensated otherwise: a no net loss policy.
3) There is no perfect restoration, which causes us all to work even more diligently to prevent spills and/or releases to the environment.
4) Diversified restoration measures are a positive means to address differing aspects of the loss, i.e., service flows.
5) "Litigation" is the last resort in Texas. In the Texas NRDA rule, the trustees and the RP must go to mediation before suit is filed. It is, however, important to perform investigations and agreements with the enforceability of the agreements in mind. Trustees are mandated to seek to protect, preserve, and restore the public trust resources. Responsible parties wish to expunge their liability in the most cost-effective manner. The public interest is best served when rapid restoration can be achieved through the most cost-efficient and scientifically sound approach.

6) Every incident teaches a lesson to trustees about what is most important to the humans that use the resources. Surveys can be constructed to give valuable information. Question: Why is it that in this instance the "willingness to pay" was a plausible survey question, yet hotly contested if used in contingent valuation? The trustees use experience, and ecological and economic science, to direct the restoration to achieve the most "bang for the buck."

In the case of Ridgeway Reservoir, Ouray, Colorado, not all of the facts were presented. Degradation of the site seemed to be due to several factors including some natural mineralization. The reduction in compensation may not be due to superior substitutes as much as the committed human-use aspect associated with flood control. Still, as trustees, we do not "write off" a degraded environment when additional enhancement at a substitute site might offer compensation for the lost use due *solely to the industrial releases*. The philosophy that if a resource is not being "used," then there is no loss is not consistent with our mandate to protect. If that were true, we would not have future use as an option for future generations. Trustees must be stewards for future human use and ecological health: again, the no-net-loss approach.

Our natural resources are finite. Trustees work to construct more habitats as natural areas are depleted; however, we are not successful in duplicating natural ecological systems. Substitutes are helpful, but only address a part of the injury. The trustees and the RPs who use objective science whenever possible and work in an atmosphere of fair-mindedness should not fear litigation. Litigation is an enforcement tool to be used only if necessary—restoration is the goal.

Acknowledgments—I wish to thank my colleagues who provided comments and critical review of this paper: Ingrid K. Hansen, Texas General Land Office, David Chapman, National Oceanographic and Atmospheric Administration, David Sager, Texas Parks and Wildlife, and my staff, Patricia M. Rives and Peter A. H. Samuels.

7d

Discussion Paper 4 on Measuring and Restoring Lost Human Uses: Two Real-World Case Studies, or Substitutes Really Do Matter

*Bruce Peacock**

The case studies presented by Birdsall et al. illustrate the difficulty trustees and potentially responsible parties face when trying to compare the value of natural resource losses to the value of compensatory restoration projects. The following comments are offered on the authors' general discussion of substitutes and the specific examples they cite.

Before these comments are presented, a preliminary note is made about the authors' stated desire to examine settlement discussions as a guide to natural resource valuation issues. The path of settlement discussions involves more than a simple search for the truth. The assessment of litigation risk also plays a major role. Positions are taken and concessions made that reflect the transactions costs involved in more elaborate preparations. The concept of reasonable assessment cost, then, acts as a constraint on the efforts taken to value natural resources. Therefore, when concerned about economic valuation per se, one must be careful to account for the influence of litigation risk when examining settlement discussions and agreements.

General discussion of substitutes

The importance of substitutes in the valuation of natural resources is not disputed. However, the ability of substitutes to replace lost uses must be clearly understood. As a first step, one should not confuse the issues of accounting for existing substitutes[1] with that of providing compensatory restoration. Existing substitutes are *fixed* by the currently available resources, while compensatory restoration projects are *selected*, *scaled*, and *implemented* to compensate the public for losses. Therefore, considerations

*Department of the Interior, Washington, DC

[1]"Existing substitutes" is taken here to mean resources that exist independently of the injury or damage recovery and are capable of providing substitute services to users and would-be users of the injured resource.

of existing substitutes are *descriptive* in nature while considerations of compensatory restoration are *prescriptive*.

The authors apparently confuse these issues when they suggest that existing substitutes may be able to fully compensate for natural resource losses. This scenario is unlikely for at least 3 reasons. First, the role of individual preferences must be acknowledged. The increased use of an existing substitute following a natural resource injury indicates a switch to a lesser preferred activity since users of the injured resource were presumably free to use the substitute resource before the injury, but chose not to instead. This switch to a lesser preferred activity implies lower use values.

The second reason why existing substitutes would be unlikely to fully compensate for natural resource injuries is congestion. The externalities associated with the increased congestion of a common-access resource imply lower-use values for all users of the resource. Therefore, congestion affects 2 groups of users. The users who preferred the existing substitute at the time of the injury will suffer lower-use values due to crowding from the influx of refugees fleeing the natural resource injury. Moreover, the increased congestion of the existing substitute will add insult to injury for the would-be users of injured resources who are forced into the lesser-preferred activity.

Finally, for completeness, the potential loss of nonuse values associated with the injured natural resources should be acknowledged. Existing substitutes, as the term is used here, exist independently of the natural resource injury. Therefore, these substitutes add nothing new for the compensation of lost nonuse values. If anything, the nonuse values attributable to existing substitutes will be diminished due to increased congestion if the public becomes aware of more crowded conditions.

Perhaps the authors had in mind compensatory restoration projects when they stated that existing substitutes may be able to fully compensate for natural resource losses. Another reason why the distinction between existing substitutes and compensatory restoration projects is important is that the *types* of services provided by each can be quite different. Services provided by existing substitutes are not necessarily the same as those lost due to a natural resource injury, whereas the services provided by compensatory restoration *should* be as closely matched as possible. This difference is illustrated by the 2 case studies described in the paper.

Upper Sacramento River case study

The authors describe the Castle View Fishing Area (CVFA) as a compensatory restoration project that was implemented to replace lost uses suffered along the Upper Sacramento River (USR). While the CVFA was in operation, surveys were conducted to determine the degree to which lost uses along the USR were replaced by the project. However, the Stage 2 survey and results apparently reflected only the responses of CVFA visitors, and therefore could not adequately measure the project's ability to compensate for all losses suffered along the USR. The type of fishing and other recreational opportunities offered at CVFA (fishing in ponds) were different from those offered along the USR before the injury (scenic "blue ribbon" trout fishing in a river). Therefore, the results of the survey were probably biased. A general population survey would seem more appropriate to compare all losses suffered along the USR with the gains provided by the CVFA.

In their implications for future cases, the authors seem to indicate a preference for restoration projects that appeal to broad segments of the population over projects that provide recreational opportunities more closely matched to the injured natural resource. Judging from the reported demographics of CVFA use, one interesting implication of this preference is that the authors ascribe nontrivial values to the participation of young (or junior) users and not just adults. Nevertheless, this preference for broad appeal can be misleading. The goal of natural resource damage assessment is to restore the injured resources and their services. Therefore, compensatory restoration projects should be selected to provide as close a match to the lost services as possible.

Idarado case study

In the Idarado case study, the authors assert little if any lost use associated with a contaminated reservoir due to the availability of higher quality fishing opportunities in the immediate area. A contact survey of anglers conducted at creeks, lakes, and rivers near the contaminated reservoir indicated a low willingness to pay for fishing at a similar, but presumably uncontaminated, reservoir. However, for purposes of valuing all lost uses of the reservoir, this survey was probably biased since the respondents included only the users of particular resources engaged in a particular activity (fishing). There may be members of the general population who would fish at the reservoir if it were not contaminated. Moreover, the fact that a reservoir is not managed for fishing does not preclude other potential uses such as picnicking and boating. The relevant services that should be replaced by compensatory restoration are those that would have been provided by the reservoir without contamination, not necessarily those that are provided by existing substitutes.

Summary

Substitutes really do matter. Because they matter, it is important not to confuse the issues of accounting for existing substitutes with that of providing compensatory restoration. The 2 sets of issues are fundamentally different. The authors' apparent enthusiasm for providing compensatory restoration for natural resource injuries is applauded. However, trustees and potentially responsible parties must clearly understand the role of substitutes in lost use valuation and recognize the goals of compensatory restoration to fairly address compensation for natural resource injuries.

7e

Discussion Paper 5 on Measuring and Restoring Lost Human Uses: Two Real-World Case Studies, or Substitutes Really Do Matter

*Neal S. Brody**

I approached each of my critiques with a focus on 2 distinct components. First, I examined the overall approach to restoration in each of the cases described by the authors. These approaches were as varied as the underlying facts in each of the cases. Second, in addition to an overall assessment, I studied the specific recommendations proposed as a result of the authors' experiences. Without exception, each author offered valuable considerations for future cases involving restoration of lost human uses.

The Birdsall paper

General response

The authors track 2 very distinctive approaches to the restoration of lost human uses of the environment. The first portion of the paper describes the Cantara Loop spill case and appears to be a model for how restoration should proceed wherever possible. Immediately following the spill, the responsible party commenced efforts to restore lost human uses of the environment. While it is not clear from the paper whether the trustees initially supported those efforts, we can reasonably conclude that at least they were not opposed to the efforts. Consequently, and to the credit of all concerned, human uses were partially restored and available to the public within 1 year of the incident. It was particularly interesting to note that rather than the parties gathering data to quantify a claim for natural resources damages, restoration was immediately undertaken, and subsequently, data were gathered to measure the success of the restoration. This is a much more effective method of restoring lost human uses of the environment.

The other experience described in the paper, the Idarado mine case, sets out quite a different situation than the Cantara Loop case. The authors seem to suggest that substantial effort has been devoted to measuring natural resource damages in the

*ARCO, Los Angeles, CA

Idarado case; however, no effort has been focused on addressing the restoration of lost human uses of the environment. In that respect, at least to some extent, it might be considered not the best way to restore lost human uses of the environment.

Recommendations

The authors offer numerous recommendations following the experiences of the Cantara Loop and Idarado mine cases. Its principle conclusion, following the Idarado mine case, is that substitutes do matter. In particular, the Idarado experience markedly illustrates the dangers and distortions of using formulaic procedures for determining natural resource damages. In virtually every case, opportunities specific to the local environment may exist for augmentation of substitutes and should be closely evaluated. In such instances, as suggested in the Mathews paper, economists and biologists should be called upon immediately to work in concert to consider the impact of substitutes and identify the opportunities they provide for early, effective resource restoration.

Following the Cantara Loop case, the authors make numerous specific recommendations. Of these, I will address two in particular. First, I will address the admonition that "the perfect is the enemy of the good." After ample reflection, I consider the phrase an apt metaphor for the natural resource restoration process. As with most generalisms, it would not be true or useful in every situation; however, it does provide some helpful guidance in the early stages of the NRDA process. In many cases, the last means of restoration that should be attempted is exact physical restoration, even if it is the only method for achieving "perfect" restoration. More importantly, trustees, responsible parties, and the public need to develop a process whereby cost-effective alternatives that fully restore lost human uses can be easily evaluated and implemented where appropriate.

The second major conclusion is that trustees and responsible parties can, and by implication should, work together. In fact, based on my experience, this conclusion can be taken even further. Not only can, and should, the parties work together, but in order to ensure prompt, effective restoration of lost human uses of the environment, the parties *must* work together. Inevitably, if they work independently, or as more often happens, if they alternatively prepare for litigation, nonproductive efforts are engaged in quantifying and documenting injury that could otherwise be utilized for restoration. Prompt, effective, and successful restoration will most often be achieved when cooperative efforts are paramount in the process.

Conclusion

Each of the papers (Chapters 6, 7, and 8) offers valuable lessons in restoring lost human uses of the environment. These lessons include clarifying the definition of human uses or services, maintaining flexibility throughout the NRDA process, considering the restoration of lost identifiable human uses early on in the NRDA process, improving the integration of economic and biological sciences, considering substitutes in the restoration decision-making process, accepting imperfect solutions, and the importance of trustees and responsible parties working together.

In addition to the specific lessons detailed previously, an overall lesson to be learned from these papers is that the approach taken to restoration really does matter. If trustees and responsible parties follow, understand, and heed the experiences of the *Valdez*, Lavaca Bay, Cantara Loop, and Idarado cases, as thoughtfully presented in these papers, win-win situations can be developed, and most importantly, the public will benefit from expedited and effective restoration of lost human uses of the environment. Finally, I propose a challenge to everyone concerned with lost human uses of natural resources to develop a process through which this occurs as a rule rather than as an exception.

8

Using Economic Models to Inform Restoration Decisions: The Lavaca Bay, Texas Experience

Kristy E. Mathews, William H. Desvousges, F. Reed Johnson, Melissa C. Ruby[1]

In this paper we present some preliminary, illustrative findings on how economic models can help inform restoration alternatives. We highlight ongoing work related to restoration alternatives for recreational fishing in Lavaca Bay, Texas. Our paper is organized as follows. First, we provide a brief description of the site. Then we describe the methodology we will use to assess both fishing losses that may have occurred as a result of a hazardous release and the gains that are associated with certain types of restoration alternatives. We then describe the survey we implemented to collect the data necessary for these economic models. Finally, we present some preliminary results and describe how such findings can help inform restoration decisions.

Site profile

Lavaca Bay is located at about the midpoint of the Texas Gulf coast between Corpus Christi and Houston. It is part of the larger Matagorda Bay system, which includes Carancahua, Turtle, and Tres Palacios Bays. The Lavaca Bay system consists of Lavaca Bay and several smaller bays such as Cox, Keller, and Chocolate Bays (see Figure 8-1). Located in Calhoun County, the Lavaca Bay system covers approximately 40,000 acres.

The Lavaca Bay system supports significant amounts of recreational fishing. It is a popular spot for local saltwater anglers, offering numerous fishing locations. There are fishing sites in Point Comfort, upper Lavaca Bay, Port Lavaca, Chocolate Bay, Magnolia Beach, and Keller Bay. These sites differ from one another in terms of facilities, access, aesthetics, and available species of fish. For example, flounder are dominant in Chocolate Bay while red drum are prevalent in Catfish Cove in upper Lavaca Bay (Pasadena Hotspot, Inc., undated).

According to Texas Parks and Wildlife Department (TPWD) creel survey data, the Lavaca Bay system draws most of its saltwater anglers from the 3 nearest counties: Calhoun, Jackson, and Victoria. From 1975 to 1991, anglers originating from these 3 counties accounted for 74% of Lavaca Bay anglers. The remaining anglers come from

[1]The authors wish to thank the following individuals: Kevin McKnight, Ron Weddell, and Kirk Gribben at Alcoa, for their support of a public viewing of this work; Sarah Holden, Jon Friesen, Karen Bourey, and Elaine Ball of TER, whose dedication to the survey made this paper possible.

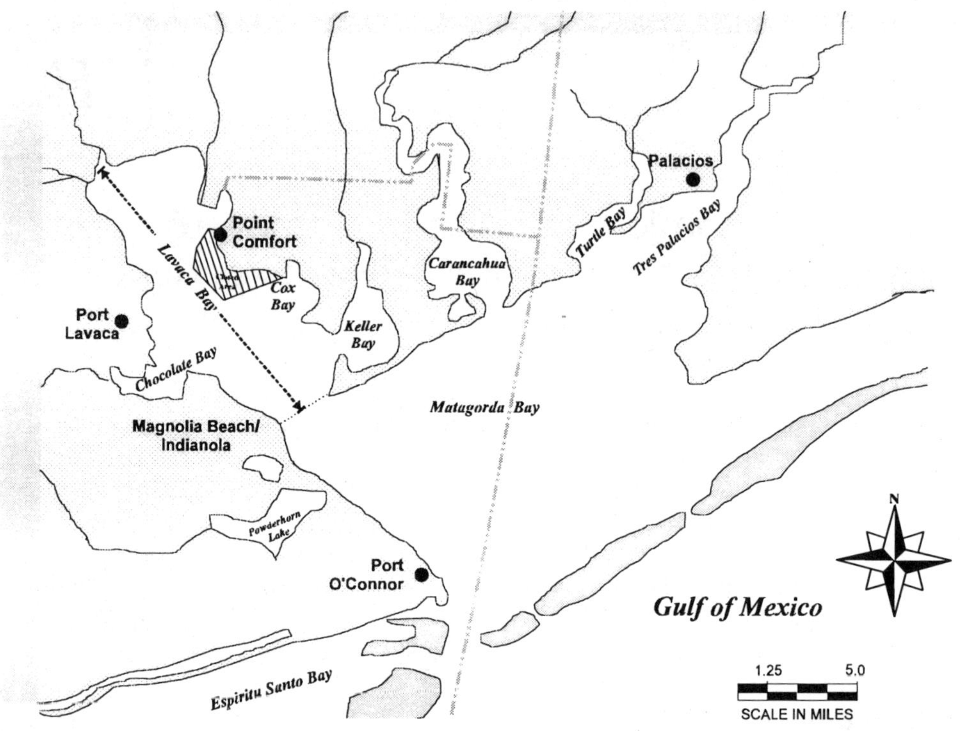

Figure 8-1 Lavaca Bay and Matagorda Bay

35 additional counties, with no single county accounting for more than 4% of Lavaca Bay anglers.

Through sampling of aquatic organisms, the Texas Department of Health (TDH) determined that mercury concentrations in certain finfish and crabs near Alcoa's Point Comfort plant are high enough to pose risks to human health. TDH thus prohibited the taking of finfish and crabs in waters around the Alcoa plant on 21 April 1988. Catch-and-release fishing in this area is permitted. As shown in Figure 8-1, the closed area covers approximately 1800 acres adjacent to the Alcoa plant. There is approximately 1 mile of shoreline that is publicly accessible to vehicular or pedestrian traffic in the closed area. The entire closed area is accessible by boat.

The Lavaca Bay site was added to the National Priorities List in 1994. The investigation of remedial actions at the site is ongoing. Here, we focus on Alcoa's study of potential recreational fishing losses.

Overview of methodology

The natural resource damage assessment (NRDA) objectives of our study are 2-fold. The first objective is to develop an estimate of the number of recreational fishing days potentially affected by the 1988 fish consumption advisory in a portion of Lavaca Bay.

This estimate will include both forgone trips and trips that still occur, but whose quality may have been reduced by the consumption advisory. The second objective is to estimate Lavaca Bay fishing days gained and enhanced under various restoration alternatives. For example, the addition of a fishing pier may enhance or increase the number of fishing days at a nearby site above baseline levels.

Our study design relies on both revealed preference (RP) and stated preference (SP) models.[2] RP models use observed site-choice behavior to estimate the probability that an individual will choose to visit a given recreation site, depending on the characteristics of that particular site and the characteristics of the other available substitute fishing sites. Fishing sites with more attractive characteristics have a higher probability of selection by anglers. These models, also known as random utility models (RUMs), incorporate the relevant number of substitution opportunities and accommodate the fact that each person may have different choices for recreation opportunities (McFadden 1974). RP models are increasingly being used to explain recreation decisions (Caulkins et al. 1986; Bockstael et al. 1989; Morey et al. 1991; Jones & Stokes Associates, Inc. 1991; Parsons and Needelman 1992; Kaoru et al. 1995) and have been used in Type B NRDAs (Hausman et al. 1993; Desvousges and Waters 1995; McFadden 1995; Desvousges et al. 1996).

In general, recreation days lost or affected can be estimated with these models by including a variable that captures the with-injury condition. Suppose that the only difference between the baseline condition of the affected site and the with-injury condition of the site is a fish consumption advisory that is specifically linked to the hazardous substance release. To estimate lost or affected days, we would first run the model including all sites and all site characteristics in the with-injury condition. Specifically, we would need to have a consumption advisory variable for all sites in the model, and the value of that variable would need to reflect the existence of an advisory for the affected site. The results of this model would estimate fishing days for each of the sites in the model, including the affected site.

Next, we would run the same model, but we would change the value of the advisory variable so that it reflects the absence of a consumption advisory. Changing this value simulates the baseline condition of the affected site because all other characteristics of the site remain the same. This second run of the model also provides an estimate of the fishing days at each site. But the number of days at the affected site now reflects the baseline number of days. The difference in the baseline number of days at the affected site and the with-injury number of days at the affected site represents lost or affected days.

A necessary feature of the data in these models is variation. Mathematically, the model can distinguish the individual influence of a single site characteristic only when sufficient variation within that characteristic exists across sites. In our application for

[2]Revealed preference models are called behavioral models in NOAA's final rule. The type of stated preference model we describe here is consistent with conjoint analysis as described in NOAA's final rule.

Lavaca Bay, the affected site is the only saltwater site in the general area with a consumption advisory. The lack of variation in this particular feature may mean that approach described above for estimating lost days is not feasible. Therefore, we may simulate the with-injury condition by excluding an advisory variable from the model and by removing the affected site as a choice. The baseline result would subsequently be estimated by including the affected site as a choice. This approach represents an overestimate because it assumes that the "closed area" is completely closed to fishing, which it is not.

SP models are based on the same conceptual framework, but describe choices among hypothetical site alternatives (Gan and Luzar 1993; Mackenzie 1993; Roe et al. 1996). Respondents repeatedly choose a preferred site from among varying groups of scenarios, the characteristics of which differ in terms of the site attributes described. In this application, for example, respondents were asked to select among 2 hypothetical fishing sites and a third alternative, discussed below. These hypothetical sites vary in terms of fishing mode (boat or shore), fish species caught, catch rate, facilities available at the fishing location (parking, restrooms, bait shop), and fish consumption advisories.

SP models use respondents' choices among different fishing scenarios to identify the most important features of a fishing experience and their relative influence in predicting site choices. Thus, SP models are well-suited for evaluating restoration alternatives because these models have the ability to identify which site attributes would increase use. Despite this ability, SP models have not been tested in an NRDA application.

Finally, our study analysis plan includes estimating a joint RP-SP model that combines actual behavioral information from the RP model on the probability of site selection and information from the SP model on the relative importance of fishing site characteristics. (See Adamowicz et al. 1994 and Adamowicz et al. 1996 as examples.) Such a joint model allows the actual choices underlying the RP model to "calibrate" the hypothetical scenarios underlying the SP model. There are 2 additional advantages to such a joint model. First, variation in site characteristics among existing sites may not include all the attributes relevant for evaluating potential restoration projects. Such variation is an integral part of the SP model design. Second, the joint model can be used to predict the number of additional fishing days associated with different restoration alternatives. Thus, the joint model provides information for scaling the restoration alternatives.

This paper is a status report on our "work in progress" on scaling restoration alternatives at the Lavaca Bay site. The model and implications shown here are preliminary. The timing of the project is such that we are unable to present the RP model and, by extension, the joint model today. We focus only on the SP model and how it can be used to identify types of restoration alternatives. Thus, the subsequent discussion on the underlying data for our model highlights the SP components of the questionnaire.

Survey overview

The data for our analysis were obtained by augmenting the questionnaire for the fish consumption study being conducted as part of the Remediation Investigation/ Feasibility Study (RI/FS) process for Alcoa's Lavaca Bay site. The fish consumption study targets recreational saltwater anglers and asks them detailed questions about where they fished and the fish they caught and consumed. Adding travel cost and site characteristic questions for the RP model and hypothetical site-choice questions for the SP model was a logical, cost-effective extension of the RI/FS study plan.[3]

This integrated questionnaire provides an important setting for the SP component of the survey. Prior to answering the SP questions, respondents are asked to identify on a map the location of fishing trips they took during November 1996. They are also asked to answer a series of questions for each trip that includes the distance traveled, the out-of-pocket expenditures associated with the trip, the number and type of fish caught and kept, and the number of meals they ate from the fish that they kept. In all of these questions, the respondent is relaying information on actual fishing trips. Thus, the hypothetical SP questions are placed in the context of actual fishing trips.

SP questionnaire highlights

The SP portion of the survey questionnaire employs several pairs of fishing site descriptions, an example of which is shown in Figure 8-2. Each site description consists of several fishing-site characteristics or attributes that correspond to variables used in the RP model.

Respondents are asked to think about what they would do if these 2 sites were available in addition to existing fishing sites. For each site pair, respondents indicate whether they would choose to fish at Site A, at Site B, or at neither for their next fishing trip.[4] The "neither" option indicates that respondents would prefer to fish at another existing fishing site, which they are asked to name.

An alternative design for the "neither" option asked respondents to assume that Site A and Site B are the only 2 sites available for their next fishing trip. Respondents who received this alternative version of the questionnaire were asked to indicate whether they would choose Site A, Site B, or not go saltwater fishing at all. The intended design splits the sample in 2, where half of the sample sees the "Neither, I will not go fishing" choice and the other half sees "Neither, I will fish at another site" choice.

Questionnaire development

Determining the relevant attributes or characteristics and the specific attribute levels used to describe the hypothetical site descriptions requires balancing several factors. First, in a joint RP-SP application, at least some of the attributes must map to variables

[3]In addition, the recreation model may be used in the baseline human-health risk assessment to predict future risk after the consumption advisory is removed.

[4]This type of stated preference question has been deemed reliable by other researchers. See, for example, Carson et al. (1994) and Louviere (1994).

	Site A	Site B	Neither
Type of Fishing	Boat	Pier	
Additional distance to fishing or launch site	30 miles from your closest saltwater fishing site	15 miles from your closest saltwater fishing site	
Catch rate	3 red drum	10 spotted sea trout	
Surroundings	View of industrial plants	No view of industrial plants	Neither Site A nor Site B
Congestion	Some people or boats in sight	Some people or boats in sight	
Facilities at site	Good parking	Limited parking	I would go saltwater fishing at another site
Fish consumption advisory	Fish should not be eaten	No advisory (Fish can be eaten)	
Check only ONE box	Prefer Site A	Prefer Site B	Prefer Another Site
			Write Name of Site Here:

Figure 8-2 Example choice questionnaire

in the RP model. Second, the attributes used in an SP design must be meaningful to respondents. For example, enhancement of marsh areas can augment fish population levels, which in turn can increase catch rates and angler utility when fishing. However, listing marsh enhancement as an attribute may not provide sufficient context for some respondents in an SP survey. They may be unable to link marsh enhancement to the satisfaction they receive from fishing at sites where fish populations are abundant. Third, the attributes must relate to practical restoration alternatives. For example, suppose that an attribute reflecting catch included 2 levels: bag limits and no bag limits.[5] Such an attribute is unrealistic because Texas has bag limits on many popular game fish for conservation reasons. It would not make sense to include this kind of an attribute in the SP design because it cannot be part of a restoration program, regardless of how this attribute may influence fishing site selection.

We developed the list of attributes and levels used in our SP design based on several different sources. We conducted a site visit, relied on our previous experience with RP

[5] Bag limits refer to a restriction, usually for conservation reasons, on the number of fish that anglers may keep.

angling models, reviewed SP recreation studies, and conducted 2 pretests. The first pretest was a one-on-one pretest with 24 anglers in Texas. The second pretest contacted 50 anglers by mail and 50 by telephone, primarily to test the mode. However, the phone version did use open-ended probes to determine if the respondents had any problems on each section of the survey, including the SP section. The majority of respondents did not indicate any problems with the SP questions.

Table 8-1 contains the final attributes and levels used in our SP survey. The first attribute is fishing mode, with "boat" and "pier" as levels. This attribute was selected because respondents have strong preferences about fishing mode and because certain types of fishing experiences are dependent on fishing from a boat or from a pier.

Table 8-1 Attributes and levels used in SP survey

Attribute	Levels
Fishing mode	Pier Boat
Additional distance to fishing or launch site	5 additional miles 15 additional miles 30 additional miles
Species and catch rate	1 Red drum 3 Red drum 2 Flounder 10 Flounder 2 Speckled trout 10 Speckled trout
Surroundings	No view of industrial plants View of industrial plants
Congestion	Many people or boats in sight Some people or boats in sight
Amenities	Limited parking Good parking Good parking and restrooms Good parking, restrooms, and bait shop
Fish consumption advisory	No advisory (Fish can be eaten) Fish should not be eaten

Furthermore, the relative importance of boat versus pier fishing can inform restoration options.

The second attribute, the additional distance to the fishing or launch site, merits some explanation. Before respondents begin answering the site-choice questions, respondents are asked the distance in miles to the saltwater fishing site nearest their home. The site-choice question instructions then explain that respondents should think about the additional distance to the hypothetical fishing sites from that nearest site when answering the site-choice questions. The specific levels were selected based on estimated distances to saltwater fishing sites from major population centers within our survey area. This attribute is included for 2 reasons. First, it maps directly into the RP models and will be important for the joint RP-SP estimation. Second, it also informs restoration options by identifying the relative importance of travel distance in restoration options.

The next attribute is the number and type of fish caught. During the pretest, we learned that target species are important in selecting fishing sites. Practical limitations required that we include only 3 game species. We also learned that bag limits for popular sport fish should be used in designing the levels for the catch-rate attribute so that the hypothetical site seems more realistic to respondents. This attribute also may help with identifying restoration options to the extent that restoration options can target specific fish species.

We include aesthetics as the fourth attribute because this characteristic captures a noticeable feature of the affected site. During the pretest we learned that congestion often is a concern to anglers, and the fifth attribute captures that facet of a fishing experience. Similarly, we learned that launch-site amenities also may influence fishing site selection, and we included that characteristic as the sixth attribute. This attribute and the associated levels are important in terms of restoration alternatives because, if influential in fishing site selection, these amenities are concrete projects that are often feasible to implement.

Finally, we include a fish consumption advisory attribute. As described above, variation in site characteristics is necessary for econometric estimation. Because we suspect there will be insufficient variation across sites with respect to a consumption advisory, we plan to supplement the RP data with SP data that reflect more variation for this particular site characteristic.

Experimental design

The specific attributes, attribute levels, and fishing site pair profiles that appear in the SP questions are called the experimental design. For any given list of attributes and attribute levels, the number of possible paired descriptions can be very large. For example, in our specific application, there are over 1 million possible pairs. Obviously, each respondent cannot evaluate all possible combinations. However, the design must contain sufficient representation across all attributes and levels to allow estimation of the model. Therefore, an experimental design must balance a respondent's abilities and the necessary statistical properties for efficient and reliable estimation.

To make the task more manageable for respondents and to achieve statistical soundness, we constructed subsets or blocks of possible combinations of sites. Based on our pretest experience, combined with our experience on other SP surveys, we determined that most respondents would be willing to answer 15 of these hypothetical, site-choice questions. Our projected number of respondents was sufficiently large to permit splitting the sample into 2 groups. Thus, the goal of the experimental design was to identify 30 site-profile pairs that would contain all the necessary combinations of attributes and levels necessary for estimating an SP model. These 30 pairs were identified using available design algorithms (Louviere and Woodworth 1983; Zwerina et al. 1996).

Sampling and survey administration

This SP questionnaire was administered to the same saltwater anglers participating in the RI/FS consumption study. The sample frame for this study included licensed saltwater anglers residing in Calhoun, Jackson, and Victoria Counties because the majority of Lavaca Bay anglers originate in these 3 counties: 50% of the anglers are from Calhoun County, 30% from Victoria County, and 20% from Jackson County. We drew a random sample of 3488 anglers from a TPWD license holder database in these same relative proportions.

The survey administration, which began in December 1996 and ended in March 1997, combined a mail and telephone mode. All anglers in the frame received via mail an introductory letter that explained the survey, a map of the Matagorda Bay system, and a booklet containing the 15 site-choice questions. Respondents were asked to identify the location of their fishing trips on the map, answer the site-choice questions in the booklet, and then wait for the telephone interview. Potential respondents then were contacted by telephone, and data on November 1996 fishing trips were collected for the consumption and RP analyses at that time.[6] In addition, the telephone interviewers also collected respondents' answers to the 15 site-choice questions.[7]

Stated-preference model and results

The model presented here is preliminary for 2 reasons. First, to have some results before May, we extracted a partial dataset prior to the completion of the survey administration. Although these partial data may be sufficiently representative of our target population, there is some potential that they may not be. For example, this subset of data does not include anglers who took more than 5 trips during November.[8] It is possible that the more avid anglers may have different underlying preferences for

[6] If an angler took more than 5 fishing trips during the month of November, he or she was classified as an "avid angler." Avid anglers were sent a mail version of the survey and asked to complete it, rather than participate in a lengthy telephone interview.

[7] The survey administration included protocols to ensure a high-quality data collection. TER staff conducted training sessions with telephone interviewers prior to administration. Respondent participation was encouraged with the use of a cash incentive and inclusion in a prize drawing. The protocols required that 10 phone calls be made to each angler before being classified as a nonparticipant.

[8] At the time of this writing, these data had not been processed.

angling. The number of respondents reflected in the model presented here is 883. Second, we have not fully explored all econometric options for this type of model. For example, we have not yet had the opportunity to classify different groups of anglers, such as boat owners, and incorporate those differences into the model.

The model used in our analysis of the SP data is a conditional-logit model, a utility-theoretic framework long used to analyze choice decisions (McFadden 1974).[9] Conditional-logit models estimate the probability of selecting a specific option, conditional on the characteristics of that option. Options with more attractive characteristics provide more utility and, therefore, have a higher probability of being selected. For example, our pretesting indicated that many Lavaca Bay anglers prefer fishing from a boat as opposed to fishing from a pier. Thus, options featuring the boat mode are expected to have a higher probability of being selected.

The variables used in our model are summarized in Table 8-2. Many of these variables are the same attributes described earlier. In addition to these attributes, we include an interaction term that captures the dual effect of the additional miles to the hypothetical fishing site and the base miles to the nearest saltwater fishing site. This interaction term allows the marginal effect of additional miles to vary by residential location of respondents.

The model also includes 2 alternative-specific constants to account for the version of the "neither" choice. Recall that about half of the respondents saw "I will not go fishing" for the neither choice while the other half saw "I will fish at another site" for the neither choice. (Hereafter, Version 1 reflects the neither choice of "I will not go fishing," and Version 2 reflects the neither choice of "I will fish at another site.") This constant is used to capture preferences for the neither choice relative to the 2 alternatives that are not captured by the other variables (Adamowicz et al. 1996).

The results of our model, which contains pooled data from the 2 versions,[10] are shown in Table 8-3. In terms of interpreting the results, we first want to assess the overall fit, or ability of the model to predict site-choice selection. Evaluating the goodness of fit for conditional-logit models is more difficult than for ordinary regression models because the dependent variable is just an indicator of whether an available alternative was chosen or not. One possibility is to compare how often the model correctly assigns the largest probability to the alternative that actually was chosen by respondents. For

[9] "Utility" is the metric that economists use when measuring individual satisfaction. See Desvousges et al. (this volume) for a more detailed discussion of utility and its role in NRDA.

[10] A standard statistical test, called the likelihood-ratio test, indicates that the pooled model is not statistically different than separate models based on the 2 different versions of the "neither" choice. However, slight differences occur between the single version models. In Version 1, RESTROOM and the interaction between base distance and additional miles are not significant. In Version 2, NOVIEW is not significant. There also are some differences in size of effects.

Table 8-2 Variables used in the SP models

Variable	Description
BOAT	1 = boat
FLNDHI	1 = 10 flounder
FLNDLO	1 = 2 flounder
REDHI	1 = 3 red drum
REDLO	1 = 1 red drum
TROUTHI	1 = 10 speckled trout
NOVIEW	1 = no view of industrial plants
CONGLO	1 = some people or boats in sight
GOODPARK	1 = good parking
RESTROOM	1 = good parking and restrooms
BAIT	1 = good parking, restrooms, and bait shop
NOADVISE	1 = fish can be eaten
MARGMILE	additional miles to fishing site
MMI*BASE	interaction term for additional miles and base miles
CDUM1, CDUM2	1 = Option C, differentiated by version

choice sets with 3 alternatives, random predictions would be correct 33% of the time. The preliminary model reported here is correct 61.8% of the time.

Alternatively, since there is some probability that any 3 of the alternatives could be selected, we could ask how well the model predicts the overall proportions of choices. Our model indicates that alternatives A, B, and C would be expected to be selected 4178, 5567, and 3500 times compared to actual selections of 4169, 5576, and 3500, respectively. Thus our overall predictions misclassify only 9 of 9745 cases.[11]

In terms of the specific results, we look next at the significance of specific variables. Significance refers to the precision of the estimated coefficient. Significant variables help to explain site-choice selection because their effect on the dependent variable is discernible. Most of the variables in our model are significant. The one exception is

[11]Various authors have suggested analogs to the R-squared statistic that sometimes are useful in comparing alternative discrete-choice models. The Madalla, McFadden, and Cragg and Uhler pseudo-R-squared statistics for this model are 0.33, 0.18, and 0.06, respectively. This preliminary model does not account for heterogeneous preferences among respondents other than those associated with distance to closest saltwater fishing site. We would expect subsequent models that incorporate individual respondent characteristics to provide better fits.

Table 8-3 SP model results

Variable	Coefficient	T-Statistic
BOAT	0.1610	11.79***
FLNDHI	0.2930	9.49***
FLNDLO	−0.2393	−7.09***
REDHI	0.1621	4.91***
REDLO	−0.3715	−10.83***
TROUTHI	0.3809	11.99***
NOVIEW	0.0323	2.39***
CONGLO	0.0567	3.87***
GOODPARK	0.1288	5.06***
RESTROOM	−0.0400	−1.60*
BAIT	0.0250	0.95
NOADVISE	0.8466	61.11***
MARGMILE	−0.0123	−8.98***
MMI*BASE	0.0001	1.90**
CDUM	−0.2501	−8.15***
CDUM	0.1257	4.37***
Log-likelihood	11,683.4	
Percent correctly predicted	61.8%	

BAIT. The insignificance of this variable suggests that the presence of a bait shop at the site does not affect site-choice selection, holding everything else constant.

We also want to look at the magnitude of the coefficients when evaluating our results. The magnitude of the coefficients reflects the relative contribution to utility. The coefficient itself can be thought of as an addition or subtraction from a utility index. The larger the coefficient, the larger is that variable's effect on utility, holding everything else constant. For example, the coefficient on FLNDHI is not quite twice the size of the coefficient on REDHI. This relative relationship suggests that in terms of the utility index, catching 10 flounder is almost twice as important as catching 3 red drum, holding everything else constant.

When evaluating magnitude, the sign on the coefficient also is important. A positive sign means that attribute increases utility while a negative sign means that attribute decreases utility. For example, the coefficient on BOAT is positive, indicating that anglers derive more utility from a boat trip than a pier trip, holding everything else constant. In terms of the other variables that have a positive effect on utility, less congestion, aesthetics, good parking, and the absence of a fishing advisory would positively affect utility. In terms of the species-catch rate combinations, the higher catch rates are positive, meaning that catching more fish of the same species is preferred to less.

The coefficient for additional miles (MARGMILE) is significant and negative. Anglers derive less utility from a fishing trip when they have to drive farther. The interaction between the additional miles and the base distance (MMI*BASE) allows residential location to affect how additional miles influence utility. The coefficient is positive and significant. This result is consistent with expectations. Additional miles have more impact on anglers living close to fishing opportunities than on anglers who have to travel farther for fishing access.

Most of the variables used in this model are a form of qualitative, or "dummy," variables. In the simplest form, a dummy variable indicates the presence or absence of a condition.[12] In our application, they take the value of 1 when the condition exists and –1 when it does not. For example, the variable NOVIEW equals 1 when the site does not offer a view of industrial facilities and –1 when industrial facilities are in sight. The significance of a dummy variable is relative to the alternative of the condition. For example, having a view of industrial plants is significantly different than not having such a view. It is these significant differences that give the model the ability to explain site selection.

Some of the dummy variables used in our model have more than 2 categories. For example, the site facilities attribute includes 4 levels, representing increasing development: 1) limited parking, 2) good parking, 3) good parking and restrooms, and 4) good parking, restrooms, and a bait shop. Statistical estimation requires that 1 of these 4 categories be omitted. In our model, we have omitted the limited parking category, leaving GOODPARK, RESTROOM, and BAIT as the dummy variables in our model. Significance of these variables is relative to the omitted category. For example, good parking is significant relative to limited parking.

Finally, the alternative-specific constants for Option C perform as expected. For Version 1, this variable is negative and significant, indicating that respondents, on average, tend to prefer one of the hypothetical sites to the alternative of not fishing at all. In contrast, the Option C constant for Version 2 is positive and significant, indicating that respondents, on average, tend to prefer an actual favorite fishing site to the hypothetical sites described. Thus, respondents clearly paid attention to the difference in Option C in the 2 versions, as we had expected.[13]

---

[12] The dummy variables in this model are "effects coded," using 1 and –1 (instead of 1 and 0) to avoid confounding the omitted categories with the third alternative, which is assigned a utility index of 0. See Adamowicz et al. (1994) and Adamowicz et al. (1996) for a discussion.

[13] While relative preferences among hypothetical site attributes were similar in the 2 versions, the difference in response to the third alternative has important implications for designing and scaling restoration plans. After restoration, real-world fishing choice sets will include some sites with current attributes and some sites with improved attributes. As our experiment indicates, many respondents

The interpretation of the coefficient on NOADVISE merits additional discussion. It is the largest coefficient in the model. Holding everything else constant, being able to eat the fish caught is most important to saltwater anglers along the central Texas coast. This result is expected. Many of the prevalent species, especially the 3 species in our design, are recognized as desirable for consumption. The fish sought by anglers in this area are not fish, such as northern pike, that are predominantly recognized as sport fish. Moreover, this type of saltwater environment has not been traditionally managed as a catch-and-release environment as many freshwater trout streams are.

It also is important to recognize that this particular attribute is only one component of the influences on utility and that it is relative to everything else. Depending on the specifics of other attributes at a particular site, and how far an angler would need to travel to that particular site, a site with a consumption advisory may yield some utility to an angler. It is the combination of all the attributes working together that determines the overall attractiveness of a particular site.

Finally, what the NOADVISE coefficient does *not* necessarily mean is that the fish consumption advisory in a small portion of Lavaca Bay has resulted in large losses in angler utility. The NOADVISE coefficient in the SP model does not reflect the large number of high-quality, existing substitute fishing sites available to anglers, including most of Lavaca Bay itself. This information is necessary to get a complete picture of what the consumption advisory means in terms of angler utility loss. Thus, the joint RP-SP model provides the full context for this assessment.

Illustrative implications for Lavaca Bay fishing restoration

The results from "solo" SP models like the one presented above can help inform restoration decisions. Specifically, these models provide the linkage between certain types of restoration alternatives and utility. Keeping in mind that the results in the above model are purely illustrative and preliminary, we more closely examine the results for information on restoration alternatives.

Relative to pier fishing, the results from this preliminary model indicate that anglers prefer boat fishing. Restoration alternatives that enhance or expand boat launching facilities would improve the utility of the "average" angler. In terms of other types of fishing facilities, good parking is preferred to limited parking by the average angler. Thus, expanding parking at existing sites is another potential restoration alternative that would increase angler utility. In contrast, however, anglers appear to be less interested in the development of facilities beyond improved parking. This result suggests that restoration alternatives of that nature would do less to augment angler utility. It also suggests that improving parking at several sites may improve utility more than adding restrooms and a bait shop at a single site.

---

would prefer fishing at their current site even if an improved site were made available. Thus, SP estimates based on a no-fishing reference alternative will produce different results than when the neither alternative is fishing at an existing site. The magnitude and direction of this difference will not be known until the joint RP-SP model is developed.

The model results on species-catch rate combinations also can inform restoration options. Recall that the results indicate that anglers prefer catching more fish relative to less fish of a given species. Restoration options that would enhance fish populations levels, such as using artificial reefs, would allow anglers to catch their limit more often, which would increase angler utility.

Some stylized examples will help illustrate these points. Suppose that an existing boat fishing site is not crowded, offers an aesthetic view, has an average catch of 1 red drum per trip, does not have a consumption advisory but has limited parking. Using the results of the SP model, the utility index of this site for the average angler is calculated to be 0.63.[14] Now suppose that a restoration option improves the parking from limited to good. As a result of this improvement, the utility index of the average angler increases to 0.87. Thus, improving parking results in an increase in angler utility.

Now suppose that at that same existing site, a restoration alternative targets increasing the population of red drum, allowing anglers to catch the bag limit of 3 fish. In this instance, the average angler utility index increases from 0.63 to 1.16. Thus, enhancing fish populations adds more to utility than does improving parking although both represent a net gain in utility.

Finally, suppose that a restoration option calls for both improving parking and enhancing red drum populations. In this instance, the average angler utility index would increase from 0.63 to 1.41.

An aside

We mentioned above that the large, positive coefficient on NOADVISE does not necessarily reflect a large loss of utility for anglers. To make that determination, we need to know more than the SP model alone reveals, namely, travel distances and the number and quality of substitute fishing sites. A simplified example helps to illustrate the role of distance and substitute sites in assessing fishing site utility. Suppose, for example, that we consider an inland angler who lives 30 miles from the nearest saltwater fishing site. Suppose that there is a site with a consumption advisory that is an additional 15 miles away. This site offers boat fishing, high catch rates for flounder, a view of an industrial plant, few people or boats in sight, and good parking. The model results indicate that the utility index for this angler is –0.22. Based on the results of our model, this angler would rather fish at this site than not go fishing. (The coefficient on the "neither, not go fishing" option is –0.25.) Thus, if this were the only fishing site available, this angler would prefer to fish at this site, even with a fishing advisory.

Now suppose that a second fishing site becomes available. This second site supports boat fishing, has an abundant population of speckled trout, is not crowded and is

[14]For purposes of this exercise, we assume that the average angler lives 20 miles away from the closest saltwater site and would drive an additional 15 miles from this particular site.

aesthetically pleasing and has good parking and no consumption advisory. This second site is only 5 additional miles away from the nearest fishing site. The utility index for this angler at this site is 1.74. Thus, this site affords the angler more utility than the first site with the consumption advisory. Between the 2 sites, this angler would select the one without the consumption advisory.

Finally, suppose that the consumption advisory is removed from the first site. The utility index is now 1.47, admittedly larger than –0.22. However, if we compare the utility index for the first site without a consumption advisory (1.47) to the utility index for the second site (1.74), the angler would prefer the second site. Thus, the existence of a consumption advisory has not affected the utility of this angler because his most preferred site affords him more utility than does the first site without a consumption advisory. This result is a direct artifact of the high-quality, closer substitute.

Broader implications for restoration

The Lavaca Bay case study experience with SP models also has implications for restoration that extend beyond this site. Perhaps most importantly, our case study shows that this approach provides a convenient, systematic way to obtain information from users about restoration. For example, the data in our model will ultimately reflect input from almost 2000 saltwater anglers who live in the general vicinity of Lavaca Bay, including more than half of the licensed anglers living in Calhoun County, which is closest to the Bay.

Moreover, SP models provide valuable information for restoration decisions by identifying the characteristics that matter to anglers and the relative importance of different characteristics that might be included in a fishing restoration program. When properly designed, these models can assess the relative merits of multiple restoration alternatives, which greatly enhances the efficiency of assessing restoration choices. Thus, the results (once we have the full dataset) provide valuable insights about the restoration preferences of anglers.

In addition, SP models of fishing choices are based on a sound economic foundation. The utility-theoretic framework focuses on the well-being of the individual. For recreation assessments, NRDAs traditionally have measured welfare losses experienced by users. This focus on utility in terms of restoration provides a consistent metric to measure losses and gains. In addition, if restoration decisions can be guided by such models, then it may be possible to identify the relative cost-effectiveness of different restoration alternatives.

Developing such models is not without challenges. One challenge is that the development and implementation of these models requires thinking about restoration early in an NRDA. This early focus is new to most NRDA practitioners but is consistent with the direction of NOAA's final rule. A second challenge is improving the integration of biology and economics early in an NRDA. These links need to be better defined to assist the public in evaluating alternatives. For example, providing additional and/or enhanced fish habitat would result in an increase in fish populations, which eventually would increase anglers' utility by increasing catch rates. Quantifying links between fish habitat enhancement and catch rates has yet to be addressed in our study. Finally, these models have no demonstrated track record in an NRDA setting.

It is also important to keep in mind that our full study plan for Lavaca Bay calls for jointly estimating SP models, which are based only on hypothetical choices with RP models that reflect anglers' actual fishing decisions in this region. We expect that the SP models are likely to be more effective when used in combination with RP models. RP models provide a sense of the real angling choices and thus help calibrate the results of an SP model.

Finally, it is important to remember that, ideally, restoration actions do not occur in a vacuum. Restoration represents the intersection of the opinions of affected members of the public, the fiduciary responsibilities of the trustees, and the costs of implementation that are borne by responsible parties. From an economic perspective, we think the overall approach described in this paper represents a useful way of providing valuable information that may yield restoration decisions that are both cost-effective and consistent with individual preferences.

References

Adamowicz W, Louviere J, Williams M. 1994. Combining revealed and stated preference methods for valuing environmental amenities. *J Environ Econ Manage* 26:271–292.

Adamowicz W, Swait J, Boxall P, Louviere J, Williams M. 1996. Perceptions versus objective measures of environmental quality in combined revealed and stated preference models of environmental valuation. Working Paper. University of Alberta.

Bockstael NE, McConnell KE, Strand IE. 1989. A random utility model for sport fishing: some preliminary results for Florida. *Marine Resource Econ* 6:245–260.

Carson RT, Louviere JJ, Anderson D, Arabie P, Bunch DS, Hensher DA, Johnson RM, Kuhfeld WF, Steinberg D, Swait J, Timmermans H, Wiley JB. 1994. Experimental analysis of choice. *Marketing Letters: Special Issue on the Duke Invitational Conference on Consumer Decision Making and Choice Behaviour* 5(4):351–368.

Caulkins PP, Bishop RC, Bouwes Sr NW. 1986. The travel cost model for lake recreation: a comparison of two methods for incorporating site quality and substitution effects. *Am J Ag Econ* 68(2):291–297.

Desvousges WH, Waters SM. 1995. Report on potential economic losses with recreation services in the Upper Clark Fork River Basin. Submitted to United States District Court, District of Montana, Helena Division in the matter of *State of Montana v. Atlantic Richfield Company*, CV-83-317-HLN-PGH.

Desvousges WH, Waters SM, Train KE. 1996. Supplemental report on potential economic losses with recreation services in the Upper Clark Fork River Basin. Submitted to United States District Court, District of Montana, Helena Division in the matter of *State of Montana v. Atlantic Richfield Company*, CV-83-317-HLN-PGH.

Gan C, Luzar EJ. 1993. Conjoint analysis of waterfowl hunting in Louisiana. *J Ag Appl Econ* 25:36–45.

Hausman JA, Leonard GK, McFadden D. 1993. Assessing use values losses caused by natural resource injury. In: Hausman JA, editor. Contingent valuation: a critical assessment. Amsterdam, The Netherlands: Elsevier.

Jones & Stokes Associates, Inc. 1991. Southeast Alaska sport fishing economic study. Final research report prepared for Alaska Department of Fish and Game, Sport Fish Division, Research and Technical Services Section, Anchorage, AK. Sacramento, CA: Jones & Stokes Associates, Inc.

Kaoru Y, Smith VK, Liu JL. 1995. Using random utility models to estimate the recreational value of estuarine resources. *Am J Ag Econ* 77:141–151.

Louviere JJ. 1994. Relating stated preference measures and models to choices in real markets: calibration of CV responses. Paper presented at the DOE/EPA workshop on using contingent valuation to measure non-market values, May 19–20, Herndon, VA.

Louviere JJ, Woodworth G. 1983. Design and analysis of simulated consumer choice or allocation experiments: an approach based on aggregate data. *J Marketing Research* 20:350–367.

Mackenzie J. 1993. A comparison of contingent preference models. *Am J Ag Econ* 75:593–603.

McFadden DL. 1995. Expert report of Daniel L. McFadden. Submitted to United States District Court, District of Montana, Helena Division in the matter of *State of Montana v. Atlantic Richfield Company*, CV-83-317-HLN-PGH.

McFadden DL. 1974. Conditional logit analysis of qualitative choice behavior. In: Zarembka P, editor. Frontiers in econometrics. New York: Academic.

Morey ER, Shaw WD, Rowe RD. 1991. A discrete-choice model of recreational participation, site choice, and activity when complete trip data are not available. *J Environ Econ Manage* 20(2):181–201.

Parsons GR, Needelman MS. 1992. Site aggregation in a random utility model of recreation. *Land Economics* 68(4):418–433.

Pasadena Hotspot, Inc. Undated. Boat fishing and wade fishing map, Matagorda Bay. Map No. F108. Pasadena, TX.

Roe B, Boyle KJ, Tiesel MF. 1996. Using conjoint analysis to derive estimates of compensating variation. *J Environ Econ Manage* 31(2):145–159.

Zwerina K, Huber J, Kuhfeld WF. 1996. A general method for constructing efficient choice designs. Working Paper. The Fuqua School of Business. Raleigh NC: Duke University.

8a

Discussion Paper I on Using Economic Models to Inform Restoration Decisions: The Lavaca Bay, Texas Experience

*Keith Eastin**

Lavaca Bay

The Texas Department of Health determined that mercury levels in the Bay near an industrial facility were unacceptably high. In 1988 they issued a Health Order prohibiting the taking of fish and crabs in the area and allowing only catch-and-release fishing. The site placed on the NPL in 1994.

The authors were retained to estimate the number of fishing days lost as a result of the Health Order and to determine the number of fishing days that might be gained or enhanced through various restoration alternatives. They attempt to determine what it is about the fishing experience that makes it valuable. To accomplish this, several alternative scenarios are propounded and submitted for anglers to value. Would they rather catch more fish or have better parking or dockside facilities? Would they prefer a fishing site that had a view of the industrial facility or not and how might that preference be quantified?

The authors' study relies on both *revealed* preference methodology and the *stated* preferences of the respondents. Put simply, revealed preference involves asking respondents about actual alternative sites and conditions. Stated preference allows the respondent to answer questions concerning preferences as between hypothetical situations. The stated preference method allows more flexibility in determining what characteristics of a resource the resource-using public prefers.

Implications of the stated preference scenarios are significant in making restoration decisions. Trustees can incorporate preferences of the public into restoration activities. The public can be given a restored resource that more closely parallels its actual desires, yielding a higher overall value experience to the public.

To the extent that actual needs and preferences are incorporated into restoration planning, the public will be better off. Incorporation of such planning into the restoration can speed the process and hopefully lower the costs involved in considering and ruminating over numerous restoration decisions.

*Deloitte & Touche LLP, Wilmington, DE

Hopefully, what could come from the authors' study might be a comprehensive and well-reasoned model from which resource decisions at other sites might be simplified. Perhaps lessons learned in Lavaca Bay might be used in other NRDA activities involving similar activities.

Conclusion

Both the Dunsmire and the Lavaca Bay scenarios may help in the expeditious return of services of damaged resources to the people. While the ponds in Dunsmuir may not mirror the quality experience of the River, the services were returned to the public quickly. At Lavaca Bay, services of the natural resources might be returned in a form that might maximize their value to the public. Both methods may herald a small step to more efficient handling of damaged natural resources.

8b

Discussion Paper 2 on Using Economic Models to Inform Restoration Decisions: The Lavaca Bay, Texas Experience

Pierre H. duVair[*1]

These authors present a conceptual analytical approach to both the assessment of lost human uses of natural resources and a means of quantitatively assisting restoration scaling and selection to address those loses. I must agree in concept that combined Stated Preference (SP)–Revealed Preference (RP) models can both aid in the assessment of damages and inform aspects of restoration planning. The authors were not able to demonstrate the validity and/or reliability of this joint approach due to status of the RP portion of the model for the Lavaca Bay case.

Unfortunately, it is difficult to provide substantive comment on the SP-model without more specific information on the survey design and implementation than was presented in the paper. While the NOAA Blue Ribbon Panel on Contingent Valuation Methods focused their attention on SP-models to assess passive-use values, the conclusions reached are also applicable to surveys that assess active human-use values. In particular, the reader cannot fully evaluate either the degree of effort or the methods used to select the 7 attributes and corresponding variable levels presented in the paper. How does one go about selecting a mix of individual attributes and levels, all practical from a planning perspective, plausible from respondent perspective, and relevant to an RP-model? The authors share at least 2 important similarities with the Birdsall paper. First, both sets of authors approach the evaluation and scaling of compensatory restoration strictly from welfare economics of the individual. Efficiency is defined solely by the maximum quantity gain in consumer surplus for the least amount of dollars expended. While maximum utility gain should be an important criterion, it is not all-encompassing to trustees with broad responsibilities for management of natural resources that generate the full range of human-use services.

A second commonality of the papers is the authors' conclusion that restoration of lost human uses is "time-critical," so much so that trustees and RPs should elevate

*California Department of Fish and Game, Sacramento, California

[1]The opinions presented herein are expressly those of the author and do not necessarily reflect the views of the Department of Fish and Game. Thanks go to Larry Espinosa and Steve Turek for their helpful insights.

quickness to an objective just below that of cost-effectiveness. Neither set of authors provide convincing arguments to support this conclusion. Birdsall et al. resort to common law tort principles and take an argumentative approach in the paper by claiming that trustees "must take or accept measures which interdict lost uses," yet fail to show by example how the public is made better off. Economic theory alone does not dictate that hastily planned and implemented projects, combined with a skeletal view of injuries, will yield cost-efficient and public maximizing restoration benefits.

I describe above a somewhat extreme view of potential problems associated with emergency restoration actions. In the CERCLA setting, often the long-term, human-use losses associated with chronic releases could be lessened by projects that have received the benefit of ample time for injury assessment and development, yet prior to the use injuries returning to baseline. In this scenario the quick action objective could be elevated in importance, but would seem to me to always remain below the objectives of effective, efficient, and fully compensatory alternatives. The authors argue that an early start is needed because of time requirements for model development and consistency with NOAA's new rule.

Several aspects of the SP model appear somewhat unusual as reported in the paper. First, it is unclear to me why the authors chose to spend a large amount of effort to capture views of local residents, while no information was gathered about the 26% that likely were systematically different and on average hold higher values for the fishing experience in Lavaca Bay. Secondly, the marginal distance and proximity to the nearest fishing site variables seem an odd way to capture the importance of any additional miles traveled to a hypothetical site. Clearly, survey respondents do not intuitively think about the marginal distance of going from point B to point C when they live at point A and can potentially envision the hypothetical point C in the opposite direction of point B. This is especially true if point B is the nearest fishing site but never visited by the respondent.

There appears to be some difficulty with the facilities variables as configured in the model results presented in Table 8-3. It is hard to imagine why people would prefer good parking relative to limited parking, but then add a restroom to the good parking and the combination be less attractive than limited parking (i.e., negative coefficient on RESTROOM)? Similarly, add a bait shop to the restroom and good parking and people are indifferent relative to a facility with limited parking (i.e., insignificant coefficient on BAIT)? As the authors note, the facilities variables can be very important to the evaluation of relative desirability of potentially "concrete projects" as compensation for lost human uses.

The authors try to downplay the very large, positive, and significant coefficient for NOADVISE by suggesting that the SP-model "does not reflect the large number of high-quality, existing substitute fishing sites" While it is difficult to estimate the effects of a split-sample on this point, it is clear that respondents answering Version 2 took significant account of available substitutes when considering whether or not to go fishing at another site. The mere presence of this option will lead respondents to expressly consider potential substitute sites.

The authors claim in a hypothetical scenario that if a person receives more utility from a site with no fish consumption advisory than what is potentially received from another site with or without such an advisory, that therefore "the existence of a consumption advisory has not affected the utility of this angler." Based upon specifics of an SP–RP joint model this may be "a direct artifact of the high-quality, closer substitute" but intuitively it is hard to imagine the angler not incurring some amount of lost option value as a result of the advisory.

In terms of restoration as an intersection, I would have used the word "preferences" rather than "opinions" of the affected public, the word "statutory" rather than "fiduciary" responsibilities of the trustees, and the costs of "assessment, planning, and successful implementation" rather than just "implementation" that are borne by responsible parties.

8c

Discussion Paper 3 on Using Economic Models to Inform Restoration Decisions: The Lavaca Bay, Texas Experience, or Natural Resource Damage Assessment: A Texas Perspective

*Diane B. Hyatt**

Purpose

Although this paper was reviewed by all Texas trustees, I am not speaking for the other trustees, and there may be differing opinions on some of the points discussed. Overall, it is the trustees' duty to restore the resources and their services. It is difficult for me to isolate the narrow interim lost human use from the whole. The human uses and other service flows from our natural resources are directly correlated to the health and diversity of the ecosystem from which the services flow. The trustees endeavor to work as a team to restore the whole. It is the goal to restore with no net losses to the system or to the users that are, in fact, part of the same system.

Using economic models to inform decisions: the Lavaca Bay, Texas experience

The state and federal trustees have signed an MOA with the RP at this industrial site in Texas in a secondary bay system. There has been a fishing closure for finfish and crabs at the site for approximately 10 years. It is the objective of the RP and trustees to work in a parallel fashion with the remedial process and expedite the restoration. Trustees are also working to reduce any residual injury at the site by participation in ecological and human-health risk assessments.

Since this is a "work in progress," the trustees have participated through an Agreed Order on Consent to comment on remedial investigation (RI) work plan drafts to incorporate as much of our data needs as possible. This paper is an illustration of that effort. Other trustee data needs that may not fit as well are addressed directly with the RP. The trustees have commented and continue to comment on the nature and extent of contamination, mass balance of contaminant input to the system, source control,

*Director, Natural Resource Damage Assessment, Texas General Land Office, Austin, Texas

remedial alternatives analysis, and risk assessments. Our goal is to restore lost service flows through enhancement and construction of viable habitats once the direct restoration (remediation) component of the injury is assured. In order to move more quickly to this compensatory restoration, the trustees are participating in the remedial decisions. A goal for the trustees is that the Record of Decision is protective (with a reopener to make sure) and the release abated. Monitoring will continue during the post-closure Operating and Maintenance phase.

The natural resource trustees reviewed and commented upon the design of the RI survey project described in this paper. The NOAA Damage Assessment Center (DAC) in Silver Springs, Maryland, and the DOI in Washington, DC. are resources for economic review. In this instance, we are working with DAC as a component of the NOAA trustee team. There are qualified economic scientists that provide the state and federal trustees the expertise required to evaluate the economic values attributable to human use.

Using the survey, the trustees and the RP wished to expedite the information-gathering related to both scaling injury and restoration. The survey is also a cost-effective mechanism to work within the RI framework. Initiated to assess risk to the recreational fishing community, the altered survey should now provide additional resource information in actual behaviors and preferences. Since the recreational fishing injury was obvious in a closure, asking direct questions (stated preference) and indirect questions through the structure of the survey (revealed preference) was a new, inventive measure for trustees to see what choices the public surveyed might make.

Some elements of the economic science are still new to trustees. Discussing the coefficient values in "utility" may be a common practice among economists, but for the general public, and to some trustees, it is confusing. Perhaps a more common term can be used to describe the effects of the variables. For instance, the NOADVISE variable might be described as "how much further would someone be willing to drive to catch eatable fish?"

At this time there is little data finalized so our interpretation will be subject to scrutiny of the economic experts. The design and the promise of using this model or ones like it in the future are positive. We believe it may be important to have a good idea of restoration options available to the trustees at the time one is developing these trade-offs through this type of modeling. It would be odd to initiate measurements of variables into the survey that may have no feasible restoration associated with it in the area. In the example that speaks to the fact that anglers prefer to catch more fish relative to less, then it will be important that the biological options of restoration are considered early in the process.

The GLO cannot agree that a closure has no effect on a consumer simply because superior alternatives exist. Otherwise we would find ourselves in the position at some point where superior alternatives would be less and less available as the resources diminish. The examples given seem to imply that if there is a nice fishing site somewhere else, then we may not have to clean up the contaminated area and, thus, remove the advisory. This would not be an acceptable restoration to the trustees as the injuries would continue.

As you can imagine, with 29 cases active, trustee resources are sorely stretched. We believe early participation is a valuable tool and the most efficient way to conduct injury scaling and restoration. The restoration of resources can be achieved in an accelerated time frame with the added benefit of an early global settlement with the responsible party. The trustees in Texas will continue to work toward this goal and use this approach in as many cases as possible.

There is a clear purpose for the natural resource trustees: to restore injured resources and the public's use and enjoyment of these resources including public trust lands, waters, and biological resources.

Acknowledgments—I wish to thank my colleagues who provided comments and critical review of this paper: Ingrid K. Hansen, Texas General Land Office, David Chapman, National Oceanographic and Atmospheric Administration, David Sager, Texas Parks and Wildlife, and my staff, Patricia M. Rives and Peter A. H. Samuels.

8d

Discussion Paper 4 on Using Economic Models to Inform Restoration Decisions: The Lavaca Bay, Texas Experience

*Bruce Peacock**

Mathews et al.'s use of a combined revealed preference and stated preference approach is new and potentially useful. The final results of this study should be interesting. However, recognizing that the study is not yet completed, this paper raises 2 issues regarding methodology and interpretation. These issues are summarized below.

Methodology

The methodological issue concerns the survey design. A split sample design was used in which half of the respondents were shown one questionnaire version while the other half was shown a second version. The first version asked respondents to choose between 2 alternative sites described in the questionnaire, Site A and Site B, and the alternative of not fishing at all. In the second version, the choices presented were between Site A, Site B, and a third site specified by the respondent. Responses from these 2 splits were then pooled in the analysis.

The concern with this approach is that there appears to be no consistent baseline with which to compare Site A and Site B. The questionnaire version that allows respondents to specify a third alternative would seem to introduce a moving baseline. Since relative comparisons are important in such analyses, the use of a self-selected baseline may make the interpretation of results difficult. One potential solution would be to include in the analysis all relevant attributes of the alternative sites specified by respondents to the second version so that differences can be statistically controlled.

Interpretation

The authors report preliminary results from the stated preference survey only. These results are expressed as relative contributions to utility associated with various site attributes. Attributes such as the availability of good parking and the absence of a fish consumption advisory are estimated to increase utility, while attributes such as low catch rates are estimated to diminish utility. As reported by the authors (Table 8-3), the greatest relative contribution to utility is obtained from the absence of a fish

*Department of the Interior, Washington, DC

consumption advisory (the "NOADVISE" attribute). This estimate is also highly significant.

Recognizing that the combined revealed preference and stated preference study has not been completed, these results are interesting by themselves. For example, these results indicate that anglers in Lavaca Bay would be willing to travel an additional 69 miles just to avoid a fish consumption advisory. In contrast, these same anglers would to be willing to travel only 24 additional miles to experience high catch rates for flounder, or only 10 additional miles for access to good parking. Clearly, the results of the stated preference study suggest that the presence of a fish consumption advisory plays an important, if not dominant, role in the behavior of Lavaca Bay anglers.

Despite the results reported in their paper, the authors appear to down play the indicated significance of a fish consumption advisory. For example, the authors state that the reported results do not reflect existing substitute fishing sites and therefore do not indicate angler impacts. However, this statement is inconsistent with the authors' description of the survey design. As noted above, the second questionnaire version in the split sample design asked respondents to choose between Site A, Site B, and a third site specified by the respondent. The specification of the third site explicitly accounts for existing substitutes. Therefore, the reported results do indeed reflect substitute fishing sites. Providing that the survey design and analysis are not flawed, then, the reported results are indicative of angler impacts and values.

A second example of down playing the indicated significance of a fish consumption advisory is given by one of the examples presented in the paper. In this example, the authors calculate the utility index of a hypothetical angler for 2 sites using the reported results. The first site has a fish consumption advisory while the second site does not. The angler's utility index is –0.22 for the first site (with an advisory) and 1.74 for the second site (with no advisory). Therefore, the stated preference model indicates a preference for the second site over the first. Next, the authors change the attributes of the first site by removing the fish consumption advisory. This increases the angler's utility index to 1.47 for the first site.

Based on these calculations, the authors conclude that the hypothetical angler suffers no loss of utility from a fish consumption advisory since the second site would be chosen even if the first site did not have an advisory. While this may be true for the authors' hypothetical angler, it may not be true for other anglers facing different circumstances. Moreover, nothing is said about the potential for increasing overall participation. It is quite possible that lifting the consumption advisory would motivate nonparticipants to fish. These other possibilities *would* indicate a loss of utility from a fish consumption advisory. The authors should recognize all possible outcomes.

Summary

The stated preference results presented in the paper are enlightening with respect to angler motivations in Lavaca Bay. In particular, these results suggest that fish consumption advisories play a very important role in the behavior of Lavaca Bay anglers. Nevertheless, certain questions are raised regarding methodology and interpretation. Hopefully, these questions can be resolved in the final analysis.

8e

Discussion Paper 5 on Using Economic Models to Inform Restoration Decisions: The Lavaca Bay, Texas Experience

*Neal S. Brody**

I approached each of my critiques with a focus on 2 distinct components. First, I examined the overall approach to restoration in each of the cases described by the authors. These approaches were as varied as the underlying facts in each of the cases. Second, in addition to an overall assessment, I studied the specific recommendations proposed as a result of the authors' experiences. Without exception, each author offered valuable considerations for future cases involving restoration of lost human uses.

The Mathews paper

General response

The authors present an interesting discussion on the measurement of lost human uses of the environment; however, it is not clear from the paper specifically how that process will contribute to the restoration of those uses. My sense is that Lavaca Bay is still in progress and, as a consequence, the authors describe more of a measurement tool being used than an approach to restoration being utilized. Therefore, like any tool, the processes described by the authors can be used correctly, incorrectly, or ignored altogether. While it probably would not be appropriate to use the tools described by the authors in every instance, in cases where it does make sense to use them, they could be extremely valuable.

Recommendations

The authors provide 2 major conclusions for the NRDA process following the Lavaca Bay experience. The first conclusion is that restoration should be considered while the NRDA process is in its infancy. This recommendation is completely consistent with my own viewpoint and experience. Too often, an instant and singular focus emerges among trustees and responsible parties related to injury quantification. As discussed in the Idarado mine case, these efforts are then used to support competing views on the extent of injuries to human uses rather than on injury restoration. Alternatively, if trustees and responsible parties focused their immediate efforts on the restoration of

*ARCO, Los Angeles, CA

identifiable lost human uses and how data collection could aid in those efforts, the efficiency of the entire process could be increased.

The authors' second major conclusion is that the disciplines of economics and biology should be better integrated in the NRDA process. This is a very important observation. These sciences are the tools through which trustees must balance the cost-effectiveness of restoration efforts with the necessary nexus to the lost human uses provided by the injured resources. Absent this integration, either substantial resources will be wasted, as restoration projects are pursued with no correlation to economics, or the restoration of natural resource injuries will devolve into a public works program as projects are pursued with no correlation to the injured resources.

The second major conclusion is that trustees and responsible parties can, and by implication should, work together. In fact, based on my experience, this conclusion can be taken even further. Not only can, and should, the parties work together, but in order to ensure prompt, effective restoration of lost human uses of the environment, the parties *must* work together. Inevitably, if they work independently, or as more often happens, if they alternatively prepare for litigation, nonproductive efforts are engaged in quantifying and documenting injury that could otherwise be utilized for restoration. Prompt, effective, and successful restoration will most often be achieved when cooperative efforts are paramount in the process.

Conclusion

Each of the papers (Chapters 6, 7, and 8) offers valuable lessons in restoring lost human uses of the environment. These lessons include clarifying the definition of human uses or services, maintaining flexibility throughout the NRDA process, considering the restoration of lost identifiable human uses early on in the NRDA process, improving the integration of economic and biological sciences, considering substitutes in the restoration decision-making process, accepting imperfect solutions, and the importance of trustees and responsible parties working together.

In addition to the specific lessons detailed previously, an overall lesson to be learned from these papers is that the approach taken to restoration really does matter. If trustees and responsible parties follow, understand, and heed the experiences of the *Valdez*, Lavaca Bay, Cantara Loop, and Idarado cases, as thoughtfully presented in these papers, win-win situations can be developed, and most importantly, the public will benefit from expedited and effective restoration of lost human uses of the environment. Finally, I propose a challenge to everyone concerned with lost human uses of natural resources to develop a process through which this occurs as a rule rather than as an exception.